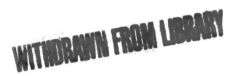

The Art and Science of
*Dance/Movement
Therapy*

The Art and Science of

Dance/Movement Therapy

Life Is Dance

EDITED BY

Sharon Chaiklin and Hilda Wengrower

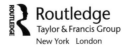

Routledge
Taylor & Francis Group
New York   London

Routledge
Taylor & Francis Group
270 Madison Avenue
New York, NY 10016

Routledge
Taylor & Francis Group
27 Church Road
Hove, East Sussex BN3 2FA

© 2009 by Sharon Chaiklin and Hilda Wengrower
Routledge is an imprint of Taylor & Francis Group, an Informa business

Printed in the United States of America on acid-free paper
10 9 8 7 6 5 4 3 2 1

International Standard Book Number: 978-0-415-99657-0 (Hardback) 978-0-415-99656-3 (Paperback)

Library of Congress Cataloging-in-Publication Data

Vida es danza. English.
   The art and science of dance/movement therapy : life is dance / [edited by] Sharon Chaiklin, Hilda Wengrower.
      p. ; cm.
   Includes bibliographical references and index.
   ISBN 978-0-415-99657-0 (hardback : alk. paper) -- ISBN 978-0-415-99656-3 (pbk. : alk. paper)
   1. Dance therapy. 2. Movement therapy. I. Chaiklin, Sharon, 1934- II. Wengrower, Hilda. III. Title.
   [DNLM: 1. Dance Therapy. WM 450.5.D2 V648a 2009a]

RC489.D3V5313 2009
616.89'1655--dc22   2009010967

Visit the Taylor & Francis Web site at
http://www.taylorandfrancis.com

and the Routledge Web site at
http://www.routledgementalhealth.com

To my dear friend Anne Wilson Wangh,
who dances her life with energy and generosity

To my family, always with me ….

Hilda

With love to Harry, Seth, Mariane, Martha, Nina
(and Matthew), Levi, Samuel, Zeke, Gabriel and
David and our dear friends who have always
been there for us. You know who you are.

Sharon

Contents

Foreword

MIRIAM ROSKIN BERGER

A unique intellectual experience awaits you as you read this book. It is a volume that will be welcomed warmly by the global dance therapy community. This is the English edition of a collection originally published in Spanish. That work was developed because there is almost no dance therapy in literature in the Spanish-speaking world even though dance therapy is rapidly growing in countries where Spanish is the mother tongue.

One of the distinctive things about this collection is that the authors are from several different countries—America, Australia, Spain, Argentina, and Israel. This brings an important cross-cultural perspective to this work. For many years, dance therapy was almost exclusively an American phenomenon, but we are now seeing that innovative methods and theory in the field are coming from all around the globe, and there are strong cross currents of influence.

Another unique attribute of this collection is that each of the included chapters has great depth. These chapters bring the reader the latest and the best that is available in dance therapy. This material goes beyond the usual survey that is presented in edited works. The authors are all experts and leaders in their particular area, and they have been able to comprehensively share their ideas with clarity. As a result, this work will be of great value to advanced clinicians and researchers, as well as to allied professionals.

The work's comprehensive stance is reflected in the organization and topics of the collection: basic concepts, theory into practice with a wide range of populations, methods of assessment, and research. The discipline of dance therapy, therefore, has been examined from all sides and within many dimensions.

Perhaps the strongest attribute of this book is reflected in its title, the *Art and Science* of dance/movement therapy. Art and science have several intersecting points; perhaps the most apparent is the exploration of patterns—patterns in time, in space, in movement. And the discovery and creation of patterns generates the understanding of meaning in both art and science. All of the authors express, in their own way, this dual focus of our profession, a most crucial focus, and one that ensures the continuing richness of dance therapy. We are indebted to the editors and their contributors for reflecting this richness in their book.

Miriam Roskin Berger, ADTR, LCAT
Chair, ADTA International Panel
Past President, ADTA
Former Director, Program in Dance Education, New York University

Preface

VALENTÍN BARENBLIT

Mental health, as a field of knowledge, is developing today as a complex combination of theories and techniques and a host of multidisciplinary experiences. Thus, a new epistemological vision is being introduced, one that is organized as an interdisciplinary terrain. A dynamics of dialectical interactions is being established that, over the last decades, has promoted the development of processes of transformation in which psychiatry as a total and hegemonic discipline is being replaced by visions that promote the compatibility and extension of different disciplines and theories regarding mental health and mental illness.

These developments promote the implementation of different types of expertise that complement each other strategically to enhance prevention, treatment, and rehabilitation in the mental health field. This having been said, it is also true that this complex interdisciplinary structure allows and upholds conceptual confrontations that might make the dynamics of producing new knowledge and corresponding actions more difficult. At the same time, stimulating factors enrich and promote the articulation of the professional resources and bring about effective transformations in the definition of the politics and application of plans and programs for mental health care.

From this perspective, the interdisciplinary team is actually the essential resource to study, research, and offer answers pertaining to treatment that are rational and effective to the problems of mental health and mental illness.

Within this conceptual framework, and from an ideological and a practical perspective of the mental health of the community, Dance/Movement Therapy (DMT) as seen within the diverse contents of this book conveys a consistent message supported by excellent theoretical and technical references. It strongly promotes the insertion of the DMT professional into interdisciplinary teams within the various networks of health care and mental health.

The text in this book is structured in relation to the premises presented in this preface, vigorously advanced by the creative and applied clinical, academic, and research activity carried out over many years by Sharon Chaiklin and Hilda Wengrower and the several authors. In my view, this book is a highly valuable contribution to the bibliography in this profession and will also be a quality reference for universities and schools of DMT as well as for health care and mental health care systems and services.

Valentín Barenblit, M.D.
Psychiatrist and psychoanalyst
President of iPsi (Center for Care, Teaching, Research and
Psychoanalytical Training), Barcelona, Spain
Honorary Professor, University of Buenos Aires, Argentina
Barcelona

Acknowledgments

The sharing of knowledge has been our primary purpose and motivation in creating this book. Many helped make this possible. We first wish to acknowledge the generosity of each author who gave of his or her time and knowledge so that dance and movement therapy might be better understood and used in aiding those with particular needs. To each of them we will always be grateful.

As co-editors we were able to complement each other's work so that the difficulty of the task was actually pleasurable. Several others encouraged us throughout the process and we would like to name just a few: Yael Barkai; Israel Hadany for his generosity in providing his art work; Marta Moldvai and Anna Moore, our editors, for their helpfulness; and Maria Sideri for her index translation. The support of family was so important, particularly our husbands, who have always both nourished and endured our endeavors. Harry Chaiklin was available to offer to read and frequently act as savior through his computer skills, while Silvio Gutkowski similarly was a consultant for ideas and smoothed out the rough times through his humor, all of which was invaluable to both of us and for which we are very appreciative.

We thank our mentors, colleagues, patients, and students, who have all been the source of our learning. The gift of their knowledge and the experiences of their lives add to the richness of the cumulative sharing that makes dance/movement therapy so special.

Hilda Wengrower
Sharon Chaiklin

Introduction

Over the past several years, there has been a gradual recognition of the importance of the interrelationship of the "bodymind" and how it affects human behavior—psychologically, physically, and socially. The concepts of *embodiment* and *attunement* are becoming commonplace in the literature of various psychotherapeutic disciplines as well as related fields. Understanding has evolved of how illness, both physical and psychological, is influenced by emotions. The body relays information—our emotional history—that remains stored in our musculature and other physiological systems. It is manifested in the individual's postures, gestures, use of space, and movements large and small. It became clear that we cannot discard the body as a source of information, whether analogical or symbolic, or ignore it in the process of healing. The *bodymind* as one entity became clear to many involved in dance in conjunction with the role of creativity as a means of bodily expression.

Dance/movement therapy evolved from this understanding early in the 1950s. The therapeutic potential of the creative process that occurs through dance and improvisation began to be formalized. Movement was no longer conceived as performance for an audience but rather was recognized as an expression of feelings and concerns. As a professional in the field of mental health, the role of the dance therapist became increasingly important within multidisciplinary settings as adjunctive therapy or as a main psychotherapeutical approach. It is through the integration of the therapeutic relationship and motoric expression that feelings, emotional history, and thoughts are uncovered with the potential of positive change occurring.

Dance/movement therapy is an interdisciplinary profession, with its own training, that evolved through the synthesis of the art of movement and dance and the science of psychology. As such, it continues to evolve based on the confluence of knowledge built upon the therapeutic and spiritual use of dance through the ages, cultural anthropology, psychodynamic theories, neuromotor sciences, the psychology of the arts, and the creative process.

Dance is the core and the roots from which the profession of dance/ movement therapy has grown. "Dance" has remained a vital part of our professional identity after many discussions and alternative suggestions. It has many meanings to people, and unfortunately some of these suggest only partial connotations such as performance or technical skill. It is the role of the dance/movement therapist to be able to explain the more basic significance of dance and how it relates to life, growth, and change.

Dance is used in the broadest sense of body movement, which may involve a small gesture or the total use of self. It lasts over time, perhaps merely a brief moment, and may use rhythms or not. It may spread out over space or use only that which one's body inhabits. However, in all cases, it is a motor action that emanates from an individual in response to internal sensations or perceived external stimuli. Even motor actions used for practical ends such as eating or bathing have a particular quality that manifests psychosocial aspects of a person.

Human beings experience the urge to move even before birth. Developmentally, we draw on movement to communicate before there is use of verbal language. A basic assumption upon which all therapy is based is that human beings have psychosocial needs as well as biological. To be able to share one's thoughts and feelings with others and be understood by them seems to be what defines humanity. Difficulty in relationships, being uncomfortable with oneself and in the world, or having experienced serious trauma are the sources of much of the therapeutic work done in any type of therapy situation.

It has been more than 40 years since dance/movement therapy organized as a profession in the United States. It is growing rapidly in many countries of the world. Therefore, it is our hope that this collection of original articles will serve as a source of important information for students and professionals of dance/movement therapy as well as other mental health and helping professions. It covers a wide range of information composed by experienced therapists who have written about their specialties. The contributors to this book come from several countries' cultures such as Spain, North and South America, Israel, and Australia. Acknowledging some of the differences of culture, the basic theories of dance/movement therapy are core to each of them as the defined concepts are the basis of all human experience. To reiterate:

1. The human being is a bodymind unity and dance/movement is its manifestation.
2. Gesture, posture, and movement express the person and allow for self knowledge and psychotherapeutical change.

3. Acknowledgment of the therapeutical effects of the creative process.
4. Dance and movement are utilized as a way to the unconscious and as a facilitator of different aspects of health and well-being.
5. There is a differentiation between the work done with an artist or dance teacher and that by a therapist. For us, dance is at the service of promoting health and change.
6. Dance therapists establish contact, plan treatment and evaluate it in terms of integrated knowledge of movement, dance, and psycho-therapy.

There are many problems that human beings face and many possibilities in understanding them theoretically and ways to respond to them. It is hoped that some of these alternatives will be illuminated for the reader through the experience and knowledge learned and shared by the several authors who have generously contributed their expertise. The common thread that unites each of them is their profound love of dance in all its meanings and the understanding of how it deeply affects our lives.

The book is divided into three sections, the first of which contains chapters related to basic concepts of dance/movement therapy. The second section contains application of dance/movement therapy theory to practice with several different populations, and the third section speaks of important learning and structures related to observation and professional considerations. In addition to theoretical background, the authors illustrate their ideas by presenting clinical examples in order to facilitate understanding and enable implementation of the information provided.

The first section includes an introductory history of dance, dance therapy and its development, and the differences between dance/movement therapy and other body therapies. The second chapter presents different psychological aspects of the creative process and artistic activity, particularly related to dance therapy. The third chapter is about the therapeutic relationship and its implementation in the profession. The author weaves the concepts of the dance therapy pioneers with contemporary psychodynamic psychotherapy as well as neuropsychological studies. The emotions and the body are then discussed from a Jungian perspective. Emotions, imagination, and movement are seen as a primary aspect in psychic life and additionally hold the potential for spiritual development when modulated and transformed by joy and interest through play and curiosity.

The second section focuses on the application of theory to practice. It is divided into two parts: the first within mental health settings and the second DMT in medical settings. Basic DMT work is fully explained in the chapter relating to working with institutionalized psychiatric patients. This includes why and how dance therapy evolves within a session. Another chapter describes the use of metaphor in treatment with neurotic patients who have chosen dance therapy as a way toward health. This is followed by a description of the use of dance/movement therapy with people with eating disorders. Systemic family therapy is discussed in the following chapter including movement observational guides for work with more than one person. The last chapter in this section is a detailed description of work with children with pervasive developmental disorders and with those hospitalized in an oncology setting.

The medical focus continues in the second section with a description of work with the elderly with Alzheimer's disease, making use of a humanistic perspective. The next chapter discusses treatment with individuals with closed head injury, its difficulties, and the potential for recuperation.

The third section studies different types of movement observation, so very important to dance therapy and other professional considerations. A discussion of Rudolph Laban's work in relation to dance therapy is offered as one way of observation of movement. This system is used widely throughout the United States, Europe, and some Latin American countries, and is referred to by several authors. The Kestenberg Movement Profile is then discussed as a different way of observing that evolved from Laban's work and is related to psychoanalytic theories. Several references to this system have been cited by professionals from various disciplines. The Paradigm devised by Yona Shahar-Levy is presented as another way to observe a person's movement expressions. This is currently in use mostly in Israel and Germany.

In addition to observational systems, there are professional issues that are important to the field. Some of these are discussed, such as matters related to cultural differences between the therapist and those with whom he or she might work. Awareness of nonverbal diversity among cultures is vital to our understanding of others. Finally, to continue to understand and build our knowledge base, it is urgent that consideration be given to the area of research. This is often thought of as a foreign way of thinking and acting for clinicians, but it is not very distant from the performance of one's clinical work and it is vital to the growth of professional proficiency.

It is hoped that this book will serve the purpose of contributing to the training of those who are in the process of becoming dance/movement therapists as well as those already working in the field who wish to deepen their knowledge. Additionally, we wish to share this information with other professionals in related fields so that they may better understand the meaning of dance and movement, and for any individual who might be interested in making use of dance/movement therapy on a personal level.

In order to simplify the reading, the term dance/movement therapy has been denoted frequently with the initials DMT. The clinician, the dance movement therapist, has been indicated by the lower-case initials dmt. Each author has provided his or her individual and relevant references.

Contributors

Cynthia Berrol, Ph.D., is ADTR Professor Emerita, California State University, Hayward, where she developed a special graduate major in Dance/Movement Therapy. She has presented at many conferences, written several articles on the topic of closed head injury and developed with another dance therapist an assessment tool used within a pilot research project called Dance/Movement Therapy with Older Individuals Who Have Sustained Neurological Insult. This was supported by a grant from the Administration on Aging, Department of Health and Human Services, Washington, D.C. She serves on the editorial boards of three professional journals and is a contributing author and co-editor of *Dance/movement therapists in action: A working guide to research*.

Patricia P. Capello, MA, ADTR, NCCP, LCAT has been senior dance/movement therapist and acting team leader for more than 27 years at Maimonides Medical Centers' Department of Psychiatry in Brooklyn, New York. She maintains a private practice specializing in working with developmentally delayed adults, has served on the faculty of New York University in its program in Dance and Dance Education, supervises clinical interns and has traveled to the United Kingdom, Taiwan and Greece to train dance/movement therapists. She has served many years on the board of directors of the American Dance Therapy Association.

Sharon Chaiklin, ADTR, is a founding member and past president of the American Dance Therapy Association. A student of Marian Chace, one of the first dance therapists in the United States, she worked for more than 34 years in psychiatric hospitals and private practice. She taught for 14 years in the Graduate Dance/Movement Therapy Program at Goucher College in Baltimore, Maryland and has authored several articles and is co-editor of the book *Foundations of dance/movement therapy: The life and work of Marian Chace*. She has been invited to teach dance/therapy in Israel, Japan, Korea, Spain, and Argentina. She currently serves as president of the Marian Chace Foundation of the American Dance Therapy Association.

Meg Chang, Ed.D. ADTR, has worked in psychiatric institutions, medical settings, shelters for women and victims of violence, hospitals and prisons. She has been on the faculty of DMT graduate programs at Lesley University (Cambridge, Massachusetts), Pratt Institute (Brooklyn, New York), and The New School in New York City. She carried out research in South Korea and Taiwan, has developed training and published on intercultural issues in DMT and facilitates Mindfulness Based Stress Reduction (MBSR). She performs with the Elaine Summers Dance and Film Company in New York, New York.

Joan Chodorow, Ph.D., ADTR, and Jungian analyst, is one of the past presidents of ADTA, author of *Dance therapy and depth psychology: The moving imagination*, and the editor of *Jung on active imagination*. Some of her early writings appear in *Authentic movement: Essays by Mary Starks Whitehouse, Janet Adler and Joan Chodorow*. Her forthcoming book is *Active imagination: healing from within*. She lectures and teaches internationally.

Varda Dascal, Tel Aviv University, is a pioneer in the implementation and development of Movement Therapy in Family Therapy settings. She has taught and conducted professional training in Brazil, Mexico, the United States, Australia, Germany, Netherlands, Slovenia, Spain, France, and Italy—in addition to Israel. Her research focuses on the relationship between movement style, personality, and non-verbal and verbal communication. She has published numerous papers, among others on the interaction between emotion and cognition, movement metaphors and their use as a clinical tool, the cross-cultural variations in expressive communication, and the interpretation of art. She received the Renoir Prize in 2008 for her work toward a culture and politics of peace in the Mediterranean.

Dianne Dulicai, Ph.D., ADTR, is a leading figure in the ADTA (American Dance Therapy Association) and other American institutions and professional organizations. She developed and directed the master's programs at Hahnemann University in Philadelphia, where she continues to teach, and at the Laban Centre of London. Her main focus in clinical practice as well as in research has been movement diagnosis in families using Labananalysis, pupils with special needs, and children exposed to lead.

Diana Fischman, Ph.D., ADTR, psychologist and educator, is director of Brecha, the Buenos Aires DMT Training Institute, and is an academic advisor and professor at the Autonomous University of National Art, the University of Buenos Aires, and a dance movement therapy master as well as in the Autonomous University of Barcelona DMT master's program. Dr. Fischman is the founder president of the Argentina Association of Dance Therapy. She created Grupo Enacción, a psychokinetic approaches company. Her dissertation for the University of Palermo was on kinesthetic empathy: the contributions of DMT in the promotion of empathy with health professionals.

Lenore Hervey, Ph.D., ADTR, is the author of the book *Artistic inquiry in dance/movement therapy.* She is active in the ADTA and is a member of the faculty at Columbia College, Chicago where she conducts and teaches research, and supervises students.

Heather Hill, Ph.D., is a professional member of the Dance Therapy Association of Australia. Her interests are in the fields of aging and of dementia. She has contributed papers, book chapters, and written the book *Invitation to the dance: Dance for people with dementia and their carers.* Dr. Hill now lectures at the Melbourne Institute for Experiential and Creative Arts Therapy, Melbourne, Australia.

Susan Kleinman, MA, ADTR, NCC, is the dance/movement therapist for residential and outpatient services at The Renfrew Center of Florida. Ms. Kleinman is a trustee of the Marian Chace Foundation, a past president of the American Dance Therapy Association and a past chair of The National Coalition for Creative Arts Therapies. She is a co-editor of The Renfrew Center Foundation's Healing through Relationship Series, and serves on the editorial board of the *Journal of Creativity in Mental Health.* She is a frequent presenter at national and international conferences.

Susan Loman, MA, ADTR, NCC, KMP analyst, is director of the Dance/Movement Therapy and Counseling Program, and professor and associate chair of the Department of Applied Psychology, Antioch University New England. She serves on the editorial board of The Arts in Psychotherapy, and is former chair of the ADTA education committee. She is the co-author of the book *The meaning of movement: Developmental and* *clinical perspectives of the Kestenberg Movement Profile* and is the author of articles, chapters and books on the KMP and DMT. She teaches the KMP and DMT at Antioch, and through the United States and abroad.

Yona Shahar-Levy, DMT, pioneer in Israel, is a former president of the Israeli Association of the Creative Therapists. She created the Emotorics system for observation and evaluation of movement, which is being taught in Israel and Germany. She is the author of the book *The visible body reveals the secrets of the mind* (Hebrew), which is now being translated into German. She has published papers in English and Hebrew.

K. Mark Sossin, Ph.D., professor of psychology, Pace University is a clinical psychologist, psychoanalyst, and KMP Analyst; clinical faculty member of the Derner Institute of Advanced Studies in Psychology, Adelphi University; a member of the New York Freudian Society and International Psychoanalytic Association; director of the Parent–Infant/Toddler Research Nursery at Pace; vice-president of Child Development Research; and on the editorial boards of the *Journal of Infant, Child and Adolescent Psychotherapy (JICAP)* and the *Journal of Early Childhood and Infant Psychology*. He is co-editor/author of *The meaning of movement: Developmental and clinical perspectives of the Kestenberg movement profile*.

Susan Tortora, Ph.D., is a licensed dance/movement psychotherapist and nonverbal communication analyst. She has extensive experience working in private practice with infants, children and their families, providing individual and group psychotherapy. Her work with pediatric cancer patients is funded by the Andréa Rizzo Foundation. Her expertise includes infant–parent dyadic nonverbal communication video analysis sessions to assist the parents in understanding how their child's and their own nonverbal cues are influencing the attachment relationship. Dr. Tortora provides training programs nationally and internationally including at the Zero to Three National Training Institute and the World Association for Infant Mental Health (WAIMH); has been featured on radio and television programs including NPR; Good Morning America, ABC-TV; Eyewitness News WABC-TV; and the *New Yorker* magazine. She is on the faculty of the postgraduate Institute for Infants, Children & Families of the Jewish Board of Family and Children's Services, and the graduate dance therapy faculty of Pratt Institute and the New School. She is a board member of the New York Zero to Three Network; and on the advisory board of MarbleJam Kids, Inc, where she is currently directing the adaptation of her Ways of Seeing program for their art, music and dance therapy programs for autistic children. She has published papers about her therapeutic and nonverbal communication analysis work with children, parent–infant dyads, and autism spectrum disorders. Dr. Tortora recently published a book, *The dancing dialogue: Using the communicative power of movement with young children.*

Hilda Wengrower, Ph.D., DMT, is academic director of the DMT master's program at IL3-University of Barcelona. She is a lecturer in the Department of Theatre Studies, Hebrew University. She has published papers and chapters on subjects related to arts therapies in educational settings, migration, qualitative research and arts therapies, and DMT.

Elissa Queyquep White, ADTR, CMA, LCAT, studied dance therapy with Marian Chace and was in the first Effort-Shape certification group taught by Irmgard Bartenieff at the Dance Notation Bureau. In 1967 she began clinical work at Bronx Psychiatric Center, was a co-founder and taught in the first master's program in dance/movement therapy held at Hunter College in New York City. She was a charter member of the American Dance Therapy Association and served as president. She currently teaches courses at Pratt Institute and the New School University in New York and studies currently with Elaine Summers in kinectic awareness.

Basic Concepts of Dance/Movement Therapy

CHAPTER 1

We Dance from the Moment Our Feet Touch the Earth

SHARON CHAIKLIN

Contents

This chapter describes the development of dance/movement therapy from its origins in primitive societies to the present day. Dance/movement therapy is a profession based on the art of dance and augmented by psychological theories involving core human processes.

Movement and breath signify the start of life. They precede language and thought. Gesture immediately emerges as the means for expressing the human need for communication. This has been true over the span of human history. Havelock Ellis writes, "If we are indifferent to the art of dancing, we have failed to understand, not merely the supreme manifestation of physical life, but also the supreme symbol of spiritual life" (Ellis, 1923, p. 36).

Within the earliest tribal communities, dance was seen as a link to understanding and directing the rhythms of the universe whether in the many manifestations of nature or as a statement of self and one's place within that world. Dances to plead for rain, for success in the hunt, or appreciation of a plentiful harvest are all examples of how dance was seen as a way to influence the gods. It took different forms in different cultures. Often, the movement structures led to trance states that enabled the individual to feel powerful and perform extraordinary feats of endurance and strength (de Mille, 1963). The rhythms of work, the rhythms used to shape nature for man's benefit, the rhythms of life's events were the rhythms that formed the cooperative community, the fundamental structure among all early people and folk societies today. The dance enabled each to feel a part of his own tribe and provided a structure for performing essential rituals related to birth, puberty, marriage, and death.

Cultural and Religious Influences

We recognize different cultural groups through the distinctive movement and dances that each has evolved relevant to its geography and way of life. These take many forms, such as the English maypole dance, Haitian voodoo dances, or Hawaiian hula. In what we call the Far East, dance has always been part of the religious and spiritual life of the people. Dancers are trained to learn the specific movements, stories, myths, and symbols of their culture. People come to watch not for mere entertainment, but for enlightenment and a religious experience. The western world had a similar belief that art was a necessary part of life and that there is magic power in the dance. In ancient Greece, all forms of art were to please the gods. The Greeks named the muse of dance Terpsichore (de Mille, 1963), a name that is still in use today. In the later years of the Middle Ages, dance was separated into two components: the earthy folk dances and those by trained dancers meant as entertainment before an audience. Dance was no longer thought of as a religious experience and was eventually banned by the Catholic Church after the dance manias of the Middle Ages. During the plague that swept through Europe, an epidemic of St. Vitus dance or tarantism (Highwater, 1978) occurred in which people obsessively danced without stopping. Whole crowds would follow each other, succumbing to the hysteria. It was likely a reaction to the death surrounding them that caused this group behavior. The Church deemed that such souls were possessed.

Those who first used dance for healing, likely shamans or witch doctors, clearly made use of the interrelationship of the body–mind–spirit. The western world lost some of that ability by dissociating the body from the spirit. The emergence of Christian religious belief during the Middle Ages and the later rational philosophy of Descartes in the 17th century tended to see the body as impure or of secondary importance. Descartes discounted the relationship of mind to the body and saw them as distinct entities, with the mind being the real self.

Roots of Dance as Therapy

Dance/movement therapy has a different philosophical stance. It sees dance as naturally therapeutic due to its physical, emotional, and spiritual components. People share a sense of community while dancing, which is why they go to public areas to share the rhythmic action of the music through the dance.

Creativity in art and, in this instance, dance, is a search for structures to express what is difficult to state. Dance/movement therapy is based on the fundamental realization that, through the dance, individuals both relate to the community they are part of on a large or smaller scale, and are simultaneously able to express their own impulses and needs within that group. There is shared energy and strength when being with others. It enables us to go beyond our personal limitations or concerns. Within the joy of moving together, we also appreciate validation of our own worth and recognition of our personal struggles.

During the early part of the 20th century, innovators such as Isadora Duncan rejected the formality of ballet and danced barefoot as herself and not someone else's character. As modern dance took hold, the individual was free to create new forms and allow the unrestrained use of the body. These dancers explored movement in ways unfamiliar until the personal dance.

Mary Wigman in Germany was another influential artist. Her improvisational and ritual use of movement, her reliance on rhythmic instruments rather than musical scores, guided the many who studied with her. Her students and those who followed have been a major precursor and influence on present-day dance/movement therapy. These different methods of learning did not diminish the discipline and preparation needed to become performing artists and create artistic meaning in the dance.

The mind–body concept has come full circle. All elements and components of a human are a set of related systems. Mind is indeed part of the body and the body affects the mind. Much research is now being done by neurophysiologists and other scientists to examine those interrelationships. When speaking of the body, we are not only describing the functional aspects of movement, but how our psyche and emotions are affected by our thinking and how movement itself effects change within them.

Scientific research now supports what has been known on an intuitive level by those involved in dance/movement therapy over the years. To connect dance and therapy, dancers begin with a deep understanding of their art. They then explore the personal meaning of dance for themselves. When one is involved in the creative aspects of any art form, it is not possible to dismiss the personal and one's individual perspective. It is the root of the creation of the product. Dancing is not merely an exercise to be accomplished, but rather a statement of one's feelings and energy and desire to externalize something from within. When one creates a dance, it is based on a concept, realistic or abstract, that needs to be communicated to others. This understanding led to the use of dance/movement therapy not only in groups but in sessions for the individual in his or her search toward self-integration.

The Pioneers

After many years of performing, choreographing, and teaching, several dancers began to observe more closely those who came to study with them. Some of these, mainly women, had gone through psychoanalysis, which was the main psychiatric form of treatment at that time. All were familiar with the psychiatric theorists emerging during and after Freud, and interpretations of how the psyche and emotions were intertwined. Due to the influences around them and their own inclinations, some learned more about psychoanalytic thinking, and others went on to study the work of H.S. Sullivan, Jung, and Adler, among others. This psychological background provided them with an understanding of human development and behavior that they then began to use to observe the movement behaviors of others. Each of the women who first pioneered the use of dance in therapy understood the power of the movement for themselves and its significance in their own lives. They had the curiosity to wonder how it affected others and what could be learned through the personal dances individuals might explore for themselves.

Marian Chace, who performed with the company of Ruth St. Denis and Ted Shawn (Denishawn) in the 1930s, choreographed and later taught in her own studio in Washington D.C. She questioned why pupils who had no intention of being professional came to take dance classes. She observed how each moved, then gradually shifted her teaching to focus on the needs of the individual. She organized classes for her students that led to an integration of the body and its movement, thus enabling personal self-harmony. As her work became known by mental health professionals in 1942, she was invited to work at St. Elizabeths Hospital, a large federal institution where many soldiers were returning from World War II. Group therapy was beginning at this time in response to the needs of so many. Dance/movement therapy fit closely into this new form of therapeutic intervention. Chace developed her concepts of treatment, working with schizophrenic and psychotic patients before the advent of psychotropic medications (Sandel et al., 1993). She trained many others and later served as the first president of the American Dance Therapy Association from 1966 until 1968. As one of those who interned with Marian Chace at St. Elizabeths Hospital (1964–1965), I was fortunate in being invited to observe her work with very regressed patients and began my own practice under her tutelage.

Marian Chace worked very deliberately and carefully. As her student, I followed her onto large ward areas, most often locked, carrying the large record player. This was before the advent of tapes and CDs. The moment the door was unlocked, attention was paid to those in view, greeting each or merely nodding. As we went into the common room used by all, Chace would notice the moods, tensions, formations of groups, or lack of them, and begin to make decisions as to how to begin a session. As patients gathered, she would greet each one and explain who she was and why she was there. She usually chose the waltz to begin as it is rather neutral and, as she noted, not likely attached to many memories. Some would join immediately in the circle she was gradually forming, others waited and she was able to allow them to take the time they needed to stand up to be part of the session. Others never joined the circle but were nevertheless recognized where they sat, so that they too took part in their own way. The session would unfold with varying degrees of energy, intensity, intimacy, laughter, and sharing. A range of emotions might be expressed through the movement and perhaps verbally. Each individual left with a different and clearer sense of self and with having related to others when they might have previously been isolated. It all occurred through sensitive awareness of the symbolic movement expressions that were offered and to which there was validation and response (Sandel et al., 1993).

Mary Whitehouse was another major figure. She evolved her own way of working during the 1950s and attributed her approach to both her background in studying dance with Mary Wigman, and her own Jungian analysis. She worked with those who were higher-functioning and had more ego strengths than did Chace, who worked primarily in institutional settings. She used the Jungian concept of active imagination as the foundation of her work. By making use of spontaneous body movement that arose from inner kinesthetic sensations, individuals recognized the symbolic nature of their communications, which then opened the door to self-awareness and possible change. She called her work Movement in Depth. This later was called Authentic Movement by her followers.

Trudi Schoop, who lived in California, as did Mary Whitehouse, had been a well known performer of dance and mime throughout Europe prior to World War II. When she settled in California, she began to work with hospitalized patients and developed her own way of thinking about this work. Making use of creative explorations and natural playfulness, she worked with fantasies and body awareness to lead to expressive movement and changing postures.

Others who added to the body of knowledge of dance/movement therapy included Blanche Evan, Liljan Espenak, Alma Hawkins, and Irmgard Bartenieff. Some, such as Norma Canner and Elizabeth Polk, primarily worked with children. Since the beginning, many have learned and carried on with their work, continuing to contribute new ideas and ways of working in many new and different settings. The work is not only in psychiatric hospitals, agencies, and private practice but in any setting where there is a need for healing. These might include working in multiple settings such as educational (autism, special needs, delayed development), prisons, outpatient settings, and with the elderly, including Alzheimer's patients. Practitioners work with those with physical disabilities such as blindness, deafness, chronic pain, anorexia, closed head injuries, Parkinson's disease, and where there is acute illness such as in oncology. Therapists work with abusers of drugs and alcohol, where there is domestic violence, and with those who have survived trauma and abuse in many situations. Dance/movement therapists use their skills and knowledge to work with people toward self-validation, resolution of past trauma, and to learn how to better relate and have positive interactions with others.

Brief Case Study

Within my dance/movement therapy private practice, I worked with a fairly well functioning middle-aged man who came because of his difficulties in relationships. It was clear to both of us that he struggled to allow himself to move freely in space and could not dance out whatever feelings he struggled with at the moment without censoring them. His movement exhibited tension and interruptions, and lacked flow or rhythmic continuity. He appeared stuck to one place on the floor. With continued therapeutic work over time that dealt with his family and his own low self-esteem, with starts and hesitations, there came a day when, after a brief verbal exchange, he moved out into space and moved through one of the most beautiful dances I had ever seen. The beauty came from the total integration of his body, his movement, and his intention to express something within himself. It had not been planned beforehand but rather emerged complete and whole at that time. He understood what had happened for himself, as did I as the therapist, and there was little need for discussion. He had accepted himself and his feelings and was willing to have them be seen. It was a complete and satisfying moment that indicated that treatment was near its end.

When the therapy is in group settings, the projections and anxieties of relating to others emerge and need to be managed. An individual may receive group support for the individual struggles, pain, and emotions that might unfold. The realization that others similarly struggle enables people to feel less isolated on their journey toward health. For example, anger is one emotion often difficult to express or to receive from others. Structuring movement that encourages but contains strong aggressive actions, and modeling various ways of acceptance and response, lessens the fears that emerge with the emotion. Similarly, expressions of loss and sadness can be shared as a universal experience. Further discussion of the practice of dance/movement therapy in several settings will be found in chapters that follow.

Professional Structures

Active in the founding of the American Dance Therapy Association (ADTA) in 1966, I served as the first vice-president when Marian Chace was president, and I then became the next president. Some of this chapter is based on what I was part of and observed. Initially, there were a few people working in very isolated situations, trying to understand what was important about the dance in therapy. Gradually they, including myself, sought out those first pioneers to learn and then to share with each other their ideas and questions. Several students of Marian Chace became convinced that it was important to form an organization for communication and continued learning. After a 2-year period of organizing, searching for those interested in the field, and deciding on the mission of the organization, the ADTA was incorporated as a non-profit association in 1966. There were 75 charter members ... some of whom still remain active. There was now a way of communicating with each other through newsletters, a directory of members, an annual conference, and eventually a professional journal. Over time, standards were set for what knowledge was needed to be a dance/movement therapist, and what ethics were to be followed. As the profession grew, treatment opportunities and knowledge continued to increase. As graduate programs were introduced in academic settings, the ADTA began to officially recognize and approve programs meeting specific standards. Similarly, individuals apply for registry (or certification process), which sets standards and thereby recognizes one's achievements in reaching those standards in order to be a professional. There was and continues to be outreach to the public and other professionals to educate them about dance/movement therapy.

Aside from understanding and having dance be part of one's life, there is much learning involved in becoming a dance/movement therapist. Theories and practice of dance/movement therapy, human development and behavior, issues over the span of life, movement observation, and group processes are a few of the courses that are covered in graduate programs leading to a master's degree in universities. Alternative programs that offer dance/movement courses are offered where there are no academic programs. Dance/movement therapy in the United States and the ADTA became a model that others around the world began to look toward as a way of learning, supporting, and evolving dance/movement therapy within their own countries. Senior therapists began to teach in other countries, either through programs or offering workshops. Students came to the United States to participate in the existing academic programs or take workshops. In this way, a program began in Israel in 1980 and since then others gradually developed. Today, there are programs, associations, or dance/movement therapists in 33 countries aside from the United States (ADTA Web site, www.adta.org). As dance/movement therapy develops in various countries, they will each need to take account of their unique cultural influences and separate understanding of the body, dance, movement, and human relationships.

With the multiplication of therapies related to the body over the past several years, it is helpful to distinguish dance/movement therapy from the many other forms such as Feldenkrais technique, Alexander technique, Reiki, massage therapy, and so many others. These all have their value, but there are some fundamental differences to be understood.

Dance/movement therapy attends to the body and its posture and how it influences perception, tensions held within the body that might inhibit action or feeling, the awareness of the breath as it is used or withheld, and the sensory use of touch. What is significant is that it is related to the art form of dance, which supports and encourages creativity through use of time and space using the body, oneself, in an active way. Improvising movements and gestures that emerge from inner impulses and that connect to rhythms natural to the dancer lead to self-expression that may or may not be cognitively understood but that nevertheless have meaning in his or her life. Improvisations are mostly self-directed and come from the unconscious or preconscious. In this way, the movement of the dance takes on symbolic meaning. Patterns may be repeated, new ways of moving may emerge, and connections to behaviors and relationships be uncovered. This material becomes part of the process through which change may occur. Verbal interactions are used to clarify, question, and support.

Conclusion

Although the world is now more socially and culturally complex than the ancient small and circumscribed tribal societies, that which was so fundamental to the life of human beings then is still basic. People need to feel integrated within themselves and be a part of a community. The use of dance is one way to enable that to happen. Dance/movement therapy overcomes discontinuity and enhances new connections. We have increased our knowledge of human behavior and how to respond to individual needs while supporting group experiences. We are no longer witch doctors, but instead call ourselves dance/movement therapists.

References

de Mille, A. (1963) *The book of the dance*. New York: Golden Press.

Ellis, H. (1923) *The dance of life*. Cambridge: Houghton Mifflin Co.

Hanna, J. L. (1979) *To dance is human: A theory of nonverbal communication*. Austin: University of Texas Press.

Highwater, J. (1978) *Dance: Rituals of experience*. New York: Alfred van der Marck Editions.

Levy, F. J. (1992) *Dance movement therapy: A healing art*. Reston, VA: National Dance Association of AAHPERD.

Sandel, S., Chaiklin, S., Ohn, A. (Ed) (1993) *Foundations of dance/movement therapy: The life and work of Marian Chace*. Columbia, MD: Marian Chace Memorial Fund.

Schoop, T. with Mitchell, P. (1974) *Won't you join the dance? A dancer's essay into the treatment of psychosis*. Palo Alto, CA: National Press Books.

Schoop, T., (2000) Motion and emotion. *American Journal of Dance Therapy*, 22 (2), 91–101.

Wallock, S. (1983) An interview with Trudi Schoop. *American Journal of Dance Therapy* (6), 5–16.

Whitehouse, M. (1970) Reflections on metamorphosis. *IMPULSE* (suppl.) 62–64.

Whitehouse, M. (1977) The transference and dance therapy. *American Journal of Dance Therapy* 1 (1) 3–7.

Whitehouse, M. (1986) Jung and dance therapy: Two major principles, in P. Lewis (Ed.) *Theoretical approaches in dance/movement therapy* Vol. I. Dubuque, IA: Kendall/Hunt.

Video

The Power of Movement (1982) Columbia MD: American Dance Therapy Association. Web site: www.adta.org.

CHAPTER 2

The Creative–Artistic Process in Dance/Movement Therapy

HILDA WENGROWER

Contents

> Creativity is one of the major means by which the human being liberates himself from the fetters not only of his conditioned responses, but also of his usual choices.

Arieti, 1976, p. 4

Introduction

This chapter deals with different aspects of the construct of creativity and their contribution to Dance/Movement Therapy (DMT). Its meanings and related concepts are introduced. This is followed by an overview of different authors' writings related to the concept of creativity and artistic involvement mainly, but not only, from the psychoanalytical perspective and the way these notions provide useful ideas for dance/movement therapy. DMT is one of the creative arts therapies; psychotherapeutic modalities that base their theories and practice on the potential for change and healing inherent to the creative process and artistic endeavor.

Professionals in the field of dance, persons dedicated to artistic and creative activities, have been those who laid the foundations of the profession of DMT in the middle of the 20th century. The multidimensional experience of the individual involved in this art was one of the main factors that led to this gestation because dance is an art that strongly integrates the physiological, cognitive, emotional, and sociocultural aspects of human beings. Psychotherapy at the end of the 20th century and the beginning of the 21st is marked by an acceptance of this multidimensionality (Fiorini, 1995; Dosamantes-Beaudry, 2003). Many colleagues include this multiplicity in their *Weltanschauung*—that is, in their world view.

Psychology, through its various approaches, has studied different aspects of the creative processes and of artistic activity, which are closely related phenomena. The most influential schools of thought in the context of our field of work are psychoanalysis and Jungian psychology. The presentation in this chapter does not mean to be exhaustive in scope but primarily concentrates on psychoanalytical contributions.

Creativity: Theme and Variations

I begin by elucidating the concept of creativity in order to relate it to the therapeutic process. Two types of creativity will be distinguished: the everyday (or ordinary) and the exceptional or eminent (Arieti, 1976, pp. 10–12). The first type is of special concern to us, because therapists are interested in the creative process of the human being asking for help, who likely is not involved in any occupation related to art.

The *Oxford English Dictionary* refers to creativity as "creative power or faculty; ability to create." As to the meaning of "create," it has a number of definitions, of which the most pertinent to our subject are the following:

1. Said of the divine agent: To bring into being, cause to exist
2. To make, cause, constitute … to cause, occasion, produce (*OED*, 1991)

Storr uses the following definition: "The ability to produce something new into existence" (Barron, 1965 in Storr, 1993, p. xv).

In DMT, in order for something to be considered new, it suffices that it is such for the individual who has connected ideas, phenomena, etc., and as a result created a new or different solution to a problem. Thus, an insight may be considered a moment of creation, or the connection established among aspects of personal life and feelings, thoughts, and modes of behaving. One of the main challenges in psychotherapy is how this can be facilitated.

The definition offered by Barron and mentioned by Storr leads us to an exposition of various concepts related to creativity. Namely, on one hand these are notions of the product of creativity and of the creative process, and on the other hand, the concepts of originality and spontaneity.

Process and Product

In verbal psychotherapy the spoken interchange is the main channel through which the therapeutic relationship flows. DMT works primarily with the nonverbal and danced expression of the patient and the therapist's movement and verbal input. The diverse purposes of these interventions may range from fostering a developmental process, assisting in the working through of a trauma, to accompany introspective, insight-focused therapy, and so forth. To achieve these, one means employed is the facilitation of a *creative process* in the therapeutic setting.

Generally, within artistic activity, a distinction is made between the process and the product, the latter being usually what is exposed to the public to be judged, although the contemporary artist tends to reveal the phases of preparation evermore. DMT does not set as a goal to elaborate a work of art as product nor to expose it in public; neither does it demand any formal or technical capacity for the person to be able to benefit from this type of therapy. Both the product and the process are seen and considered as fully as possible within the context of a dialog between a professional and a patient. How this is carried out will be seen over the succeeding chapters. What many dmts have learned from their experience as dancers and what psychoanalytical knowledge has added, is that creative process and results are psychologically meaningful and healing for the person engaged in them. Carol Press considered that psychoanalysis and creativity are not interchangeable, that the working-through processes cannot be replaced by artistic undertakings (2005, p. 119). In dance/movement therapy, we integrate them. This is possible when knowing psychodynamic theories about facets of the artistic endeavor.

Originality and Spontaneity

Originality and spontaneity are associated concepts within the theme of creativity. Storr, Arieti, and others are of the opinion that originality and spontaneity are not synonymous with creativity, even if they are related phenomena. Both are revealed in the fluidity of images, ideas, and actions. The technique of free-association of words that Freud used in treating his patients is based on the notion that spontaneous expression allows unconscious aspects to appear, decreasing their repressive control. Therefore, spontaneity can be part of the creative process, but as we shall see, it is not enough.

In DMT, this lack of restraint may be enjoyed by some groups of patients through improvisation. This is a rich and complex technique. From the beginning of the 20th century it flourished, strongly influenced by Freud's writings. Improvisation encourages the mover to detach from typical or stereotyped reactions and connotations, so that new psychophysical forms may emerge and be explored. At times, a person may even choose as a therapeutic goal the desire to be able to develop spontaneity as a way of feeling better with himself and his relationships. Lack of this trait of spontaneity often seems to be associated with difficulty in emotional expression or feeling unsafe. In other situations, as with some children with attention and hyperactivity disorder (ADHD), the therapeutic goal might be to develop awareness and control of their spontaneity, which is connected to impulsiveness.

Originality is manifested in various ways. Guilford (1968) used the term "divergent thinking" referring to unusual answers, when a solution, a response, or an option is sought. Nevertheless, Arieti does not fully value it, because Guilford stated that its purpose is to look for functional solutions; however, we have to consider that it may beget new narratives, understandings, and answers to situations of stagnation. Arieti's view is that originality includes spontaneity, even admitting that one often reaches an unusual reflection after intensive work. Thoughts of a psychotic patient will possibly be original, divergent, and unique, and their expression spontaneous, but they are associated with a bizarre trait removed from creativity. Arieti examines dreams in order to clarify the difference between originality, spontaneity and creativity. Although dreams are original and undoubtedly spontaneous, they are basically products of the primary process, the working mode of the unconscious.[1]

In DMT we are interested in subjective originality, in those changes the individual can explore for himself. Sometimes, the patient will embark on a process of experimentation with qualities of movement that are original to her characteristic style of movement in order to test new possibilities such as changes in body image, or his perspective/experience/understanding of a conflict. Fiorini (1995), a *verbal* psychotherapist, conceptualizes psychopathology as a trap of repetition and creation as a search for new options. Arieti suggests something similar (see quote at the beginning of this chapter).

Psychology, Art, and Creativity

Art and creativity have been subjects of study in psychoanalysis. Some of the aspects analyzed are: the person of the artist, the sources of his or her talent or motivation, the meaning expressed in the work of art, the unconscious psychological processes enabled by artistic activity, the creativity of geniuses and everyday creativity, and types of mental activity involved. Psychoanalysts of different schools have examined these subjects in relation to their theories, using examples from different fields of art: literature, visual arts, and music (Arieti 1976; Fiorini, 1995; Freud, 1908, 1914 and others; Klein, 1929; Kris, 1952; Storr, 1993). No one has related dance to a theory or used it as an example, which underscores what Anzieu has stated:

> In or about the period between 1950 to 1975, the great absentee, the unknown, the one relegated by teaching, by everyday life, by the expansion of Structuralism, of the psychologies of many therapists (...) was (and to a great degree still is) the body as a vital dimension of human reality, as a global pre-sexual and irreducible datum, as that in which the psychic structures find their support." (Anzieu, 1989/1998: 33, my translation)

It appears that psychoanalysts do not acknowledge an art in which the body of the artist is the message as well as the transmitter. Freud told Roman Rolland that he did not refer to music since it is related to the *oceanic feeling*, thus admitting lack of affinity with it. Dance, as music, is a nonverbal art, markedly sensorial, which can be very emotional for the performer and the viewer. It is a *temporal art*: movements and body shapes are performed and gone instantly, "the development over the whole length of a dance is based mostly on units of visual-kinesthetic time patterns; in other words, their duration, repetitions, similarities, contrasts, and relationships are revealed over time" (Nadel & Strauss, 2003, p. 272). The emphasis by psychoanalysis on verbal expression may be one of the reasons for the omission of dance from this field when researching art and creativity. The innovations presented in the work of Daniel Stern and others are a welcomed beginning.[2]

What follows is a brief synthesis of ideas that elaborate concepts related to art and creativity that I consider most noteworthy, as they are part of the theoretical base of DMT. While C.G. Jung has influenced DMT through his writings on art and the use of creative expression by patients in therapy, I will not discuss his ideas within this chapter. (For further reading see Chodorow, 1991.)

I will illustrate each theory with a brief clinical example that will be preceded by an asterisk. Because they are presented out of context, the reader might find more than one connotation for them or, if for the same person, the creative expression may have more than one discrete meaning. The human being is a complex creature, dealing simultaneously with various conflicts, issues, or developmental tasks. The movement/dance that discloses itself in the session may convey a style of interpersonal (*object*) relations, a sense of self or some adaptive/defensive modality (Govoni et al., 2007). Instead of presenting one single possible meaning, I include alternative interpretations. Creativity implies openness of the therapist as well, being aware of what may best explain the patient and help develop his of her process toward growth or change.

The creative process that unfolds during the session as part of the therapeutic process becomes integrated within DMT. The therapist encourages the expressive creative process and intervenes in ways that further acknowledge and accept it (Winnicott, 1979a).

Freud: Artistic Activity as Expression of Desires and Sublimation

Freud basically studied works by great artists; his writings on literary and visual art works are well known. He appraised them as revealing the unconscious, as symbolic expressions of desires, of the sexual drive, or as the direct satisfaction of these desires and drives—in other words, as a product of sublimation.[3] Despite an ambivalent position, especially regarding artists, and notwithstanding his expressed lack of knowledge as to aesthetics and the means to produce beauty, Freud established the basis upon which the psychoanalytic study of art and the artist was developed, including the art of laymen. Some of his ideas are currently disputed.

One of the problems in Freud's treatment of art is the segmentation he sometimes established between form and content. He said that he did not know about aesthetics but was interested in the significance of the work of art. However, when analyzing visual art, he definitely referred to forms as meaningful (Schneider Adams, 1993). Art criticism has shown that form carries meaning, and furthermore, that form itself *is* meaning. In dance, this is especially crucial, and therefore in DMT as well. Any reader can see that a jump, light and graceful, as an experience and emotion, is very different compared with a slow movement of dragging the body with a great deal of effort.

In his 1908 article Creative Writers and Daydreaming, Freud conceptualized artistic activity as a way of expressing desires and a means of realizing them, in both cases symbolically. He draws a comparison between the common features of the artist's activity and that of child's play. Both create a fantasy world and relate to it in a very serious manner, even as they are able to discern it from reality. The work of art yields a degree of enjoyment and appreciation that would be impossible without its aesthetic appearance or if the unconscious elements that are its roots were to be uncovered. Similarly, feelings that would otherwise be painful to withstand can be tolerated due to their presentation in a symbolic form. The artist unfolds aspects of psychic life while camouflaging them in the aesthetic form.

Rank (1907/1973) added that by publicly exposing her work, the artist achieves an unconscious pleasure: she expresses her desires and unconsciously shares the hidden meanings of her undertaking with the public. The open acceptance achieved through the display alleviates the guilt caused by these desires. In DMT, the therapist or the group sometimes functions as the audience.

> Therefore, according to Freud, a child who puts a cape on his shoulders and jumps and moves, crossing the space in a room, could be symbolically exhibiting desires of power and conquering, or his drive of penetration. The acceptance of this action frees the child from unconscious guilt and allows him to sublimate his desires through the game and the physical activity, thus taking his developmental process further.
>
> A group of adults in a day center of the public mental health system mark the rhythm with their feet while dancing in a circle, and comment that this reminds them of stepping on ants. They can thus express aggression, anger, or a similar emotion in a way that does not cause them anguish by means of symbolic thought. To summarize: "… in fact, the work can be a much more valid piece of self-expression than what is revealed in action or conversation in *real* life." (Storr, 1993, p. 109)

Artistic Expression as a Way of Approaching Reality

The similarity established by Freud, in particular, between the work of art and daydreams does not distinguish between levels of complexity and elaboration in the creative process and its product (Trilling in Storr, 1993). Storr considers that there is literature that constitutes the realization of desires or a catharsis, by both the author and by the reader, as in the novels by Ian Fleming with his character James Bond, or in romantic narratives. But these cannot be equaled to the works of Tolstoy, Proust, and other great writers, through which the reader acquires a subtler understanding of life and obtains the possibility of measuring him- or herself with more complex characters.

In DMT, we often find ourselves witnessing a game or a dance that expresses a desire, but this is not the only function fulfilled. When a girl dances "like a queen," we know that through this experience she tries out feminine forms of movement and action, and by doing so she is identifying with her mother or other women. She embodies and constructs her gender identity, develops self-perception and her bodily image. (Schilder, 1950)[4]

This girl may remind us of prehistoric man, who, with his mimetic dance, would move about wearing an animal's skin in order to obtain, in his fantasy, the powers of that creature that he might later confront while hunting. Therefore, we see not only an expression of desires, but a phenomenon of identification, inspiration, and training of social roles and aspects of the self. We could also think about Oedipal dynamics taking place. (Freud, 1900, 1910)

In the previous chapter we saw the connection between art and ritual. Frobenius (in Read, 1955), Lewis Bernstein (1979), and Wosien (1992) describe ceremonies that are performed before hunting. Their function was to allow a better knowledge of the animal that was to be pursued. Read adds that the human being felt and feels unsure and perplexed in facing the complexities and uncertainties of life and the cosmos; man desires a better comprehension of reality, a sharpening of those faculties that will aid him in fighting for his existence. Mimetic dance served this objective of increasing knowledge of the feared or adored animal. Art is not a pastime that employs free psychic energy but has been necessary for survival since the earliest days of humanity (Read, 1955:65). Dance, especially, has been used to find out what is furthest from understanding and communication (Béjart, 1973).

A girl, eight years old, with behavioral disorders with whom I worked individually in a special education school, approached me in one session imitating/parodying me: she smiled and talked gently, quite an opposite mode from her customary habit. From there we engaged playfully in a dance that adopted my style, allowing her to try to introject another embodiment.

If we further consider the analogy between play and the creative process stated by Freud, we must remember E. Erikson, who established that child's play has functions of adaptation and integration in his or her development, which is naturally asynchronous (Erikson, 1963). Play activity allows the harmonization of these asynchronic changes of different orders, physical, psychological, and social, through a fantasy put into action.

In DMT with children, the distinction between dance-movement and playacting is often blurred. In accordance with my statement that therapists have to be open to capture more than one meaning in one creative expression, the following example will be interpreted in three ways that may complement each other.

When 10-year-old Jackie plays soccer during a session, he possibly will be preparing himself to be more effective when engaged with his friends, or he may be showing his therapist his abilities and not only his difficulties. He might be trying to get her admiration and satisfy his need to feel recognized, seen as valuable and appreciated (Kohut, 1977; Winnicott, 1979). It is also possible that he is delineating the concrete and symbolic territories of each of the persons in the room. As time passes and he reduces the width of the goals, he may be saying he can also reduce his defenses within the relationship and that he feels less vulnerable and more trusting with himself as well as with the therapist. This possible meaning of Jackie's playing leads us into another function of creative involvement.

Creative Activity as a Defense against Anxiety

Storr (1993) studied the unconscious motivations and processes of the artist and the scientist, who are both committed to creative pursuits; what moves them to create, what do they seek with their endeavor? Many of his ideas can be implemented in order to understand patients and the artistic process carried out by them during therapy. One of the pillars on which this psychiatrist bases his work is the idea that creative activity is particularly suitable for protecting the human being from unconscious anxieties, and that some people turn to it out of this motive. Basing his ideas on concepts defined by Klein (1929), he works on the premise of two basic kinds of anxiety, the schizoid and the depressive. Regardless of theoretical perspective, the emotional characteristics of the schizoid or depressive individual can be distinguished.

These ideas stem from two factors:

1. Knowing the type of anxiety prevailing in the patient may allow formulation of a beneficial and creative action in exploratory or a supportive therapy. The objective may be different in each case.
2. The way in which a person commits him or herself in the creative process is indicative of the dominant anxieties and allows us to better understand the artistic expression.

Creating Control and Order

The schizoid style is introverted and eludes the possibilities of establishing affective relationships, which are unconsciously experienced as dangerous and untrustworthy. This avoidance carries with it a feeling of futility, of life lacking any sense, because emotional involvement is a factor that bestows meaning (Storr, 1993, p. 70). Another characteristic of the schizoid personality is the paradoxical combination of feelings of omnipotence and sentiments of vulnerability that are also characteristic in infants and children. Thus, a vicious circle develops, because the less satisfaction the person obtains from relationships, the more they are avoided, incrementing the tendency to focus on fantasies or the internal world. A person with strong schizoid traits has not been able to build a coherent image of the world, of the relationship between cause and effect and of the persons who are significant for growth.

For such individuals, their creative actions are on behalf of the purpose of control and to establish order. It is easier for them to be revealed through an artistic expression than in the course of a relationship. Fairbairn (1952/1994) saw this exhibitionist tendency as compensatory for difficulties in bonding.

Similarly, someone with high levels of anxiety, overwhelming life experiences, or a chaotic reality, may use art or play to achieve imaginary control.

> Lidia is a 32-year-old patient with schizoid characteristics. She prefers to move to classical music, making ballet movements while never having studied this style. Lidia enjoys the calmness, the slow movement, and the symmetrical harmony she finds in classical dance. She thought she would never explore the style of modern or contemporary dance, which she associates with dislocation and strong emotions. In DMT, the therapeutic relationship is not the only potential privileged space of treatment (Winnicott, 1979); but the creative process and its manifestation in the patient's work is another essential pillar in therapy. Therefore, the professional has to know not only psychology and psychotherapy and be aware of transference and countertransference processes, but must also have a wide and varied training in "languages of movement." This means diverse forms and styles of dance, body techniques, an awareness of personal movement as well as a *mastering* of the body. The dmt not only offers dance/movement ideas for exploration, but, in specific groups of patients, moves and dances with them. The therapist has to be open to and perceptive of small details, able to improvise, respond, and know how different movement and actions might be kinesthetically and emotionally experienced.

Achieving Recognition and Repairing Fantasized Inflicted Damage

A person with manic-depressive characteristics fears losing the affection and approval of others. Thus, we often see such an individual will adjust to meet the expectations of others, sacrificing his own. A manic state may manifest the contrary, a lack of interest in others. Storr found that artistic undertaking "eases the emotional problems of those who suffer a predominantly depressive psychopathology" (1993, p. 106).

One problem is that many times respect and consideration are not enough to fill the void the person feels. The recognition obtained is not a lasting experience. The person thus finds himself in a constant search for praise. For some, the fruit of their work is more important than themselves. They hope to obtain acknowledgment through the artistic product in which they are intensely invested. Yet, precisely due to the high emotional value assigned to it and the lack of differentiation between the work and the artist, it is sometimes difficult to conclude and expose it. Exhibiting it is tantamount to displaying one's innermost depths. An additional function of artistic creation may be the repair of suffered or inflicted aggression. This has special significance in the case of dance, where the differentiation between the artist and his or her work of art is less clear.

Winnicott: Life as Creation

The most influential contributions in DMT are those of D. W. Winnicott. Most important are the closely linked concepts of transitional phenomena, play, and creativity. Furthermore, he stipulates that the creative apperception (attitude) of life is "what makes the individual feel that life is worth living" (Winnicott, 1979, pp. 93–94).

These ideas fit wonderfully within the context of DMT and other arts therapies. Winnicott refers to the process of creation not as merely a vocational activity but as fundamental to the development of the individual and his or her relationships. The baby has the illusion of having created the object (an emotionally significant other) that, paradoxically, has been presented and offered by that same person in order to be created and used by the infant. For the sake of mitigating the absence of this caregiver, the baby also creates the first symbol that represents and substitutes for this person. The infant creates what Winnicott calls a transitional object, generally a blanket, part of a blanket, or a doll. Both Freud and Winnicott note that this absence, within a tolerable degree, based on a bond established with the caregiver, is what brings about the birth of symbols. The representation of the absent person is one of the main factors in the development of the individual through entering the world of symbols. This yearning leads to new meanings in life and we continue to create in order to substitute or cope with it.[5]

If Winnicott describes psychotherapy as the overlapping of the areas of play of the patient and the therapist, this is often quite evident in DMT, especially when working with children. It is true that he confers ample meaning to the concept of play in the therapeutic relationship, including associations, humor, and mental games. All of these are present in DMT and, additionally, we have parallels in movement, images, and metaphors. As Robbins said, it's about two minds trying to establish contact on a pre-logic level (Robbins, 1980, p. 27).

In my work with children, I discovered the precision of Winnicott's words when he said that if a patient does not play, our task is to help him do so. Introducing patients to the world of symbolization or of sublimation has often been one of the main objectives of treatment—and not only with children. My experience has shown that depressed persons, people with high levels of anxiety, rigid, highly impulsive, or hyperactive patients, have benefited from the work that the creative process of DMT allows to occur.

Psychotherapy as a Space of Creativity

There has been extensive writing about creativity in psychotherapy, psychology, and sociology, and about the task of continuous construction of the individual's identity. Some psychodynamic theorists, connecting philosophy and sociology, trust the possibility of evading the pitfall of the psychical determinism of personal history, and even the trap of trauma (Aulagnier, 1980; Castoriadis 1992; Cyrulnik, 2003; Fiorini, 1995; Strenger, 1998, 2003; Winnicott, 1979b).

Fiorini begins his book about what he considers the *creative psyche* and drive, the drive to create, with a reflection about the fundamental modes of being according to the philosopher E. Trías. These modes are (1) what one wishes to be; (2) what one has to be; (3) what one is; and (4) what one can be (p. 11). Fiorini affirms that psychology in all its trends has been occupied with the first three phases. He proposes the construct he calls *creative psyche* as a central element in an epistemology where the present is not consolidated, but is one of many possibilities of becoming. The *creative psyche* comes about in actions that alter the given, subvert what is codified and immobilized in the person and his narrative. I would add that the actions of change produced creatively may be behaviors of different orders such as mental, verbal, physiological, or movement (Bleger, 1970). Fiorini proposes new forms of conceptualizing some aspects in psycho-pathology and clinical practice, calling on the fields of creative processes and artistic production. He proposes the activation of the individual's creativity, which might be confined in what can be called *loops of enclosure in images and narratives* that are frustrating and limiting,[6] in order to look for ways of exiting them and bringing about new models of symbolization in the *tertiary order*. This concept will be further explained. One of his definitions of creation is confronting contradictions and tensions in order to bring about a new situation that may contain them in processes of change. With persons who suffer neurotic psychopathology, he suggests working with those contradictions and conflicts so that they transform into new constellations.

Fiorini takes up and innovates the concept of tertiary process, elaborated earlier by others, each of them adding his own input to the term. Arieti (1976) has defined this as the integration of the primary processes of thought that are characteristic of the unconscious level and the secondary processes used in everyday conscious logic. Therefore, they constitute a combination between the rational and the irrational, between the Principle of Pleasure and the Principle of Reality, which enables innovation. Green's explanation is that tertiary processes are "those processes which bring about a relation between the primary and the secondary processes in such a way that the primary limit the saturation of the secondary and the secondary limit the saturation of the primary" (Green, 1996).

To this statement we add that creativity and creation are "universal unconscious potentials," an expression of the tertiary processes that are developed in intersubjective links (Zukerfeld & Zukerfeld, 2005), thus including the importance of relationships and context in the process of change or innovation.

Some patients, mainly those with psychoses, may need help to develop the abilities of secondary process through movement and creation. Others may require an unblocking or a mobilization of that process. When a dmt fosters the patient's body awareness, body action in the here and now of the session or enactment of daily activities in harmony with group members, she is promoting experiences related to secondary process.

Allow me to introduce a brief linguistic digression. In addition to the categories of everyday creativity (Arieti, 1976), and the eminent one (that of the great artists), we also encounter the difference between creation *ex nihilo*, that is, the divine act of originating something from nothing, and the human act of creation. The romance languages as well as English do not have different words for these phenomena, while Hebrew, the language of the Bible, does. These different meanings can contribute to our subject. The biblical text starts with a cosmogonic narrative. The divine creation is called *briah*. In fact, this verb is used only for creation *ex nihilo*. Yet, when alluding to an act of creation carried out by a human, the term employed is *litzor*, whose linguistic root is suggestively the same as the words for "instinct" and "production." Hebrew *knows* that human creation is the conjunction between drive and the harsh task of adjusting to reality, of thinking, acting, and producing. The only creation that *generates* is the divine one, while the human creative process is of a tertiary order.

Returning to the ideas of Fiorini, Trias, and Winnicott, the dance movement therapist tries to enable the person who comes to the session to delve into the paths of what he might be, to try out new possibilities, to play with them. Toward this goal, DMT relates not only to the present body, the body that can be observed, but to the symbolic and metaphoric body as well.

> A certain individual's arm is not only an upper extremity moving in a restricted manner in space and remaining close to the torso. It is probable that this arm is fantasized as capable to hit, or that upon extending would make itself present, thus earning disapproval and rejection. One of these images could be the reason for the limited gesturing. Depending on the particular case, a therapeutic intervention would be to look for the meaning of this configuration, to go back in history, through movement, to situations and relationships related to the restricted gesture. This process would begin by exploring the presenting movement or posture. Accordingly, the patient will search for the emotion that the particular gesture expresses or suppresses. The procedure has similarities with verbal psychotherapy. Phenomena of transference and counter-transference would be treated, and further, the body and its emotional baggage are present, active, and acknowledged throughout the entire process.

In DMT we promote the tertiary process, discovering new meanings and experiences of self, as we propose exploration of movements, images, metaphors, often in nonlinear paths of thought and action. In addition, we create a space of therapeutic relationship where the patient can embark on a process of introspection and integration. He or she can also try out different ways of being, actual and potential. To elaborate on this last point, I will turn to the theory of communication.

The Analogical Characteristic of Dance/Movement

Watzlawick et al. (1967) distinguished between two modes of communication: the digital mode and the analogical mode. The first mode is mainly verbal language in which the relationship between significant and signified is a matter of convention. It has rich and complex syntax, but alone is less efficient in expressing emotions or conveying relationships, and in this aspect is semantically limited. In contrast, the analogical mode is more closely related to the signified; it is based on similitude and equivalence, has more freedom from conventions, but is far from being univocal. This is the case of gestures, movements, body posture, the use of space and interpersonal distance (proxemics), and the nonverbal aspects of speech (speed, modulation etc.)

Various authors agree that analogical patterns are the privileged mode of emotional expression. Nowadays we don't maintain this as a strict division, especially when we deal with artistic expression, and approach art as communication. In poetry, words can be used in an analogical manner and elsewhere, movement can be used in a very cognitive way. Another interesting point is that the shift from one kind of language to another implies the loss of information, to which Daniel Stern (1985) would agree, as he wrote that language acquisition by the infant implies simultaneously the attainment of one language and the loss of another.

"Analogic communication can be more readily referred to the thing it stands for ... has its roots in far more archaic periods of evolution and is, therefore, of much more general validity than the relatively recent, and far more abstract, digital mode of verbal communication" (Watzlawick et al., 1967, p. 62). Buck and VanLear (2002) distinguish between spontaneous and pseudo-spontaneous nonverbal behavior. The first one is based on very ancient biological, nonintentional, and nonconscious shared systems. In spontaneous nonverbal behavior the inner state is directly associated with its display, so, "... it makes no sense to inquire whether they are true or false, for if the internal state did not exist, the signs would not exist" (p. 525).

> An example of the analogical features of movement is that of a person whose muscles are very contracted, the torso is shrunken, movements are contained, slow, and lacking a focus in space, breathing flows in a limited manner. This individual has a very different experience of self and the environment compared with another who is relaxed, breathes deeply, and moves fluently.

In DMT one of the methods of intervention in the above example may be to offer the client the chance to experiment with different types of movement, to feel herself and the environment with these new qualities, exploring associations and the connotations they yield. As Stanton-Jones (1992) said, movement generates a new experience of *being in the world*. In DMT we relate to the basic kinesthetic, emotional, and symbolic aspects of movement, while the functional is on a secondary level.

Some Aspects of Improvisation in DMT

In DMT, one of the tools through which the therapeutic/creative process may take place with the purposes stated above is improvisation. It was stated earlier that improvisation may bypass repression and diminish repetition. It favors disconnection from usual meanings and responses, looking at them from different perspectives and offering opportunities for exploration of unknown styles and movements, opening the way for change or innovation. Its main tool is the body, its relations to others or to props. Movement dynamics are "the full range of human attributes including the physical, conceptual and emotional resources embodied.... With improvisation there is the hope that one will discover something that could not be found in a systematic preconceived process" (Carter, 2000: pp. 181–182) It opens the possibilities of leaving the loops of enclosure, stagnation, and iteration. This method clearly illustrates the reciprocal influences between dance as an art and its relation to psychology that contributed to the formation of DMT and gave name to this book.

An element the therapist observes, aside from the aspects already discussed, is the time the person requires to begin or to sustain the improvisation. I will present two examples to demonstrate that it is not only the movement, the dance, or the creative activity that determines the process and what is observed, but also the way they are carried out and the therapeutic relationship established. Psychodynamically, form is meaning and content.

> Lidia, whom I mentioned earlier, would end her improvisations very quickly and would immediately tell me what she had experienced. In her case, there was difficulty in containing her experiences and staying with them.
>
> Ruth, a 33-year-old woman, would improvise for very short periods of time and would move with her eyes open, very quickly getting "solutions" or answers. After several months working together, I suggested she spread a blanket on the floor, lie down on it and start to move only when she had some sort of sensation or feeling in her body. When she finished her work and I asked her to share her experience with me, the first thing Ruth talked about was her wondering whether I had been watching her or doing anything without being attentive to her. I was utterly astonished at her suggestion until I remembered that Ruth had grown up in a kibbutz, where she used to sleep in the "children's home," away from her parents and sharing the space as well as the attention of the caretaker with nine other children. For this woman, Ruth had no special meaning and the young child did not see herself reflected in her eyes (Winnicott, 1979a). From that day on, it was clear that one of the most therapeutic elements was the meeting of our gaze at the very moment when she would finish an improvisation. From then on, this encounter had a deeper quality. Ruth could enhance her "ability to be alone" and to trust my attentive and careful look (Winnicott, 1981).

From these examples we learn that there might be hindrances toward engaging in a profound creative process. This is left for another time.

Conclusion

The purpose of this chapter has been to highlight the meanings and functions the creative process has for mental health and their contribution for psychotherapy through dance/movement. Toward this end, I have presented various topics and theories regarding creativity that have been developed in psychology and psychoanalysis.

I adhere to the integrating position of Noy (1969), who recommends not to blindly adopt a specific school of thought but to be aware of the process and its vicissitudes, and to try to understand them within the context. This choice does not imply eclecticism; it is the result of many years of work that have taught us to adopt a basic position, but one that is flexible and attentive to specifics.

The ability to tolerate uncertainty is one that a dmt has to develop, remembering that "the most complex activities of thought can come to be without the conscience having taken part in them" (Freud, 1900). The dance movement therapist has not only to have gone through his or her own therapy, supervision, and continuous training in areas of psychology, but also has to dance, to be acquainted with movement techniques, and to be up to date regarding the history of dance and contemporary developments in this art.

Endnotes

1. Primary process: see in Laplanche and Pontalis, 1973.
2. Several researchers of early development stated that the first interpersonal relationships have characteristics similar to those of the temporal arts. They describe the first interactions as *performance*, in which sound, facial gesture, and movement create communication and attachment (Dissanayake, 2001; Español, 2006; Stern, 1985, 2004; Trevarthen 1982, Wengrower, 2009). Stern (1985) acknowledges KMP and other systems of movement observation that dance therapists use (p. 159).
3. A definition of sublimation: "the drive is sublimated, in as much as it is derived towards a new, non-sexual end, and points towards socially valued objects." (Laplanche and Pontalis, 1973). Freud referred to artistic activity and to scientific investigation as activities of primordial sublimation. He also alluded to the drive for aggression as a source of this process. Sublimation can be seen as a transaction between the instincts and social norms (Homs, 2000).
4. Schilder remains a pioneer with his study of body image and the influence of movement and physical activity on it.
5. For the reader not acquainted with these ideas, I recommend Winnicott's seminal book *Playing and Reality* (1971).
6. This statement may be compared with some authors writing about the Narrative Approach (Richert, 2006; White, 2008).

References

Anzieu, D. (1998). *El Yo-Piel*. Madrid: Biblioteca Nueva. Trans. S. Vidarrazaga Zimmermann. (In English, 1989, *The skin ego*, New Haven: Yale University Press.)

Arieti, S. (1976). *Creativity: The magic synthesis.* New York: Basic Books.

Aulagnier, P. (1980). *El sentido perdido.* Buenos Aires: Trieb.

Béjart, M. (1973). Préface. In R. Garaudy, *Danser sa vie.* Paris: Seuil.

Bleger, J. (1970). *Psicología de la Conducta.* Buenos Aires: Centro Editor de América Latina.

Buck, R., & VanLear, C.A. (2002). Verbal and nonverbal communication: Distinguishing symbolic, spontaneous and pseudo-spontaneous behavior. *Journal of Communication,* 52 (3), 522–541.

Carter, C. (2000). Improvisation in dance. *The Journal of Aesthetics and Art Criticism,* 58 (2), 181–190.

Castoriadis, C. (1992). *El Psicoanálisis, Proyecto y Elucidación.* Buenos Aires: Nueva Visión.

Chodorow, J. (1991). *Dance therapy and depth psychology: The moving imagination.* London: Routledge.

Cyrulnik, B. (2003). *Los patitos feos.* Trans. T. Fernández Aúz and B. Eguibar. Barcelona: Gedisa.

Dissanayake, E. (2001). Becoming *Homo Aestheticus:* Sources of aesthetic imagination in mother–infant interactions. *SubStance,* 94/95, 85–103.

Dosamantes-Beaudry, I. (2003). *The arts in contemporary healing.* Westport, CT: Praeger Publishers.

Erikson, E. (1963). Toys and reasons. In *Childhood and society.* New York: W.W. Norton.

Español, S. (2006). Las artes del tiempo en Psicología. Actas de la V Reunión de SACCoM. 9–25.

Fairbairn, W.R. (1952/1994). *Psychoanalytic studies of the personality.* London: Routledge.

Fiorini, H. (1995). *El psiquismo creador.* Buenos Aires: Paidós.

Freud, S. (1900/1953). Typical dreams in the interpretation of dreams. *Standard edition of the complete psychological works of Sigmund Freud.* London: Hogarth Press. 4: 241–276.

Freud, S. (1908/1973). Creative writers and daydreaming. *Standard edition of the complete psychological works of Sigmund Freud.* New York, International Universities Press, 9. 141–155.

Freud, S. (1910/1953). A special type of object choice. *Standard edition of the complete psychological works of Sigmund Freud.* London: Hogarth Press, 11. 166–175.

Freud, S. (1914/1968). El Moisés de Miguel Angel. *Obras completas.* Trans. L. Lopez Ballesteros. Madrid: Biblioteca Nuevo 1069–1082.

Govoni, R.M., & Piccioli Weatherhogg, A. (2007). The body as theatre of passions and conflicts: Affects, emotions, and defenses. *Body, Movement and Dance in Psychotherapy,* 2 (2) 109–121.

Green, A. (1996) Notas sobre procesos terciarios. In *La metapsicología revisitada.* Buenos Aires: Eudeba. 185–189

Guilford, J.P. (1968). *Intelligence, creativity, and their educational implications.* San Diego, CA: R.R. Knapp.

Homs, J. (2000). El arte, o lo inefable de la representación. *Tres al Cuarto,* 1, 14–17.

Klein, M. (1929). Infantile anxiety situations reflected in a work of art and in the creative impulse. *International Journal of Psychoanalysis,* 10, 439–444.

Kohut, H. (1977). *The restoration of the self.* New York: International Universities Press.

Kris, E. (1952). *Psychoanalytic explorations in art.* New York: International Universities Press.

Laplanche, J., & Pontalis, B. (1973). *The language of psychoanalysis.* Oxford, England: W.W. Norton.

Lewis Bernstein, P. (1979). Historical Perspective in DMT. In *Eight theoretical approaches in dance-movement therapy.* Dubuque, IA: Kendall Hunt. 3–6.

Nadel, M., & Strauss, M. (2003). *The dance experience. Insights into history, culture and creativity.* Highstone, NJ: Princeton Books.

Noy, P. (1969). A theory of art and aesthetic experience. *Psychoanalytical Review,* 55, 623–645.

Oxford English Dictionary (full edition), 1991.

Press, C. (2005). Psychoanalysis, creativity and hope: Forward edge strivings in the life and work of choreographer Paul Taylor. *Journal of the American Academy of Psychoanalysis and Dynamic Psychiatry,* 33(1), 119–136.

Rank, O. (1907/1973). *Art and artist: Creative urge and personality development.* New York: A. A. Knopf.

Read, H. (1965). *Icon and idea. The function of art in the development of human consciousness.* New York: Shocken.

Richert, A. J. (2006). Narrative psychology and psychotherapy integration. *Journal of Psychotherapy Integration,* 16(1), 84–110.

Robbins, S. (1980). *Expressive therapy.* New York: Human Sciences Press.

Schilder P. (1950). *The image and appearance of the human body,* New York: International Universities Press.

Schneider Adams, L. (1993). *Art and psychoanalysis.* New York: Harper Collins.

Stanton-Jones, K. (1992). *Dance movement therapy in psychiatry.* London: Routledge.

Stern, D. (1985). *The interpersonal world of the infant.* New York: Basic Books.

Stern, D. (2004). *The present moment in psychotherapy and everyday life.* New York: W. W. Norton.

Storr, A. (1972/1993). *The dynamics of creation.* New York: Ballantine Books.

Strenger, C. (1998). *Individuality, the impossible project: Psychoanalysis and self-creation.* Madison, CT: International Universities Press.

Strenger, C. (2003). The self as perpetual experiment: Psychodynamic comments on some aspects of contemporary urban culture. *Psychoanalytic-Psychology,* 20(3), 425–440.

Trevarthen, C. (1982). The primary motives for cooperative understanding. In G. Butterworth and P. Ligth (Eds.), *Social cognition.* Brighton, U.K.: Harvester.

Watzlawick, P., Beavin, H., & Jackson, D. (1967). *Pragmatics of human communication, a study of interactional patterns, pathologies and paradoxes.* New York: Norton.

Wengrower, H. (in press). Dance then and now; in history and in the individual. Why dance in therapy. In S. Scoble, M. Ross, & C. Lapoujade (Eds.) *Arts in arts therapies: A European perspective.* Plymouth, U.K.: University of Plymouth Press.

White, M. An outline of narrative therapy. http://www.massey.ac.nz/~alock/virtual/white.htm (Accessed 12 Nov 2008).

Winnicott, D.W. (1971). *Playing and reality.* New York: Basic Books.

Winnicott, D.W. (1979a). Papel de espejo de la madre y la familia en el desarrollo del niño. In *Realidad y juego*. Barcelona: Gedisa. 147–156.

Winnicott, D.W. (1979b). *Realidad y Juego*. Trans. F. Mazía. Barcelona, Gedisa.

Winnicott, D.W. (1981). La capacidad de estar a solas. In *El Proceso de Maduración en el Niño*. Barcelona: Laia. 31–40.

Wosien, M.G. (1992). *Sacred dance: An encounter with the gods*. London: Thames and Hudson.

Zukerfeld, R., & Zukerfeld, R.Z. (2005). *Procesos Terciarios. De la vulnerabilidad a la resiliencia*. Buenos Aires: Lugar.

CHAPTER 3

Therapeutic Relationships and Kinesthetic Empathy

DIANA FISCHMAN

Contents

Introduction

Kinesthetic empathy is a core concept that has long been mentioned in dance movement therapy (DMT) literature and implemented in dance/movement therapy practice. Empathy is the ability of one person to understand another. It attempts to experience somebody else's inner life and implies knowing what the other one feels, having information about the other's situation and acting accordingly. It arises out of elements that are common in the experience of both individuals who are involved in the empathy process. Considered one of DMT's major contributions to psychotherapy (Levy, 1992), this construct synthesizes an approach of the dynamics of the therapeutic relationship that includes non-verbal communication, bodily movement, dancing and verbal expression. Through the use of kinesthetic empathy, the dance therapist facilitates the self-development of a client when the process has been blocked or interrupted. It demands that each therapist be open to his or her inner sensations and feelings and be aware of what is familiar in his or her own movement. Understanding, acknowledging, and interpreting are functions inherent in therapeutic processes that aim to relieve human suffering. The ways in which these operations are defined determine different practices in psychotherapy. Dance movement therapy focuses on the experience of movement sensing and how movement makes sense. The dance therapist gets empathically involved in an intersubjective experience that is rooted in the body.

This chapter illustrates how these concepts can be integrated into DMT practice. To understand this approach it is necessary to describe first the epistemological frame of reference that explains psychotherapeutic practices oriented to somatic and relational expressions.

Psychoanalysis and psychotherapies have been influenced by the new paradigms of contemporary scientific postmodern thinking. The truth is no longer conceived as essential and unique but diverse, partial, implying different perspectives that undergo a continuous transformation. Pure objectivity is an illusion. Reality is a consensual construction. Laws and truths that pretend to be absolute collapse. Meanings are contextually related. Today, a therapeutic relationship is considered the encounter of subjectivities, two perspectives meeting for the goal of comprehending one.

Influenced by Sullivan's thinking (Levy, 1992), Marian Chace conceives DMT as a relational therapeutic modality that intervenes in response to the patient's movement patterns. Therapists reflect through their own movements the clients' experience. The dance therapist, acting as a partner, begins a dialogue of movement. Communication is established through all available sensorimotor channels, favoring both nonverbal and verbal expression. Chace empathically involved herself in the subjective experience of the patient, joining him "where and how he is." They jointly create an environment of trust and safety that helps in unwinding defensive behaviors, exploring conflictive aspects of the patient's life, and allowing spontaneous expressive movement to emerge. In this way the dance therapist is able to facilitate fluid communication with the most cut-off aspects of the client's self, facilitating awareness of being and becoming alive that gradually enables a socialization process.

DMT is essentially a discipline that is continually evolving. A variety of dance and psychotherapy approaches are interwoven in the construction of this practice. Today, neurosciences, early developmental research, Self Psychology, Relational psychoanalysis, and certain concepts of post-rationalist cognitive science such as embodied mind and enaction (Varela et al. 1991) contribute to explaining what dance movement therapists (dmts) early understood on an intuitive level.

DMT can be seen as an enactive approach. What does this neologism mean? It means that "we can only know by doing" (Maturana, 1984). Classical cognitive science conceived that an inner mind represents an outer world using symbols. In its development, cognitive science arrived at a newer concept that views mental processes as embodied in the sensori-motor activity of the organism and embedded in the environment. This viewpoint has come to be known as enactive or embodied cognitive science (Varela et al., 1991) The basic principles of the enactive approach state that "the mind is not located in the head, but is embodied in the whole organism embedded in its environment"; "Embodied cognition is constituted by emergent and self-organized processes that span and interconnect the brain, the body, and the environment"; "In social creatures, embodied cognition emerges from the dynamic co-determination of self and other" (Thompson, 2001, pp. 1–32).

Affect and emotion that had been seen for decades as interferences in cognition are now considered as the basis of the mind (Damasio, 2000; 2001). Neuroscientists describe affects as prototypical whole-organism events; Thompson (2001) goes further and says that much of affect is a prototypical two-organism, self–other event. In this way empathy becomes an evolved human biological capacity.

Enaction and Embodiment

We will describe a way of thinking that strives to overcome the dualistic mind-body separation.

Enaction is a word that comes from the verb to enact, which means "to start doing" as well as "to perform" or "to act" (Varela, 2002). It entails an epistemology of complexity that considers knowledge to be a constructive organic experience; in a single act something is perceived, created, and transformed. This perspective integrates action, perception, emotion, and cognition. The term enaction synthesizes the effectiveness of DMT, as it operates on the repertoire of the patient's movement patterns, bringing them to a conscious level, and offers an unprecedented opportunity to expand this range through new intersubjective experiences.

Human movement patterns involve emotional tonalities that have intrinsic meaning. Laban (1987) and Bartenieff (1980) hold that movements or effort dynamics that have been developed by different animal species shape their body structure, limiting and enabling an action repertoire, while the body structure determines the species' movement habits. In the same way, human bodies have been shaped by the effort habits they have developed in their relationship to the environment through the ages. The subjective experience is indissolubly tied to its own structure, according to Maturana (1984). Our clinical practice endorses this theory every time we come across patients whose limits and possibilities are anchored to their past experiences, to their history. Their ways of being become actualized in every action, and each new experience becomes an opportunity of finding something different through a new intertwining of self, other, and the environment. We also know that change is genuine when it becomes part of our own spontaneous movement repertoire and this may happen when we get our safety needs met.

Enaction theory conceives knowledge as action in the world, therefore as movement, a living cognition emerges as it manifests in every vital moment. The world in which we live emerges or is molded; it is not defined a priori. Enaction is an epistemological background with which I conceive DMT; individuals know the world through their own actions. This occurs at the same time they co-create the worlds in which they live, generating their everyday life. By this process people transform themselves and their world, at the same time the world transforms them (Varela et al., 1997; Najmanovich, 2005).

DMT is a therapeutic modality in which the patient and the therapist compose,[1] taking into account the developmental needs of the patient, which at the same time is reciprocally determined as the task unfolds. Co-determination doesn't mean absence of the sense of self-determination, owning sense of agency of each participant of the dyad. Both know their role, needs and intentions, and at the same time they regulate their behaviors intersubjectively. This means that they affect each other consciously and unconsciously.

The literature has described a diversity of aspects and perspectives from which this therapeutic relation phenomenon can be accessed. I have chosen the concepts co-determination (Thompson, 2005), compose (Deleuze, 2004), affective attunement (Stern, 1996), and kinesthetic empathy (Berger, 1972), to consider how their nuances relate to DMT clinical practice. The same consideration will be given to the terms grounding (Lowen, 1991) and embodying (Johnson, 1991; Lakoff & Johnson, 1998) considering that both are used to describe the idea of "inhabiting the body."

To Inhabit the Body or Life Is Elsewhere

The causes that induce us to separate ourselves from our body are complex and diverse. One of DMT's main goals is to revitalize the body, reestablishing the connection that has been blocked.[2] Motherly care, physical manipulation, the introduction and support of the world as an object, modulate the processes of integration, personalization, and the sense of existential continuity in an infant (Winnicott, 1979). The sense of core self (Stern, 1996) is the result of a healthy condition. The flaws in the constitution of the self are related to a deficit in early care. Winnicott describes holding as the mother's ability to contain each and every one of the states (hunger, sleep, cold, tiredness, interest, excitement, calm, and attention) the baby experiences during the day. Holding is related to the temporal process within which the infant develops and thereby permits it to experience existential continuity. Handling and contact refer to the ways in which the baby is touched, rocked, carried, and moved.

The early relational patterns are influenced by the way these operations are performed and can be described according to time, space, intensity, degree of activation, and hedonic tone. The caregiver participates actively in the self-regulation of the dyad itself.

Winnicott (1979) believes that the flaws introduced by erratic maternal behavior produce hyperactivity in mental functioning which becomes reactive. The mind-body opposition is born here. Cognition starts moving away from the intimate relationship it had with the psychosoma. Each infant has different qualities. Therefore, observing the dyad as a whole, one can see how they affect each other and reciprocally regulate their interaction (Stern, 1996). As dance therapists we draw on Winnicott's concepts that underlie his outlook on the integration processes that lead to the construction of the self as psychesoma, as well as for shedding light on the importance of the way actions or caretaking are performed.

The self, meaning awareness of our own existence, is not there from the very beginning. It is a lifelong construction resulting from the development of intersubjective experiences. The sense of self as a separate being is determined by our primary experiences. Stern states that the ability to recognize oneself as the performer of one's actions implies:

1. To have volition, to have control over the generated action.
2. To be consistent, to have a sense of being a non-fragmented physical entity, with boundaries and integrated actions both when moving and standing still.
3. To have affections, to experience qualities.
4. To have a personal story, a sense of permanence and continuity with one's past, so that one can change and yet remain oneself (1996, p. 95).

This core sense of the self as being an agent is the foundation of all the other more elaborate domains of the self such as the awareness of our own subjectivity and others.

The primordial self is shaped in the preverbal stages of development, whereas the possibility of naming and telling the story of one's experiences is added later on with the addition of the verbal domain (Stern, 1996). The exploration of different combinations and ranges of movements, sounds, and touch as intervention modes including words, make DMT the ideal approach to access non-integrated or undeveloped aspects of the nonverbal domains of the self that need to be restored.

Failures and misunderstandings occurring in the original mother–infant dyad shape the self accordingly, and result in a partially developed or false self. Winnicott (1979) refers to the feeling of nonexistence. This description relates to the phenomena of dissociation, split personality, non-integration, and disintegration of the self that we observe in our clinical practices. When the sense of existential continuity is interrupted or absent, the perception of temporality manifests itself in particular ways: a timeless life, in a dream world, discontinuous, accelerated, or slowed down. In depersonalization processes the body and its actions may be experienced as something strange, as an enemy. Taking action may not be recognized as one's own. The body is felt as if it falls forever or is injured in a psychotic disintegration. As an example, I remember a physically healthy woman who argued that she had marital problems because "her spine was broken."

Whoever has gone through a traumatic situation has experienced the dissociation implied in abandoning the body to avoid feeling pain, denying the experience. A disconnection from oneself occurs. The connection with the body is lost in the attempt to interrupt the flow of information coming from the perceptive channels. Pain is blocked and so are all other feelings such as anger, fear, and so many other affects considered to be negative or dangerous. Even pleasure can be segregated. There are families and cultures that deny or prohibit some emotions among their repertoire. Emotional expression is thus limited to a minimally accepted spectrum. Expanding the movement repertoire goes with expanding the range of emotions. Embodiment implies revitalizing the body, reestablishing the enactive sensoriperceptive connection and recovering the possibility of accessing the emotional wealth present in the unfolding of life.

Case Study: From Survival to the Experience of Existence

I will illustrate the transition from survival to the sense of existence from a clinical report.

Pablo, about to turn 50, seeks help to solve his grief from a broken love affair that he anticipates as endless. He is down, devastated, with no interest in life. Having almost no hope in his chance to heal, he starts therapy submissively trying to do what he is told. He begins each session pouring out his grief and pain, complaining and going into a long and detailed account of his frustrated relationship. This is repeated during each session in a monotone manner, methodically, with a discourse that shows no change. It appears as a traumatic repetition containing no elaboration. He seems to need to be heard, to let his pain be known. It seems that he could repeat the story hundreds of times as a way of getting back together with his lover; the love of his dreams being more real than all the other aspects of his life. Pablo lives in his own mind. He is hardly aware of my presence and my hearing; it appears that "his life is elsewhere."

Pablo lost his mother when he was 4, and from then onward he lived in different boarding houses. He chose a military career where respect and absolute obedience meant survival. His linear, thin, and emaciated body shows an extreme level of stress. After listening to the daily story, and when my own body no longer tolerated being unknown as a presence, I invited Pablo to lie down on a mat and watch his own breathing, to discover which parts of his body move under the effect of the circulating air. He balances and discovers the floor that holds him and explores his limited and painful possibilities of moving. Gradually, and through a slow process, Pablo begins to perceive. After quite a few sessions he manages to recognize his rigidity and he discovers how he has lived in armor as a way to avoid feeling life. He begins to learn of his survival. Through contact with my hand, his chest expands, he makes sounds, he finds his pain, he cries like a disconsolate child while curling into a fetal position, which allows me to find a way of holding him by touching his head and tail bone. I meet the child inside the man. We are moved. He ends the experience and recovers his usual posture, but he and I know that there is something else, a new affective tone that impregnates everything. There are many monotonous and repetitive sessions that take turns with those other ones where a moment of contact arises, where closeness and encounter with another existing human being is possible. Through such instances of decisive experience of recognition, new relational patterns will be built in which a new variant appears. These "human warmth" experiences of finding new ways of relating, contribute over a long term to allow his body to be a livable space.

Movement and Emotion

Movement involves affective tonalities that are inevitably expressed, although on occasions they remain at an unconscious level for the mover. A complex system of processes and degrees of muscular tension relaxation allows affects to emerge. The inhibition, repression, or suppression of emotions (by means of extreme tensions, sometimes chronic ones) and at the opposite end, the explosion, outburst, or loss of emotional control, make up the range of expression.

Dmts invite patients to experience new combinations of muscular and respiratory activities. They offer an opportunity to record alternatives in the bodily emotional expression within a supportive environment that helps to regulate and modulate emotions. DMT's effectiveness is related to working with the awareness of bodily experiences when they emerge, are recreated, or repeated.[3] DMT operates where sensation and meaning come together. Freud (1916) believes one of the aspects of the therapeutic process is to reconnect affect and meaning when they have been separated. Focusing and working with the body and movement enhances the integration of the psychosoma (Winnicott, 1979).

The dmt, in the role of an observer who participates, becomes the necessary relationship within which new emotional experiences can develop in a safe environment of respect and trust. DMT posits that the integration of sensations, perceptions, affective tonality and cognition in the intrapersonal, interpersonal, and transpersonal domains promote development.

During clinical practice with children, adolescents, and adults, the operative specificity of DMT is related to implicit messages. Dmts grasp and meet the needs of those aspects of the self that are disadvantaged, split, or frozen. They understand within their bodies as they echo with that of the patient. Therapists structure movement exploration in accordance with the particular mobility qualities of the patient to elicit movements, sounds, and sensations that were missing in the patient's original experience.

Transitional space, as Donald Winnicott describes it, is an area developed between self and other inner and outer worlds, mother and infant, which allows primary creativity, meaning the sensing of self-existence. It is a potential space in which it is not important who does what, it is a place for relaxation, of freedom, where spontaneity arises. Through movement interactions, DMT creates transitional spaces between the dance therapist and the patient through which an inner world is unfolded and shared. Welcoming the patient's movement qualities becomes the key to get to movement spontaneity. DMT operates by processing, on a body level, experiences from the past that could have been profound intersubjective misunderstandings. In this way, it takes care of the aspects of the self that were neglected and therefore injured.

Relational interactions can be analyzed as relational patterns. Acknowledging Laban movement analysis categories and Stern's (1996, 1998) summary of transmodal qualities involved in emotional attunement, we can enumerate and group qualities as follows:

1. Related to time: speed, rhythm, duration
2. Related to space: origin-path-goal, edges or boundaries, axes and coordinates
3. Related to energy: intensity, strength, weight, fluidity
4. Related to support: degrees of rigidity and flexibility
5. Related to physical contact and different handling modes
6. Related to the ways objects are presented: lack or excess of stimulation, spectrum of qualities presented
7. Related to the range of actions and concomitant affects: intersubjective emotional regulation

All these abstract sensed qualities can be combined and in their complexity become actions and phrases. DMT process focuses through a wide range, beginning with abstract simple qualities being in the process of organization, to complicated scenes, memories, and stories with highly dramatic dynamic contents. Enabling this spectrum allows integration of different domains of the self.[4]

Transference in DMT

This approach focuses and underlines presymbolic intersubjective features in relation to transference. Besides recognizing the classic psychoanalytical theories of drives, symbolic, representational, and verbal models, the enacting model alludes to emerging processes that include repetition and restraint. It argues that when contextual changes take place, a quantum of modification happens in the self; when this amount increases, a qualitative behavioral transformation occurs.

New procedures designed "to be with" destabilize the preexisting behavioral organization and work like a change engine to make more coherent and flexible forms. Repeated encounters give rise to increasing complexity and articulation of relational procedures.

Relational psychoanalysis focuses the attention on implicit forms of knowledge that involve procedures, actions, and skills. It suggests that besides verbalization and recovery of memories to bring the unconscious to consciousness, it pays attention to affective–perceptive and spatial–temporal experiences. Changes in this operational modality do not always become symbolized. This does not deny the value of words and narration of lived experiences. It maintains that they are two parallel and interlinked ways of operating, one verbal and the other one preverbal, and untranslatable one into the other (Lyons-Ruth, 1999).

Changes that happen in the intersubjective plane do so thanks to what Stern (2004) calls moments of encounter. The concept of moment captures the subjective experience of a sudden (here and now) change in the implicit relational knowledge for both parts of the dyad. Mutual regulation of this state is based on the interaction or exchange of information through perceptual systems, demonstration of affect, and how they are appreciated and correspond with the process that implies bi-directional influence (Stern, 1998).

During the development of the sense of oneself and of the other, from the self psychology perspective, Kohut (1990) maintains that the driving force of the therapeutic process is determined by the reactivation of frustrated needs of the self in the transference through repetition. The patient searches unconsciously for a new chance to restore his damaged self through a new encounter with somebody who responds more empathically than those relations experienced originally. He points out the three fundamental aspects involved in transference:

1. Mirror transference: transference relative to personal ambition, trying to cause within the self and in the other confirmatory and approving responses, looking for appreciation.
2. Idealization transference: patients seek, from their injured ideals, that the self and the other one tolerate being idealized. It is related to the feeling of grandiosity.
3. Twin transference: transference referring to talents and skills that seek an encounter with the peer or fellow man. It is related to sharing, in opposition to isolation (Kohut, 1990).

These three ways involve the basic needs of individuals who all through their lives search for acceptance, relationship and personal worth. Meeting somebody virtually similar, who mirrors and reflects back what the person experiences, is a concept supported by Winnicott (1982), Lacan (1988), and Chace (Chaiklin & Schmais, 1986). This eagerness for empathic encounter evolves from suffering emptiness, loneliness and devaluation.

DMT proposes a theoretical-clinical system that operates when words are not a sufficient form of contact and encounter. It favors the establishment of a type of transference that operates at a psycho-corporeal level, recovering the experiences that were frozen in the body through chronic spasms and tensions that have inhibited movement, and the intensively longed for and unlived spontaneous interactions. Empathetic mirroring or kinesthetic empathy facilitates the expressiveness of the self and enables a response that differs from the original, restoring the damaged self and succeeding in developing richer and more meaningful interactions.

Kinesthetic Empathy

In his history of empathy, Wispé (1994) points out that in 1873 in a paper by Vischerin related to aesthetic perception, the concept "Einfühlung" meant feeling with the artist, admiring his work. This indicates that empathy as a concept is a very recent achievement of culture.

Dance therapists were influenced by contemporary thinkers such as Rogers, Adler, Sullivan and Jung, among others. They all were interested in the suffering of people and how to relieve them from their excessive pain and trauma during the postwar period of the 1940s and 50s.

At the University of Chicago, many well known philosophers and psychologists with different perspectives converged, with their ideas contributing to the development of empathy as a concept and as a technique implemented in psychotherapy. Each emphasizes some aspect involved in this ability. George Mead, Bruno Bettleheim, Heinz Kohut, Martin Buber, and Carl Rogers are among them (Shlien, 1997).

Today, empathy is thought of as a collectively developed concept that is continuously revisited and renewed. Neuroscience (Gallese, 2003; Iacobini, 2008), early developmental research (Stern, 1998; Meltzoff, 2002) and post-rationalist cognitive science (Varela, 2001; Thompson, 2002) provide strong support in the deepening of the field of empathy.

Dance/movement therapists evolved movement and nonverbal communication aware that they essentially involve emotion and embodied cognition. Marian Chace describes empathic mirroring coming from her own intuitive experience of reflecting her patients in her intent to get into their idiosyncratic worlds. Communication was her goal. She let them know that she was available and interested in their feelings, movements, and thoughts. By making the spontaneous movements of the patients her own, acceptance showed in her body. Mary Whitehouse worked in a different setting— the transformed dance studio, where more highly developed movers and dancers were eager to be in contact with their inner worlds. Through the richness of the collective unconscious, active imagination, and creativity, she became a special witness for their processes by allowing herself to resonate and letting her body be moved by the experience of others.

Mirroring and resonating, both faces of the same coin, the first externally oriented and the second inner directed, are implemented during movement sessions as main tools of deeply understanding others' experience. Through movement and dance, perception, understanding, and intervention, dance therapists are able to relate to both inner and outer worlds. They understand that empathy enables intimacy and human closeness. The process involves elements that are common in the experiences of both individuals so that recognition of differences is therefore tolerable.

Freud (1982), in *The Psychology for Neurologists*, describes a psychic system that works toward searching identities and establishing differences. The subject compares the current experience with the original mnemonic imprinting, and through this quasi-mathematical and deeply unconscious process, he builds a perceptive reality, providing categories to the world of significant objects. This operation happens in an intersubjective matrix.

In the research "Dance Movement Therapy as a medium of improving empathy levels of educators and health working professionals" (Fischman, 2006), I maintain that the common factors in the intersubjective experience imply twinlike conditions, closeness, fusion, consensus, while discrepancies refer to that belonging to somebody else, difference, otherness, strangeness. Total agreement disallows subjectivity, while total discrepancy disconnects. Kinesthetic empathy implies one and the other in varying proportions but with a positive balance favoring similarities.

It is a co-relational, descriptive research design that relates different variables or issues. The participants were professional women working in Buenos Aires as educators, psychotherapists, and midwives. Forty subjects divided into four groups attended eight DMT sessions of 2 hours each. The average age was 41 years old. None had dance training. The content of the workshops: "DMT, emotions and professionalism" consisted of exploration of space, time, flow, and weight. These movement activities led the group to move, be moved, and talk about their experiences related to themselves and issues in their work.

Several research scales were used that compared affective tones, movement, and relational qualities between duos during their improvised dance interactions. With a tool created for the purpose, participants marked their perception of enumerated qualities involved in their own movement experience, in their partners, and how they imagined their partners viewed them. Comparing scores from a first interaction to a second evaluation made eight sessions later, we found that perception of relational qualities (such as sensation of comfort, being molded, individuation, fusion, freedom, discomfort, pleasure, displeasure, being followed when initiating, willing to follow when other initiates, shared interests) diminished differences among partners; perception of affective tones diminished differences comparing their own to their partners; and perception of movement qualities diminished differences of self perception and of others in quantitative terms. Analyzing item by item told more about improvement of differentiation levels between self and the partner.

Some conclusions found through the research were

1. Modified movement, affective tones and relational qualities are considered as kinesthetic empathy factors.
2. Positive affects increased while negative ones diminished. Emotional intelligence, empathy, psychological well-being, and life satisfaction levels improved.
3. Changes in movement repertoire relate to psychological changes.

Some meaningful associations between health indicators and kinesthetic empathy results were as follows: differences in the *perception of Time* comparing how each perceives himself and the partner perception had a positive correlation with negative affects such as difficulties in describing another's feelings. Not sharing a similar perception of time as a movement quality brings discomfort, misunderstanding, and negative affects. As an example of this, we only need to think of a hurrying mother walking with a slow toddler on their way to kindergarten.

Differences in perception of weight during movement interaction had a very meaningful negative correlation with emphatic concern. Use of weight suggests strength and weakness. The wider the perceived difference of use of weight seems to diminish the will to attend to others' needs. As an example, we can imagine a strong man meeting a weak one. How do they behave and feel about each other? We would hope that both might be open to and understanding of the other. If this is so, there is empathy, which is an achievement in the evolution of humankind. But we also painfully know that sometimes being alive means the survival of the strongest. Fortunately, we don't depend only on our use of weight as strength; humans have a wider range of resources.

To understand other human beings sometimes implies overcoming distance through mechanisms such as: simulation, imitation, echoing or using our imagination whereby we build theories matching our own and somebody else's experiences. This manner of understanding empathy implies that not everyone empathizes with everybody. It is the inter-subjective matching that makes a therapeutic couple work. This concept becomes graphic when we ask our colleagues about the choice of the population with which they prefer to work. We are sure to find common affinities between the experiences of therapists and their patients. The empathetic possibility is relational and selective. One of the basic goals in DMT is to expand movement repertoire so that it will lead to a wide variety of experiences and resources which allow us to accept, respect and understand different human feelings and ways of living in the world.

Both Chace and Whitehouse stress the corporality of the empathetic phenomenon; the former by mirroring through the use of her own movement and the latter by resonating internal movement, felt or imaginary, while witnessing somebody else's experience. Both forms imply some degree of communion with the group or patient through the dance therapist's own felt body experience.

Whitehouse (1999), imbued with Jung's thinking, uses the concept of active imagination to create an introspective investigation. Unfolding the spontaneous expressive movement that appears driven from deep inside the human being in touch with the collective unconscious provides a source of riches and wisdom (Chodorow, 1991, 1997). She describes making use of the active imagination, which makes it possible for the unconscious to emerge through free association, by implementing diverse expressive forms, among them painting, dance, sculpture, games, and words. This implies interruption of critical and rational faculties with the aim of giving way to fantasy, getting in touch with the emptiness or silence inside in order to reach the unconscious. In other words, we integrate the emerging processes within the self. The aforementioned description can be attributed to an empathetic process, where in the presence of a witness acting as a vital other receives the contents of the unconscious like a caring midwife receives the newly born. Picking up its vital strength and its delicate fragility, and allowing time for it to develop, concedes that at some time this development will take its own shape, clear and consistent.

Janet Adler (1999) writes in depth of the roles of "mover" and "witness." She points out that empathy happens in the bodies of witnesses when watching the dance of the dancer while focused on their own corporeal experience. Dancers resonate with what they see, hear, feel in their own bodies, picking up and understanding the other from their own felt experience. The material registered by the mover and the witness, added to the verbalization of the experience, will engender a process of empathetic accompaniment in revealing unconscious contents.

Chace interacts with patients with the conviction that movement expression tears down verbal barriers and defenses. In this way, she manages to draw them out from their psychotic isolation (Levy, 1992). "Mirroring" or reflecting shows a strong correspondence with the concept of "transmodal affective attunement" (Stern, 1996, pp. 99–173). Stern describes an intersubjective domain of self that involves communication, like a mother and baby understanding each other. Sharing affective states comes from matching qualities. Each partner takes part in the interaction, sharing elements of the other's manifest behavior, by imitating, mirroring, introducing "modifying imitations" that maximize or minimize some features of the other's behavior and giving continuity to the communicative-expressive-emotional process. The matching is produced by a correspondence of the intensity, of the temporal or spatial modality present in the conduct of both participants.

Caregivers and infants mutually create chains and sequences of reciprocal behaviors that make up the social dialogue of the baby's first 9 months of life. Attunement suggests mother–baby's affective exchanges. It has to do with active accompaniment from the caretaker. Stern (1996) points out that these communicative modes do not get lost but become working forms of the self during one's entire life. Attunement implies affects that are always the transmodal coin involved in sounds, movement, touch, and any experience related to pleasure–displeasure that leads to approach and avoidance as human basic movement.

Consciousness of oneself as an embodied individual in the world is founded on empathy—on one's empathic cognition of others, and others' empathic cognition of oneself (Thompson, 2001).

Some Contributions from Neuroscience

Neurologists have validated empathy as a physical phenomenon. The concept of the "imitative mind" (Meltzoff, 2002) and the findings describing the function of "mirror neurons" account for the neurological bases of intersubjectivity and the organic roots of empathy. The ability to understand others is rooted in the nature of our interactions. A pre-reflexive form to understand other individuals is based on the strong identity that binds us as human beings. We share with our fellow human beings a multiplicity of states that include actions, sensations, and emotions. Gallese (2003) thinks that it is through this shared diversity that communication, intentional understanding, and recognition of others as our fellow human beings are possible. Similar neuronal structures are activated in the processing and control of actions, perceived sensations, and emotions when the same are perceived in others. Mirror neurons, originally discovered in relation to actions, may be considered a basic organizational form of our brain that enables the rich diversity of intersubjective experiences.

Through imitation we are able to feel what others feel. Different schools of thought have investigated imitation, emotional contagion, and analogy phenomena. (Iacobini et al., 1999; Hatfield, Cacciopo & Rapson, 1994; Holyoak & Thagard, 1995). These phenomena, despite their great conceptual difference, are here considered a continuum where there is a variation in the degree to which identical and different characteristics manifest themselves. Full identity is also a conceptual ideal as no two dogs, two canaries, or two spoons are ever "absolutely" identical. But, from my point of view, seeing these differences may be caused by many circumstances such as the distance of the observer, personal background, previous interactive experiences, knowledge, and particular interest at the time of the observation, the context, attitude, the movement, the object state, and other variables. The concepts of similarity and difference are always relational.

Processes within DMT

DMT focuses on the most elementary aspects of interactions through minimum variations, almost homeopathic doses of the qualities involved in the emergence of the behavioral phenomenon such as changes in the concrete management of time (speed, duration, rhythm, continuity–discontinuity), of weight (degree of force—softness, strength), of space (direction, levels, spatial planes), flow (degree of activity—quietness, high energy) and body parts involved (whole body, the limbs, the trunk, the head). The phenomenon is complex; while a glance is quick and avoidant, the hands may be warm and grasp. While the abdomen is relaxed, the chest might be tense, reducing the expansive capacity of the plexus during inspiration and increasing that of the abdomen. The system implements multiple compensations in order to live or survive according to context.

Kinesthetic empathy implies identification and differentiation. Identification basically connects, binds, reflects, or resounds. Differentiation brings novelty, uniqueness, otherness, distance, separation, strangeness (Fischman, 2006). Therapeutic sessions imply the patient's and dance therapist's cultures meeting. By acknowledging differences, exchange becomes possible. It is a complex process, in which a patient sometimes resists change while the therapist reserves the time and space waiting for the patient to work through defenses to allow such change.

To include movement and dance in psychotherapy reminds us that we are continuously evolving and therefore we are, by being. The dance, like a metaphor, reminds us that we are permanently changing, even though we may not always nor immediately achieve the changes we long for.

Kinesthetic empathy is a form of knowledge, of contact and shared construction that may take many forms. It might appear through direct mirroring and affective attunement in the dance therapist's movements— the forms, qualities and tones of the body language. It might also make use of analogy, metaphor, the telling of a semantically isomorphic story with movement or the patient's verbalization.

Movement explorations are designed by capturing themes or issues patients show in their postures, gestures, attitudes, movement, and speech. The patient's behavior expresses itself in different modes. The dance therapist acts in transmodal forms—through diverse sensorimotor channels (auditive, kinetic, visual, and tactile). In this way, a dialogue among different channels begins where similarity and the matching of qualities and meanings will prevail. Inevitably, differences that contribute toward facilitating the approach and confrontation with reality will also emerge with a maximum of shared reality and a degree of difference, a nourishing and stimulating diversity.

We believe that any new element should be gradually presented so that it is not experienced as unacceptable, strange, and disruptive. Identity may be felt to be at risk. To develop, the self requires going through the experience of omnipotence, which implies feeling as the creator; having the illusion of being one and the same with the object and feeling as the discoverer of its world. This experience should be "good enough" so as to later be able to tolerate disappointments that set the limits of the personal domain (Winnicott, 1979, 1982).

The therapeutic process is seen as an affective—cognitive—creative experience that implies a shared adventure. Recognizing a patient's need, dmts are ready to be available objects known by their perceptible personal qualities. Here is where the paradox exists of the therapists accepting shared intimacy and closeness and at the same time, abstaining from participating in the patients' personal life. They thus become a substantial part of the patients' lives and at the same time, are not included in it. Therapists authenticate the patients' perceptions, reestablishing their basic confidence as a perceptive affective organism.

Again, paradoxically, the therapeutic relationship is real and virtual at the same time. The dmts play intersubjective roles that are imposed on them as transference needs, accepting the assigned role, assuming the role, character, or attribute the patients need them to be. It is in the combination of both the virtuality of the performed movement and the reality of each of the participants that the relational change occurs.

To Meet the Patient's Needs

The following clinical vignette illustrates how affective attunement operates in providing understanding.

Susana is a successful lawyer. She dazzles with the richness of her language and the clarity of her arguments. She seems to have everything under control, except for her home, husband, children and even the dog, who do not meet her expectations in the least. Her headaches begin when she enters her house, where she usually loses her temper, arguing with all the members of her family. She says they make her life miserable and that the only solution is to move to her law firm. She sets aside all the annoying aspects of life by projecting them on her close relatives, who in turn do not feel loved, and thus frees herself for a moment from what she dislikes.

When she started attending her sessions, she enjoyed moving with intensity. She preferred music with "gay and quick" rhythms, to which she moved frantically. Her discourse and the quantity of associations were endless. Did she expect to receive an award or acknowledgment? Did she expect that, finally, someone would tell her that she was so very good? Very slowly, Susana became aware of the attention and care she was receiving during the session, and at the same time, she started recognizing amiable attitudes from her family.

Susana discovered the floor and found unconditional support on which she investigated different possibilities for contact. When exhausted from her own intensive movement, she explored slowness until she finally found stillness. At this point, she became aware of her daily life rhythm and speed. She said she did not deserve so much care. She recognized her primitive cruelty and started worrying about the effects of her actions. How are others feeling? What did I do to them? How is it that they are still with me, needing me? Susana started to alternatively integrate movement and stillness as valuable resources. Through experiencing a whole range in between these polarities, she started to tolerate the love and hate coexisting inside her. She lost part of her identity as "Mrs. Successful" but started feeling less lonely. She managed to value other aspects of her life. According to her, the experience of finding her own dance allowed her to "get rid of what I had in excess and to have access to unknown feelings," to get rid of old demands, which became manifest in her own self abuse through her addiction to work. Internalized original relationships with which she identified were causing her terrible pain that she turned into hatred against herself and her family. The DMT process where she could move according to her needs, the sustained presence of the therapist, kinesthetic empathy expressed in the most subtle contacts, in the music selected for her experiences, the tone of the dialogues, made it possible for her defenses to give way. Her degree of denial and projection started to decrease; her defensive intellectualization started to turn into an embodied rationality connected to her feelings and emotions. She stopped depending on herself alone and began trusting in human relationships.

Conclusion

This approach describes a way of understanding that emerges from the practice of human encounter rather than from critical judgment. Empathy as it evolves through the therapeutic relationship is at the heart of DMT and it is the basis of this therapeutic model.

Endnotes

1. Term used in the Spanish translation of Deleuze's *En medio de Spinoza* to refer to a joint creation or construction of that which is becoming (Deleuze, 2004).
2. Several authors warn us not to take "life in the body" for granted (Berman, 1990, 1992; Caldwell, 1999; Winnicott, 1979; Lowen, 1990, 1991) *Life is somewhere else* alludes to Milan Kundera's novel of that title (Kundera, 2001).
3. The approach coincides with Damasio's description (2000) of the emergence of mental patterns he calls *images of an object* and Johnson (1991) describes as *image sketches*, referring to periodic and dynamic patterns of perceptive interactions and motor programs that structure and add consistency to the experience.
4. Daniel Stern's description of self, focusing on different domains of Self and Other as relational and individual developments, is useful to understand for the range of levels, aspects and experiences DMT covers. The domains are sense of emergent self, core self, subjective self, and verbal self.

References

Adler, J. (1999): Who is the witness? A description of authentic movement. In Whitehouse, M. J. Adler, & J. Chodorow. *Authentic movement*. London. Jessica Kinsley.

Barnes, A., & Thagard, P. (1997). Empathy and analogy. University of Waterloo Philosophy Department. http://cogprints.org/620/00/Empathy.html. Accessed 2/19/09.

Bartenieff, I. (1980). *Body movement: Coping with the environment.* New York: Gordon and Breach Science Publishers.

Berger, M. R. (1972). Bodily experience and expression of emotion, *American Journal of Dance Therapy*, 24(1), 27–33.

Berman, M. (1990). *El reencantamiento del mundo.* Santiago, Chile: Cuatro Vientos.

Berman, M. (1992). *Cuerpo y Espíritu.* Santiago, Chile: Cuatro Vientos.

Caldwell, C. (1999). *Habitar el Cuerpo.* Santiago, Chile: Ediciones Urano.

Casullo, M., & Castro Solano, A. (2000). Evaluación del Bienestar Psicológico en Estudiantes Adolescentes Argentinos. *Revista de Psicología.* Pontificia Universidad Católica del Perú, XVIII (I), 35–68.

Chaiklin, S., & Schmais, C. (1986). The Chace approach to dance therapy. In Lewis, P. *Theoretical approaches in dance therapy.* Vol. I. Dubuque, IA: Kendall/Hunt.

Chodorow, J. (1991). *Dance therapy and depth psychology: The moving imagination.* London: Routledge.

Chodorow, J. (1997). Jung on active imagination. In *Encountering Jung.* Princeton, NJ: Princeton University Press.

Deleuze, G. (2004). *En medio de Spinoza.* Buenos Aires: Cactus.

Damasio, A. (2000). Sentir lo que sucede. Cuerpo y emoción en la fábrica de la consciencia. Chile: Andrés Bello.

Damasio, A. (2001). *El error de Descartes.* Barcelona: Crítica.

Damasio, A. (2003). *Looking for Spinoza: Joy, sorrow, and the feeling brain.* Orlando, FL: Houghton Mifflin Harcourt Inc.

Davis, M. (1983). An introduction to the Davis Nonverbal Communication Analysis System (DaNCAS). *American Journal of Dance Therapy*, 6, 49–73.

Diener, E. (1994). Assessing subjective well-being: Progress and opportunities. *Social Indicators Research*, 28, 225–243.

Fischman, D. (2006). La mejora de la capacidad empática en profesionales de la salud y la educación a través de talleres de Danza Movimiento Terapia. Buenos Aires. Tesis Doctoral. Biblioteca Universidad de Palermo.

Freud, S. (1916). *Lecciones introductorias al psicoanálisis: Teoría general de las neurosis.* Obras Completas. (1972) Tomo IV, Madrid: Biblioteca Nueva.

Freud, S.(1982). *Proyecto de una psicología para neurólogos.* Obras Completas. Buenos Aires: Amorrortu.

Gallese, V. (2003). The roots of empathy: The shared manifold hypothesis and neural basis of intersubjectivity. *Psychopathology*, 36, 171–180.

Hatfield, E., Cacioppo, J., & Rapson, R. (1994). *Emotional contagion: Studies in emotion and social interaction.* New York: Cambridge University Press.

Holyoak, K. J., & Thagard, P. (1995). *Mental leaps: Analogy in creative thought.* Cambridge, MA. MIT Press/Bradford Books.

Iacobini, M. (2008). *Mirroring people: The new science of how we connect with others.* New York: Farrar, Straus and Giroux.

Iacobini, M., Woods, R., Brass, M., Bekkering, H., Mazziota, J., & Rizzolatti, G. (1999). Cortical mechanisms of human imitation. *Science,* 286, 2526–2528.

Johnson, M. (1991). *El cuerpo en la mente.* Madrid: Rogar.

Johnson, M., & Lakoff, G. (1998). *Metáforas de la vida Cotidiana.* Madrid: Ediciones Cátedra.

Jung, C. G. (1999). *Recuerdos, Sueños y Pensamientos.* Barcelona: Editorial Seix Barral.

Kohut, H. (1971). *The analysis of the self.* New York: International Universities Press.

Kohut, H. (1990). *¿Cómo cura el análisis?* Buenos Aires: Paidos.

Kundera, M. (2001). *La vida está en otra parte.* Biblioteca Breve. Barcelona: Seix Barral.

Laban, R. (1987). *El dominio del movimiento.* Madrid: Fundamentos.

Lacan, J. (1988). *Mas allá del principio de realidad,* Buenos Aires: Siglo XXI, p. 84.

Lakoff, G., & M. Johnson (1999); *Philosophy in the flesh. The embodied mind and its challenge to western thought.* New York: Basic Books.

Levy, F. J. (1992). *Dance movement therapy: A healing art.* Reston, VA: National Dance Association, American Alliance for Health, Physical Education, Recreation and Dance.

Lewis, P. (1986). *Theoretical approaches in dance movement therapy.* Vol. 1. Dubuque, IA: Kendall-Hunt.

Lowen, A. (1990). *La Depression y el cuerpo.* Madrid: Allianz.

Lowen, A. (1991). *Bioenergética.* Méjico DF: Diana.

Lyons-Ruth, K. (1999). The two-person unconscious. Intersubjective dialogue, enactive relational representation and the emergence of new forms of relational organization. Trans. Manuel Esbert con autorización de Analytic Inc. Press. *Psychoanalytic Inquiry,* 19, 576–617.

Maturana,H, (1984). *El árbol del conocimiento.* Santiago, Chile: Universitaria.

Meltzoff, A. (2002). *The imitative mind. Development, evolution and brain bases.* London: Cambridge University Press.

Najmanovich, D. (2005). *El juego de los vínculos.* Buenos Aires: Biblos.

Paez, D., & Casullo, M. (2000). *Cultura y Alexitimia.* Buenos Aires: Piados.

Rogers, C. R. (1957). The necessary and sufficient conditions of therapeutic personality change. *Journal of Consulting Psychology,* 21, 95–103.

Salovey, P., Mayer, J. D., Goldman, S. L., Turvey, C., & Palfai, T.P. (1995). Emotional attention, clarity and repair. exploring emotional intelligence using the trait meta-mood scale. In J.W. Pennebaker (Ed.) *Emotion, disclosure & health.* Washington, DC.: American Psychological Association, pp. 125–154.

Sandel, S., Chaiklin, S., & Lohn, A. (1993). *Foundations of dance movement therapy. The life and work of Marian Chace.* Columbia, MD: The Marian Chace Memorial Fund of the American Dance Therapy Association.

Sealers, H. (1980). *Escritos sobre Esquizofrenia.* Barcelona: Gedisa.

Shlien, J. (1997). Empathy in psychotherapy. A vital mechanism? Yes. Therapist's conceit? All too often. By itself enough? No. In A. Bohart & L. Greenberg (Eds.), *Empathy reconsidered. New directions in psychotherapy.* Washington, DC: American Psychological Association, pp. 63–80.

Stern, D. (1996). *El mundo interpersonal del infante.* Buenos Aires: Paidós.

Stern, D. (2004). *The present moment in psychotherapy and every day life*. New York: Norton & Co., Inc.

Stern, D. et al. (1998). Non-interpretative mechanisms in psychoanalytical therapy. The "something more" than interpretation. *International Journal of Psychoanalysis*. 79, 903.

Thompson, E. (2001). Empathy and consciousness. *Journal of Consciousness Studies*, 8, (5–7), 1–32.

Thompson, E. (2005). Sensorimotor subjectivity and the enactive approach to experience. *Phenomenology and the Cognitive Sciences*, 4, 407–207.

Varela, F. (2002). *Conocer*. Barcelona: Gedisa.

Varela, F., Thompson, E., & Rosch, E. (1997). *De cuerpo presente, las ciencias cognitivas y la experiencia humana*. Barcelona: Gedisa. (The embodied mind, cognitive science and human experience, Cambridge, MA: MIT. http//mitpress.mit.edu.)

Whitehouse, M., Adler, J., & Chodorow, J. (1999). *Authentic movement*. Pallaro, P. (Ed.). London: J.K.P.

Whitehouse, M. (1999). Creative expression in physical movement is language without words. In *Authentic movement*. Pallaro, P. (Ed.), p. 33. London: J.K.P.

Williamson, G., & Anzalone, M. (1997). Sensory integration: A key component of evaluation and treatment of young children with severe difficulties in relating and communicating. Washington, DC. *Zero to Three*, 17, 1997.

Winnicott, D. W. (l979). *Escritos de pediatría y psicoanálisis*. Barcelona: Editorial Laia.

Winnicott, D. W. (l982). *Realidad y Juego*. Barcelona: Gedisa.

Wispé, L. (1994). History of the concept of empathy. In N. Eisenberg & J. Strayer (Eds.), *Empathy and its development*. Cambridge, U.K.: Cambridge University Press.

CHAPTER 4

Dance Therapy, Motion and Emotion

JOAN CHODOROW

Contents

Introduction

This chapter speaks about the ongoing interwoven relationship between the emotions and the imagination.* In addition to distinctive patterns of felt bodily sensations and expressive physical actions, emotions have their own

---

* This chapter is adapted from The Marian Chace Foundation Annual Lecture, "The Moving Imagination" published in the *American Journal of Dance Therapy*, vol. 22, no. 1: 5–27.

potential patterns of imaginative development. I will give special attention to a limited number of basic emotions as they intermingle and combine with each other, transforming into a sensitive network of feelings and emotionally toned complexes and ultimately the highest values of human culture. Emotions and their forms of facial and bodily expression have always been important to dance/movement therapy studies. However, for many years, American academic psychology considered the study of emotion and imagination to be unreliable, unscientific, and even disreputable. Only a few became interested in the individual emotions or in the possible interactions of emotions with each other, or in the relation between the emotions and other functions of the psyche. Things finally began to turn around in the mid-1980s and since then there continues to be an increasingly strong interest in the emotions and their development across many fields of study, including interest in the relationship between emotions and imagination. Hopefully, this paper will contribute to a more differentiated understanding of dance movement therapy as a comprehensive method of psychotherapy that draws in a natural way from the intrinsic forms of imagination, particularly the aesthetic, the religious, the philosophic/scientific, the social, and the central, self-reflective psychological imagination.

In this new millennium, it is useful to pause and reflect on historical resources. This material is largely informed by an elegant and useful theoretical synthesis proposed by Jungian analyst Louis Stewart. I offer it as a way to strengthen a continuing process of creative development. His differentiated understanding of the relationship between affect and archetype and his contribution of the archetypal affect system is relevant to Dance Therapy as well as Analytical Psychology because it is all about the body, the imagination and the emotions.

Stewart's archetypal affect system is a multidisciplinary synthesis, drawing from a wide range of classic and contemporary sources highlighting the contributions of C. G. Jung and Silvan S. Tomkins. For Tomkins (1962, 1963), the affects are the primary, innate, biological motivational system of the higher mammals, including human beings. The drives and other responses are secondary. Emotion not only amplifies the drives, but it motivates memory, perception, thought, and action as well. In this aspect of his theory, Tomkins was restating the same theory that had been proposed by Jung as early as 1907: "The essential basis of our personality is affectivity. Thought and action are, as it were, only symptoms of affectivity" (CW 3:38, par. 78). For Jung, emotions are the source of value (1951, CW 9-II:27–28, par. 52; and pp. 32–33, par. 61), imagery (1961:177), energy and new consciousness (1938, CW 9-I:96, par. 179). What Tomkins had to offer that was new was a carefully developed hypothesis of the evolution of the affects that specified a particular set of emotions and their particular functions.

I'm using the terms affect and emotion interchangeably. I use several terms to describe the inherited emotions, for example, primal, archetypal, primordial, innate, primary, basic, fundamental, etc. Moods and feelings are understood as myriad complex mixtures, modulations, and transmutations of a limited number of basic emotion themes.

Louis Stewart's first paper on the affects was written in collaboration with his brother Charles Stewart. Stewart and Stewart (1979) proposed a system of seven inherited affects. They built on the idea that every basic emotion has its own symbolic stimulus that is partly conscious and partly unconscious. The conscious part consists of certain typical life situations that are likely to stir a similar reaction in most people, for example: Loss (sadness), the Unknown (fear), Restriction of autonomy (anger), Rejection (disgust), the Unexpected (startle), the Familiar (joy), and Novelty (interest). The unconscious part, then, would have to be primordial image-imprints at the foundation of the psyche that mirror these typical or existential situations of life. For example, the primordial image-imprint that corresponds to loss would have to be something like archetypal emptiness, the void. When the inner void meets the life situation of loss, the two parts unite to form a symbolic stimulus that releases emotion along a range of intensity, in this case, distress or sadness, or grief or anguish, depending on the kind of loss and the individual situation.

Trudi Schoop, one of the pioneers of dance therapy described something like this many years ago when she used the German word *ur* to identify the primal or archetypal experiences of life. She said there are two kinds of fear. There is the basic *ur* fear or archetypal fear that is always there as an unconscious potential. And then there are the conscious fears that can be named. In speaking of her own childhood fears, she remembered each of them distinctly. The conscious fears "were reminders which tapped the ur fear inside" (Schoop, 1978, p. 96). Another way of saying this: When the *ur* or archetypal image is mirrored by a corresponding life situation, there is a mutual recognition or reverberation in psyche's body that releases a particular emotion.

The Biological Substratum

Images of reverberation are described in the book *Molecules of emotion* (Pert, 1997). Ever since her early discovery of the opiate receptor, Candace Pert has been engaged with the neurochemical aspect of emotion. Her description of the biological process that draws a particular chemical to a particular receptor offers a way to imagine the affect releasing function at the molecular level. There may be millions of receptors on the surface of a typical nerve cell, of at least seventy different types. In her words, the receptors

… hover in the membranes of your cells, dancing and vibrating, waiting to pick up messages carried by other vibrating little creatures, also made out of amino acids, which come cruising along—*diffusing* is the technical word—through the fluids surrounding each cell. We like to describe these receptors as "key holes" although that is not an altogether precise term for something that is constantly moving, dancing in a rhythmic, vibratory way. …

Though a key fitting into a lock is the standard image, a more dynamic description of this process might be two voices—ligand and receptor—striking the same note and producing a vibration … to open the doorway to the cell. (Pert, 1997, p. 23–24)

Ethologists seem to describe a similar process when they speak of the "innate releasing mechanism" (Tinbergen) or the "key tumbler" structures that release patterns of instinctive behavior in animals and humans (Stevens, 1983, pp. 56–58). In his 2003 study *Emotions Revealed;* Paul Ekman describes his early use of the term "autoappraisers," which must exist within each individual. Autoappraisers constantly scan the environment to receive and evaluate input from every sensory organ, often in milliseconds, below the threshold of consciousness.

In recent years, neuroscientists have turned their attention to "mirror neurons," a new classification of neurons involved with processing and controlling actions, sensations, and emotions. Vittorio Gallese speaks of a mirror-matching mechanism (made up of different kinds of mirror neurons) that "could well be a *basic* organizational feature of our brain, enabling our rich and diversified intersubjective experiences" (2003, p. 171). An outstanding contribution by Cynthia Berrol "examines aspects of the neurobiological mechanisms and evolving theoretical constructs of mirror neurons and then views them through the qualitative lens of the therapeutic process vis-à-vis DM/T and empathy" (2006, p. 303).

The formation of neural connections throughout the brain/mind/body is largely movement-dependent (interactive and self-motion), not only in infancy and childhood, but over the life span. Even when we seem to be still, every breath, every thought and every feeling has a neuromuscular component. Through the use of noninvasive neuroimaging techniques, mainstream science gains a better understanding of brain plasticity; implicit (somatic) memory; neural aspects of actions, sensations and emotions (mirror neurons); imitation learning; affect attunement; affect regulation; creative and destructive aspects of projection; and other embodied experiences. It is an exciting time to be alive as insights emerging from the field of neuroscience support and enrich dance therapy, depth psychology, and related fields of study.

For Louis Stewart, a symbolic stimulus or process releases an emotion or mood. It involves a coming together, a union of conscious and unconscious domains: "The conscious stimuli of 'life experiences' must be 'met' so to speak, by unconscious, innate image/imprints, or the potential for such image/imprints" (1986, p. 200).

Seven Primordial Image-Imprints

In his search for what the innate image-imprints might be, Stewart found that certain images of pre-creation appear and reappear in myth and symbol as well as in the paintings and dances and visions and sandtrays of "active imagination" (Chodorow 1997). In describing the primordial image-imprints, Louis Stewart uses the language of poetic metaphor:

> In the "beginning"—in truth before the "beginning"—myth and religion identify a matrix of protean images, "pre-creation" symbols we may call them, which hold the potential for all that is to be created. These are the Abyss, the Void, Chaos, Alienation, and Darkness which enshrouds them all; and, of course, a Creator. These images reverberate with experiences of the world: the deep abyss of time, the caverns and depth of the sea, and the starry sky; the void of the vacant ocean and the vastness of empty space; the confusing multitudinous nature of life spawning life; the icy cold of the empty, lifeless cosmic space of the alien universe; and the deeps of the night and the loss of orientation. Meditation on these aspects of the world inevitably brings us to the inner world of the Self: to its depth and voids; its chaotic fantasies and alienating emotions; and its labyrinthine corridors of the dream. Myth is a product of such meditations.
>
> These symbols are primordial symbols of the Self. And each of them represents the Self in one of its manifestations. They are the culture spirit that has evolved in its forms as the religious, the aesthetic, the philosophic, and the social/moral. And the primordial symbols are the source of basic emotions. It takes no great stretch of the imagination to place oneself in the Abyss of Hell in the presence of demons and devils. When this is the dream, we experience terror. Yet if we safely pass through that Abyss we come out at Dante's Holy Mountain. And so it is with each of these symbols of the Self, their opposites are the symbols of healing and wholeness. (1997, p. 1)

Let us take a moment to reflect on these images that are at the same time experiences of the primal affects. It may be helpful to remember that an image is not only visual, rather, images are experienced and imagined through all of the senses. To experience the *void* is the actual, empty feeling in the body of loss, sadness, and grief. To be at the edge of the *abyss*—or to fall into it—is the actual gasp of fear as the ground drops away from under you. To experience *chaos* is the feeling of being tied up in knots, that is, the confusing muddle and tangle and frustration of anger. To experience *alienation* is the actual withering rejection we feel in disgust. When disgust is turned toward the self, we call it shame. When disgust is turned toward the other, we call it contempt. Either way, both sides are alienated. The experience of sudden *darkness* is that startling, unexpected, suspended moment of total disorientation.

In addition to the void of sadness, the abyss of fear, the chaos of anger, the alienation of disgust (contempt/shame), and the darkness of startle, there is, of course, a Creator represented as two forms of *light*. In human experience, these are the affects of life enhancement, joy, and interest. The *light of diffuse illumination* is surely the playful, blissful, all-embracing experience of joy. The *light of focused insight* holds within itself the intense, pinpointed concentration of interest and excitement.

Darwin (1882/1998) distinguished between the innate emotions with their clear, recognizable patterns of behavior, and the complex emotions. Darwin's complex emotions are universally known, yet they lack distinctive patterns of facial expression or bodily action. Darwin's complex emotions include jealousy, envy, admiration, respect, greed, generosity, and many others. Louis Stewart coined the term "complex family emotions" to describe alchemical mixtures, modulations and transmutations that develop in the family (1992, p. 93).

There are seven basic emotion themes, each expressed along a continuum of intensity. In addition, there are many subtle and complex affect combinations and affect sequences. With its range of intensity as well as subtle mixtures and modulations, each basic emotion can be understood as a theme with variations. Emotion themes are innate, while variations of the theme tend to be shaped by culture and family (Ekman's "display rules," see Ekman's Afterword in Darwin, 1882/1998, pp. 383, 385, 386, 391–92).

Seven Basic Emotion Themes

All of the emotions are essential, but for development to occur, much depends on joy and interest as they interact with each other and with all of the other affects. Joy is the affective source of play, imagination, and ultimately the development of *Eros-mythical consciousness*. Interest is the affective source of curiosity, exploration, and ultimately the development of *Logos-linguistic consciousness*. Building on Jung and on Henderson's concept of the cultural unconscious (Henderson, 1984), Stewart's hypothesis came to be that all of the higher functions of the psyche—including the ego functions and the symbolic cultural attitudes—have evolved from joy and interest as they modulate and transform the affects of crisis and survival (grief, fear, anger, disgust) and the affect of reorientation (startle).

The pages that follow will describe facial and bodily expressions of seven inherited emotions, including certain potential patterns of imaginative development.

Beginning with the life enhancing emotions (joy and interest), I'll then introduce the affect of centering and new orientation (startle). This section closes with four affects of crisis and survival (grief, fear, anger and disgust), including patterns of expression and transformation. As you read the descriptions, I invite you to imagine and remember your own experiences.

Enjoyment–Joy–Ecstasy

The life situation that evokes joy is the well known, the beloved, *the familiar.* As the eyes grow bright, the lips widen up and out. The felt bodily sensations are light hearted and expansive. With laughter, the arms may open wide. At a peak moment, we leap and jump for joy. But whether the expression is the prototypical "jump for joy," or rolling, rollicking laughter, or an all-embracing blissful state of being, joy is the affective source of play, imagination, mythical consciousness, divine relatedness. What I'll always remember about Trudi Schoop is how fully she expressed all of the emotions, but especially joy. She understood and fully embodied "a healthy, joyous lightness that contains a recollection of ground and weight to support it" (Schoop, 1978, p. 95).

What might be the pattern of imagination corresponding to the experience of pure joy? Joy is expressed through play and fantasy. Its nature and condition are utter spontaneity. No thought is "unthinkable." Nothing is "unimaginable." And that is why joyful play and imagination tend to put us in touch with material that is ordinarily repressed.

Sooner or later, the archetypal imagination will take us to the emotional core of any complex. But instead of, or in addition to, direct experience of raw emotion, imagination creates symbolic images and stories that somehow make the unbearable bearable. The compensatory nature of the psyche is part of this, producing images and experiences that may completely transform an emotion, feeling, or mood.

Carolyn Grant Fay, a dance therapist, describes such an experience. In the following narrative, the inner-directed movement process takes her back to painful feelings of emptiness and loss many years ago when her mother died.

> I lay for what seemed like a long time, listening inwardly to myself. My throat brought itself to my attention. It hurt and felt constricted and tense, so I let my throat lead me into movement. It led me up to kneeling, then forward, and then slowly across the floor in a sort of

crouching position. In my imagination I became aware as I concentrated on the throat that it was red with blood. The heart area was also aching and bloody. Finally my throat brought me up to standing and propelled me farther along. It stopped me suddenly, and I just stood there. At this point I collapsed onto the floor and lay there motionless. There was no movement … not an image … nothing.

After a while I became aware that the color red from the blood was there at my throat and breast. Little by little it became many shades of red from light pink to deep crimson. A rose began to take shape, rising out of the throat and heart through movements of my arms up, out, and around. The rest of my body down from that area seemed, in the fantasy, to be forming the stem and leaves of the flower. All sorts of superlatives come to me now as I try to express how I felt at that moment: warm, happy, fulfilled, in order, at one with myself."

Reflecting on the meaning of her experience, she wrote:

"The collapse onto the floor, and the nothingness that followed, seemed to symbolize a death of what had been wounded. I think of a dream I had … in which a woman, bleeding at the throat and breast, and ragged and grey from centuries of neglect, appeared. I associated this woman to myself at eighteen when my mother died. The reawakening to the color and the forming of the rose, with all the concomitant feelings of well-being, I associated with rebirth. (Fay, 1977, p. 27)

Imagination is largely energized and shaped by joy as it modulates and transforms the emotions of crisis. As described by Carolyn Grant Fay, the archetypal theme that emerged was loss, leading to a symbolic experience of death and rebirth, expressed and transformed through movement. Obviously, this kind of inner-directed experience is not directed by the ego, rather, it is energized and shaped by the archetypal imagination itself. Another way to say it, whether we are children or adults, the archetypal imagination involves the ongoing dialectical relationship between the life enhancing emotions joy and interest—expressed through play and curiosity—modulating and transforming the emotions of crisis and survival. Children play for the fun of it, yet as we know, the content of play is often about difficult, upsetting, even blood curdling experiences. It seems useful to differentiate here between the content of play and imagination (which often involves a recapitulation of wounding experiences) and the function of play and imagination that is about integration and healing.

Just as the archetypal imagination may lead us from joyful spontaneous play to the emotional core of a troublesome complex, Carolyn Fay's description of a death–rebirth experience shows it may also work the other way around. There are many examples of this: in every culture, throughout human history, people report spontaneous visions of light that typically come in the midst of a very dark time.

Interest–Excitement

The life situation that evokes interest is *novelty*. The distinctive facial expression is: sustained focus, eyebrows slightly drawn together, mouth softly opened or pursed lips. We track and look and listen. In excitement, there may be a "breathless" moment, as we are fascinated and engaged with every detail of an ever-changing world.

There is a reciprocal interplay between joy and interest, as each potentiates the other. While joy is expressed through play and imagination, interest is expressed through curiosity and exploration. When encountering something new, it is part of human nature to be curious, to want to explore it. With exploration, the novel experience at some point becomes familiar and we begin to play with it and weave fantasies of who we are around it. The fantasies go on then, until we discover another new facet, which is then explored, and so on and on. In dance therapy, there is an ongoing, interwoven relationship between interest and imagination: interest in the body the way it is, and fantasies of what the body might be about (Fay, 1996; Fleischer, 2004; Mendez, 2005; Panhofer, 2005; Stromsted, 2007).

As part of my discussion of Interest–Excitement, I include Jung's ego functions (Sensation, Thinking, Feeling and Intuition). Following a brief quote by Jung, I will ask the reader to give some thought to an evolutionary and developmental idea. Could it be that interest—expressed through curiosity and exploration—infuses, modulates, and transforms each of the crisis affects, moving from raw affect toward modulated affect and the ego-orienting functions? Jung's ego functions have much to do with orientation. For example, imagine walking in the woods (with a companion or alone) and finding a stream. Will you cross the stream? Or pause and reflect? Or find another way? How do you decide?

> These four functional types correspond to the obvious means by which consciousness obtains its orientation. *Sensation* (or sense perception) tells you that something exists; *thinking* tells you what it is; *feeling* tells you whether it is agreeable or not; and *intuition* tells you where it comes from and where it is going. (Jung, 1961/1964, CW 18, p. 219, par. 503)

The feeling function has sometimes been confused with emotions and emotionality in general. However, Jung's feeling function is an evaluative function. It evaluates the emotional atmosphere.

On one hand, interest has its own dialectical relationship with joy. On the other hand, as interest connects us to the world and the Self, it engages and infuses any or all of the other emotions or moods. Consider the idea that Jung's ego functions (Jung, 1921, CW 6) have evolved mainly through the affect theme interest-excitement as it modulates and transforms specific affects of crisis. For example:

> *Thinking.* In anger, we perceive that something is the matter and all attention is fiercely focused on how to identify the problem and attack it. A thinking person is likely to be interested in this domain.
>
> *Feeling.* As disgust (contempt/shame) forces us to grapple with the bitter experience of alienation, we develop sensibilities that help us evaluate the intricate network of human relationships. Interest in the emotional atmosphere seems to be an early stage of the feeling function.
>
> *Sensation.* In sadness, our constant longing is for the embodied presence of the one we miss. Interest in the physical, tangible world is essential to a well-developed sensation function.
>
> *Intuition.* In fear we sense the presence of myriad intangibles, unknown possibilities. An intuitive person is likely to be interested in this realm.
>
> From the twin streams of life enhancement (enjoyment–joy–ecstasy and interest–excitement), I turn now toward surprise-startle, the affect theme of centering and new orientation.

Surprise–Startle

When something happens that is completely *unexpected*, we are surprised, astonished, startled. The facial expression is eyebrows raised and eyes open wide, with open mouth. The affect theme surprise-startle is the primal expression of disorientation. It serves to center consciousness and leads to reorientation. In Louis Stewart's words, startle

> leads to a centering of the total organism, which imposes an immediate and total cessation of any movement or sound; breathing ceases, and even the beat of the heart may be momentarily interrupted. At that moment all of the other affects are, in a very real sense, functioning as its opposite. That is, their energy is totally in abeyance, although in a state of readiness to be sure, since we know that immediately following the startle response, ego consciousness is quickly restored to a particular function, and moreover, a specific archetypal affect may take over in response to whatever it was that led to the startle response. Startle's survival function then is to prevent, if possible, the occurrence of an inappropriate response before the threat has been evaluated (one cannot help but wonder about a relationship between startle and the physiological shock reaction). (1987, pp. 41–42)

Pioneer dance therapist Mary Whitehouse describes movement that comes from an inner impulse: "The experience ... always carries an element of surprise—it is unexpected and seems to happen quite of itself" (1963, in Pallaro, 2000, p. 54). Her simple yet profound observation brings an introverted perspective to surprise-startle: we may be surprised or startled in response to unexpected inner events. Internally generated movement may emerge, with surprising results. An unexpected fantasy may float up, or a passing thought or insight, and one is surprised. Could it be that noticing the surprising nature of inner events is the beginning of self-reflective consciousness?

The shadow aspect of startle is when there has been too much of it, it may become habitual, as if frozen into the musculature (the extreme example of a person who is catatonic comes to mind). But normally, surprise-startle is a remarkable and wondrous affect. Ordinarily expressed in a split second, it marks a palpable moment of reorientation that is essential to psychological development.

At the primal level, the felt bodily sensation is shock, ranging from mild to intense. The image comes of a deer that freezes, until something shifts and it is released. When we can be conscious of and present to a state of disorientation, the psyche is likely to produce exactly the images and experiences that are needed to move us through it. One of Jung's studies makes this process visible through a marvelous series of paintings created by a highly educated, cultivated woman in her mid-50s. Discussing her second painting in this series, he describes a bolt of lightning that releases a dark stone and kindles a light at its core: "Lightning signifies a sudden, unexpected, and overpowering change of psychic condition" (Jung, 1933, p. 295, par. 533). It has an "illuminating, vivifying fertilizing, transforming and healing function" (Jung, 1933, p. 314, par 558). In an alchemical text, lightning causes the royal pair to come alive; in Jewish tradition, "the Messiah appears as lightning" (Jung, 1933, p. 295, par. 533, note 7). In dance therapy, surprise-startle might be as subtle as a passing expression on the face, or it might be a spontaneous physical action that seems to jolt the mover from within, or it might be a dream or fantasy or dance about lightning. All of these and countless other symbolic experiences are related to surprise-startle and the evolution of self reflective consciousness.

From surprise-startle—the affect theme of centering and new orientation—we shall now look at the basic existential affect themes of crisis and survival (grief, fear, anger, and disgust), approaching each from two overlapping perspectives: expression and transformation.

Distress–Sadness–Grief–Anguish

When we experience *loss*, the inner corners of the eyebrows are raised at an oblique angle and the corners of the mouth are drawn down. With intense grief and anguish there is wailing and sobbing. With eyelids tightly closed, the muscles around the eyeballs contract, often pulling the mouth open into a square-like or rectangular shape of grief.

In loss, the bodily sensation may be the feeling of emptiness, dead weight, or both. If the one we miss is not there, the person who mourns may move back and forth between identification with the lost beloved (dead weight) and experiencing the emptiness of the world, which has turned into a barren wasteland. The heart is heavy, it hurts and aches. Sometimes it feels as if it is being ripped or torn apart. Heart rending experiences are culturally mirrored in traditions of mourning that require tearing a garment or piece of cloth when a loved one dies.

To approach his study of sadness and grief, Louis Stewart wondered. What could be the use of such a punishing affect? At the level of survival, the affect themes of fear, anger, and disgust are understandable as self-protective responses to different kinds of danger. But how can we understand the survival function of sadness and grief? To say it another way: What would the world be like without sadness? One can only imagine the bland, indifferent quality of life if the typical response to the loss of a beloved person were something like: "Oh well, too bad. Here today, gone tomorrow." Sadness connects us not only to the significance to us of those we love, but to the beauty of nature, the element earth, and the tangible world.

Wherever humans experience the full impact of loss, the traditional rhythmic, rocking expressions of grief can be seen. Grief is universal and recognizable, even when modified and shaped by different cultures. In addition to the rhythmic movements of the body, humans in a natural way are drawn to create and re-create, with beautiful fresh flowers and shrines and idealized images of the beloved person who has died. The AIDS quilt (created by families and friends to remember loved ones who died of the auto-immune disease syndrome), the quilt of tears (created by schoolchildren to remember friends and neighbors who died from the random violence of "drive-by" shootings), and so many other memorials show this process clearly. Each is at once an expression of grief—and a memorial of beauty.

If we consider the form or category of imagination that has evolved from sadness and grief, we are led to the imagination of beauty expressed through rhythmic harmony. As the rhythmic, rocking expressions of grief interact with joyful memories and other experiences, lamentations have developed into songs, music, poetry, dances, paintings, and sculpture. From the beginning, the mixture of joy with sadness has evolved and continues to evolve through the imagination of beauty, expressed through the arts.

Anxiety–Fear–Terror

In contrast to the compressed eyes of sadness and grief, the eyes of fear are wide open. Sadness, grief and anguish can go on for a long time and crying may bring release and relief. But even when we tremble, it is not a simple thing to discharge fear. At bottom, fear is an encounter with the *unknown*. The facial expression is: eyes opened wide, eyebrows raised and drawn together; the lower eyelid is tensed, and the lips are stretched horizontally.

In its lower range of intensity, the survival function of fear may be to ensure that we approach an unknown situation with caution. In anxiety, there may be nervous twitching of the hands, feet, or legs, as if preparing for an emergency. In the extreme intensity of panic and terror, one may be faced with death, or the living death of drastic injury. Death is the ultimate unknown. In a life-threatening emergency, the survival action of fear is to freeze, faint, or flee. Uncontrollable repetitive actions include trembling, headlong flight, jumpiness, gasping, recoil, cowering, motionlessness. Felt bodily sensations include heart pounding, cold sweat, loose bowels, weak knees, and the dry mouth of fear.

Many years ago when I was studying with Trudi Schoop, she asked the question: How do you move when you're afraid? Each of us took turns moving one after another across the room, imagining and remembering a fearful life experience and our response to it. Most of us expressed the lower intensities of fear; mainly we expressed anxiety and nervousness, alternating between tension and tremor. Trudi then developed the image further by inviting us to imagine fear in the history of humans on this planet: "It is many thousands of years ago," she said. "You are the first humans on earth. Can you imagine what you would feel and what you would do if, for the first time, without warning, you hear the sound of thunder?" Trudi's drum became the crack of thunder and when I heard it, I didn't plan anything, but my body fell to the ground. In that moment, I first experienced the link between fear and the voice of God.

Fear has both a survival function and a spiritual dimension. Imagination of the *Mysteries* is a particular form or category of the archetypal imagination. As we encounter the dreaded unknown, the primal expression is uncontrollable repetitive action. Whether obsessive rituals to ward off demons, or the ceremonial actions of prayer and worship, the expressive behavior of fear is ritual.

Ceremonial enactment may include trembling, shivering, shaking, whispering, and chanting. And, it may include repetitive actions of quiet calm, for example, lighting candles, making offerings. But whether the repetitive action is hair-raising or contemplative, the process allows us to concentrate on certain well-known physical actions that may protect us from a direct encounter with the dreaded Unknown. In *The idea of the holy,*

Rudolf Otto (1923) shows how all of the great religious traditions of the world have evolved from the archaic experience of daemonic dread. I imagine Otto might agree that the development he describes could not have come from fear alone, but rather from a subtle and complex mixture, especially fear and joy.

A question comes to mind about the similarities and differences between the repetitive quality of ritual and the rhythmic quality of dance. Each is grounded in its own affective source, yet there is a special relationship between ritual and rhythm, the sacred and the beautiful. Each seems to flow naturally into the other.

Frustration–Anger–Rage

The life situation that evokes anger is *restriction*, restriction of autonomy. The facial expression of anger is: eyebrows frown, eyelids raised, eyes fixed, nostrils dilate. The mouth opens to show teeth, or it is closed with a clenched jaw. Heart rate increases; the skin is hot and blood flows to the hands. The expressive behavior of anger is threat and attack, an extremely primitive form of reason. If we consider the category of the imagination that has evolved from anger, one is led from chaos toward a compensatory image/experience of order. With the development of consciousness, one learns to attack a problem symbolically, identifying the cause of the frustration and developing strategies to put things back in order. Many games, for example, are all about the development of strategic thought and symbolic attack. Other examples that come to mind are the emphatic gestures that punctuate scholarly discourse. A beautifully written passage in Chaim Potok's novel *The chosen* describes a passionate scholarly argument between an orthodox Rabbi and his brilliant 15-year-old son:

> Danny and his father fought through their points with loud voices and wild gestures of their hands almost to where I thought they might come to blows. Danny caught his father in a misquote, ran to get a Talmud from a shelf, and triumphantly showed his father where he had been wrong. His father checked the margin of the page … and showed Danny that he had been quoting from the corrected text. Then they went on to another tractate, fought over another passage, and this time Reb Saunders agreed, his face glowing, that his son was correct. I sat quietly for a long time, watching them battle. (1967/1982, p. 155)

With insistent gestures and fiercely focused attention, anger, combined with joy (imagination) and interest (curiosity) is the affective source of scholarly, philosophic imagination. The compensatory ideal of the ordered cosmos has evolved from the chaos of frustration, anger and rage.

The following quote describes the inner-directed movement process of a gifted, young, intelligent, hard-working, professional woman. Arriving for one of her weekly individual dance therapy sessions, she seemed somewhat agitated and told me she felt hyperactive and uncomfortable. I invited her to use her body to express what she was feeling. She was eager to open herself to the embodied world of felt sensations, impulses, and images. On this day, she chose not to use music. Spontaneous movement emerged as she followed her inner rhythms.

She started moving in many different ways, but it was disjointed and chaotic. Something would start and then it would seem to get cut off. Then something else would start. But nothing came together—she just looked increasingly irritable and at odds with herself. But gradually, as she became more conscious of feeling pressure and frustration, a form began to emerge. She began to move with clarity and purpose, creating a space for herself. Her movement began spontaneously to integrate with her breathing and she began to attend to the process of what her body was doing. At the very end, she was sitting on the floor, legs folded, spine easily stretched upwards, as she made smaller and smaller circles with the top of her head, using the base of her spine as a fulcrum. These last movements were very subtle and centered; she was breathing easily and looked peaceful and grounded. When she opened her eyes, she had a string of insights that included a realization that her hyperactive mood had been a mask of avoidance. From the movement experience, she realized that she had been feeling pressured and restricted by certain people in her life. When she was able to let herself feel the terrible frustration, she could identify the problem and begin to do something about it. Her imaginative solution was to become more definite and assertive with herself and others—to metaphorically claim her own space. The self-directed movement process also reflected an archetypal theme. It took her through chaos to a new sense of order. (Chodorow, 1991, p. 35).

This narrative is included to illustrate a theme I have witnessed many times in dance/movement therapy involving the expression, modulation, and transformation of frustration and anger. As this competent, self-reflective young woman symbolically expressed a disjointed, chaotic mood in the presence of a trusted dance therapist, something shifted. It was as if the self-regulating nature of the living body led her to discover a new center, followed by spontaneous insights and a new experience of order and meaning.

Sometimes it happens the other way around; for example, when an individual is frustrated but unable to express irritation, frustration, or anger, it sometimes feels like a calm before the storm. Titrating the expression of intense affect is a natural part of dance therapy. Rena Kornblum, for example, a dance therapist who works with children, sometimes invites dances of gentle breezes that gradually increase in intensity all the way to the chaos of a hurricane, and then as the storm passes, to gradually decrease intensity, returning to gentle breezes and perhaps stillness.

Disgust (Contempt/Shame)

The life situation that evokes disgust is *rejection*. The facial expression is: lips curl, noses wrinkle, eyes crinkle. In scorn or contempt, we turn up our noses and lower our eyelids, as if pulling away from a dirty, smelly object. In embarrassment and shame, we may blush and squirm, hang the head, avert the eyes, and wish the ground would open up and swallow us.

As a survival function, disgust uses the senses of smell and taste to identify a noxious, potentially poisonous substance. We turn away from a bad smell, or reject rotten food by spitting it out. In early infancy, this acute evaluative function is carried out with only a mild emotional twinge. If disgust were limited to the rejection of bad food, it would remain a relatively uncomplicated affective reflex, but it is not so simple. As the infant develops, the expression of disgust differentiates through the "stranger reaction" around seven to nine months of age toward the developing binary (two-part) affect contempt/shame, in which the object of disgust is no longer limited to offensive smells and tastes. We move now from the evaluation of food toward the evaluation of human beings.

The question whether an experience is contempt or shame depends on whether rejection is turned toward the other, or toward the self. Either way, one is alienated. At the barnyard level, the antecedent to contempt/shame is expressed through a "pecking order." The dominance and submission behavior of many mammals is similarly related to maintaining a hierarchical social structure. Every child has to grapple with feelings about being included or excluded, and has fantasies about how to get along with others. Social customs differ from one culture to another, but all are concerned with status, deference and the mediation of human relationship.

Contempt/shame forces full attention to one's place in the human community. This punishing affect is always expressed within the context of a relationship, whether an interaction in the present, or intrapsychic reflections on the past.

In shame, the self may be "split in two, with one part of the self a judge, and other the offender" (Tomkins, 1963, p. 152). Depending on the nature and development of an individual, the inner conflict may be contained and eventually integrated. When an individual cannot bear the tension, the split tends to be acted out by projecting shadow—the archetypal image of the stranger within—onto some other individual, group or nation. A development from the alienation of contempt/shame toward the ideal of social justice can be seen in the wide range of customs that mediate human relationships. There is a world of difference between a custom that subjects an individual to painful humiliation and a custom that embodies mutual respect between humans.

Due to its two-part nature, contempt/shame may be the most complicated of the emotions. As joy (imagination) and interest (curiosity) are turned toward the variety of human experiences involving rejection, we may experience "imagination of relationship," encompassing awareness of right and wrong, good and evil, leading ultimately toward the capacity for social, moral, ethical, empathic imagination.

Conclusion

I have tried to present a vision of the Self as it evolves from the primordial depths of the unconscious toward the highest values of human culture. Reviewing the seven archetypal affect themes, we looked at *joy* and *interest*, expressed through play/imagination and curiosity/exploration. While each basic emotion is essential, psychological development depends especially on the two life enhancement affects as they potentiate each other and as they intermingle with, modulate, and transform all of the other affects. After joy and interest, we considered *surprise-startle*, the affect of centering and new orientation. Finally, we looked at each of the fourfold affects of crisis and survival: *grief, fear, anger, disgust*. In addition to felt bodily sensations and expressive physical actions, emotions have their own potential patterns of imaginative development.

For those who might be interested in further developments of this material, Charles Stewart has continued to develop the archetypal affect system, as he investigates the affects, symbols, and conditions that shape (and block) development and healing (Stewart, C. T., 2001; 2008).

As dance/movement therapists, we are engaged with all of the intrinsic categories of the imagination. Different forms of imagination will be prominent in the work of different individuals, depending in part on tastes, talents, inclinations, and typology. Even so, given the nature of our work, it seems inevitable that every dance therapist is engaged with the aesthetic imagination, *imagination of beauty* expressed through the arts, especially dance. Similarly, every dance therapist is engaged with *imagination of the mysteries* expressed as ritual enactments, rites of entry and exit, the ceremonial and meditative aspects of dance therapy that may lead toward an ongoing dialogue with the god (or gods) within.

We are also engaged with the philosophic, scientific, *scholarly imagination*, as we trace the links from movement experience to an early memory, or wonder about the meaning of a symbolic image that floats up in the midst of movement. And scholarly imagination motivates research as we seek a better understanding of dance therapy—why we work the way we do (Cruz & Berrol, 2004; Fischman, 2006; Goodill, 2005). Dance therapy is completely interwoven with social imagination, the *imagination of relationship,* interactive experiences, work with the dynamics of shadow projection and other projections in the mutual transference. This is the realm of empathic imagination and the whole world of fantasies that people have about each other. Finally, dance therapy leads us inevitably toward the central, self-reflective *psychological imagination,* which is a quintessence of the other four, shaped by the age-old value inscribed at the Delphic Oracle: Know Thyself.

References

Berrol, C. (2006). Neuroscience meets dance/movement therapy: Mirror neurons, the therapeutic process and empathy. *The Arts in Psychotherapy* 33: 302–315.

Chodorow, J. (1991). *Dance therapy and depth psychology: The moving imagination.* London: Routledge.

Chodorow, J. (Ed.). (1997). *Jung on active imagination.* London: Routledge, and Princeton, NJ: Princeton University Press.

Cruz, R., & C. Berrol, (Eds.). (2004). *Dance/movement therapists in action: A working guide to research options,* Foreword by Joan Chodorow. Springfield, IL: Charles C. Thomas.

Darwin, C. (1882/1998). *The expression of the emotions in Man and animals.* 3rd ed., P. Ekman, Ed. Oxford: Oxford University Press.

Ekman, P. (2003). *Emotions revealed.* New York: Henry Holt.

Fay, C. (1977). Movement and fantasy: A dance therapy model based on the psychology of C. G. Jung. Master's thesis, Goddard College, Plainfield, VT.

Fay, C. (1996). At the Threshold: A Journey to the sacred through the integration of the psychology of C. G. Jung and the expressive arts, with Carolyn Grant Fay, videotape and DVD. The Jung Center of Houston, TX. www.junghouston.org.

Fischman, D. (2006). La mejora de la capacidad empática a través de talleres de Danza Movimiento Terapia en profesionales de la salud y la educación. Ph.D. thesis, Universidad de Palermo. Buenos Aires.

Fleischer, K. (2004). Una experiencia en movimiento autentico: entre lo individual y lo colectivo. *Campo Grupal (Buenos Aires),* 7/61, 12–13.

Gallese, V. (2003.) The roots of empathy: The shared manifold hypothesis and the neural basis of intersubjectivity. *Psychopathology,* 36, 171–180.

Goodill, S. W. (2005). *An introduction to medical dance/movement therapy.* London: Jessica Kingsley.

Henderson, J. (1984). *Cultural attitudes in psychological perspective.* Toronto: Inner City Books.

Jung, C. G. (1907). *The psychology of dementia praecox. Collected Works 3.* Princeton: Princeton University Press, 1960 (2nd printing with corrections, 1972):1–151.

Jung, C. G. (1921). *Psychological types. Collected Works 6.* Princeton: Princeton University Press, 1971.

Jung, C. G. (1933). Study in the process of individuation. *Collected works 9-I.* Princeton: Princeton University Press, 2nd edition with corrections and minor revisions, 1968 (new material copyright, 1969:290–354.

Jung, C. G. (1938). Psychological aspects of the mother archetype. *Collected works 9-I*. Princeton: Princeton University Press, 2nd edition with corrections and minor revisions, 1968 (new material copyright 1969):75–110.

Jung, C. G. (1951). *Aion: Researches into the phenomenology of the self. Collected works 9-II*. Princeton: Princeton University Press, 2nd edition with corrections and minor revisions, 1968.

Jung, C. G. (1961). *Memories, dreams, reflections*. New York: Random House—Vintage Books, 1965.

Jung, C. G. (1961/1964). Symbols and the interpretation of dreams. *Collected works 18*. Princeton: Princeton University Press, 1976:183–264.

Mendez, M. (2005). Desde los huesos: Apuntes de simbolismo corporal. Revista Venezolana de Psicologia Arquetipos, Caracas-Venezuela, No. 1:15–21.

Otto, R. (1923). *The idea of the holy*. London: Oxford University Press, 1981.

Panhofer, H. (Ed.). (2005). *El cuerpo en psicoterapia: Teoría y práctica de la danza movimiento terapia*. Barcelona: Gedisa.

Pert, C. (1997). *Molecules of emotion*. New York: Scribner.

Potok, C. (1967). *The chosen*. New York: Ballantine Books, 1982.

Schoop, T. (1978). Motion and emotion, Reprint, *American Journal of Dance Therapy* 22/2, 2000:91–101.

Stevens, A. (1983). *Archetypes: A natural history of the self*. New York: Quill.

Stewart, C. T. (2001). *The symbolic impetus: How creative fantasy motivates development*. London: Free Association Books.

Stewart, C. T. (2008). *Dire emotions and lethal behaviors: Eclipse of the life instinct*. London: Routledge.

Stewart, L. H. (1986). Work in progress: Affect and archetype. In *The body in analysis*, N. Schwartz-Salant and M. Stein, Eds. Wilmette, IL: Chiron Publications:183–203.

Stewart, L. H. (1987). A brief report: Affect and archetype. *Journal of Analytical Psychology* 32/1:36–46.

Stewart, L. H. (1992). *Changemakers: A Jungian perspective on sibling position and the family atmosphere*. London: Routledge.

Stewart, L. H., & C. T. Stewart. (1979). Play, games, and the affects. In *Play as context: Proceedings of the Association for the Anthropological Study of Play*, Alice T. Cheska, Ed. West Point, NY: Leisure Press: 42–52.

Stromsted, T. (2007). The dancing body in psychotherapy. *Authentic movement: A collection of essays*. Vol. 2, P. Pallaro, Ed. London: Jessica Kingsley. 202–220.

Tinbergen, N. (1951). *The study of instinct*. London: Oxford University Press.

Tomkins, S. (1962). *Affect, imagery, consciousness*. Vol. I. NY: Springer.

Tomkins, S. (1963). *Affect, imagery, consciousness*. Vol. II. NY: Springer.

Whitehouse, M. (1963). Physical movement and personality. In *Authentic movement: Essays by Mary Starks Whitehouse, Janet Adler and Joan Chodorow*. Vol. 1, P. Pallaro, Ed. London: Jessica Kingsley, 1999. Second impression 2000 [with photo errors corrected]:51–57.

The Path from Theory to Practice

CHAPTER 5

BASCICS

An Intra/Interactional Model of DMT with the Adult Psychiatric Patient

PATRICIA P. CAPELLO

Contents

Introduction

This chapter is an overview of a system that identifies the fundamentals necessary for effective, meaningful, and creative dance/movement therapy (DMT) sessions designed specifically for those challenged by both acute and chronic mental illness.

The structure of this model is divided into two related and reciprocal systems: Intra-actional and Interactional. The *Intra-Actional System* deals with concepts related to the individual and his or her perception of body and self (specifically, Body Attitude and Selfhood). The *Interactional System* is concerned with concepts related to individuals and their capacity to relate to the world as social beings (specifically, Communication and Interpersonal Dynamics). The combination of the Intra/Interactional System or **B**ody **A**ttitude—**S**elfhood—**C**ommunication—**I**nterpersonal Dynam**ics** will be referred to by the acronym BASCICS.

As diagrammed in Figure 5.1, the two systems and their specific categories interact and co-relate. Rather than being a true sequence or step-system, it is more of a "relay system," with each aspect influencing and supporting the other. The conceptualization of this particular system attempts to reveal a moving, flowing relationship rather than cause and effect. Given the potential scope of this BASCICS system it has been necessary to focus only on the fundamentals for each area indicated. Furthermore, the system makes use of case examples and describes techniques suitable for adult psychiatric inpatients and outpatients. However, it is adaptable for use within a wide diagnostic range and for most age categories.

Finally, it attempts to be a true *dance/movement* model, focusing on the limitless creative capacities and aesthetic qualities of the moving body using force/time/space/flow as a unique and specific fundamental for therapeutic process.

The Intra-Actional System

Body Attitude: How We Experience the Human Body

Every human experience is connected with the sensation of one's own body (Schilder, 1950). We can relate only to weight, space, force, or time in terms of their relationship to and influence on the body. As infants, our bodily needs are cared for with the utmost attention and scrutiny and we respond to this caretaking with bodily gestures of pain or pleasure. As Berger (1972) succinctly states: "The fact is that the body is the only means we have through which to experience life and to respond to it" (p. 224) It seems logical, then, as we view the body as the personal reference point, to begin with the concept of Body Attitude.

Body Image   One aspect of this body attitude is *body image*. Body image is defined as the memory of experience with the body recorded in the form of images (Schilder, 1950). In agreement with this author, Leventhal (1974) states that the body image is a three-dimensional image formed from the tactile, visual, and kinesthetic receptors, resulting from both internal and external stimuli. The body image refers to the body as a psychological

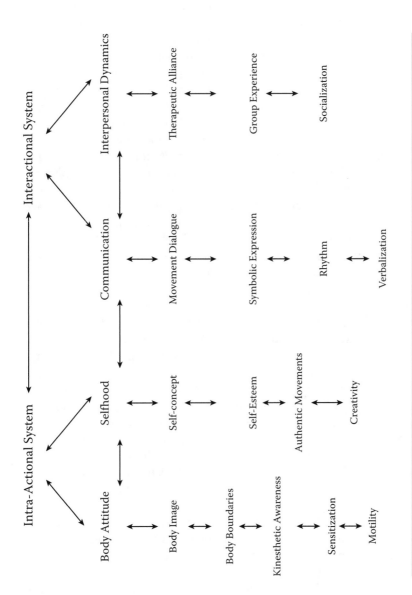

Figure 5.1 An intra/interactional model of dance/movement therapy.

experience; it focuses on the individual's feelings and attitudes toward his or her own body (Fisher & Cleveland, 1968).

In 1927 Freud wrote that the ego is ultimately derived from bodily sensations and chiefly from those springing from the surface of the body. The ego may thus be regarded as a mental projection of the surface of the body. According to Freud (1927) infants at birth are completely self-oriented, to the extent that they are unable to differentiate themselves from their surrounding environment. Because of this preoccupation with the self, children perceive their mothers and others in the environment merely as extensions of themselves. Their existence, as seen by children at this stage, is to function solely to satisfy their needs for food and comfort.

It is through the process of differentiation that infants begin to see themelves as something apart from their environment. At this point, according to Davis (1964), children must form a clear, undistorted image of their physical bodies. Through self-exploration and stimulation of body parts (i.e., hand to mouth, touching toes) children develop a mental image or body image of their physical structures. Body image is of utmost importance in the development of a satisfactory concept of one's self (Davis, 1964).

As dance/movement therapists we often see patients with a limited, distorted, or often non-existent knowledge of their bodies. Fisher (1973) contends that the schizophrenic who has lost some of his or her inhibitions and controls "seeks openly to find in the mirror a clear picture of the body world that has probably never made sense to him" (p. 8). Perhaps, Fisher believes, the excited schizophrenic woman who exposes her naked body is merely trying to "make contact with the world of her body which has previously been hidden or denied to her direct awareness" (p. 9).

It is at this primary level of self-discovery that the dance/movement therapist, using tactile stimulation, movement reflecting, and breathing can make initial contact and intervention. For the extremely regressed or chronic patient, identification of body parts, joint articulation, and constructive use of muscles is a first step toward redefining the body image. Often, as a result of regression, schizophrenics' reality testing mechanisms are no longer functioning; therefore they may develop bizarre ideas about their bodies (i.e., depersonalization). In the here and now of DMT sessions, confirmation of reality and restructuring of the body image is possible. The therapist must recognize that there are fluctuations in body image and how culture and religious beliefs have an influence on the perception of the body.

Body image work could include exercises with visual and auditory perception within the warm-up period of a DMT session. This provides the opportunity to make initial body contacts. As therapists prepare the physical space where the session will take place, patients can be engaged in assisting in moving chairs or setting up a table for musical equipment. Thus, the environment of the hospital setting can be adjusted into a therapeutic space specific for dance. Gathering the group for warm-up in the central space also changes the individual's visual perception, preparing patients to focus on their bodies as tools for therapy. With the first "welcome" to the session, through eye contact and greeting everyone by name, the group members are encouraged to practice both watching and listening skills. Further attunement to the sounds and lyrics of musical selections and making a personal choice in songs engages them even further.

Beginning with a breath or sigh allows group members to hear both their own and others' sounds and voices. Practicing fuller breathing by concentrating on inhaling through the nose and exhaling through the mouth helps to activate the face and lungs more fully. Using sounds such as "ohhh ..." or "ahhh ..." with the breath on the exhale works to sustain and deepen breathing. As therapists begin to observe and follow movement cues, they reflect the subtle changes and offer new ways to expand the patients' use of muscles, joints, and limbs. Therapists can also direct some simple self-touch experiences such as patting down and up the body, clapping the hands, and tapping the feet. Body image is further explored through body part identification ("roll your shoulders," or "nod your head") and bending and stretching (sinking the body down toward the floor and alternately lifting up onto the toes with arms toward the ceiling). Use of lateral movements of swinging the body from side to side or crossing one's arms and holding the adjacent person's hands while in a circle help fragmented or disorganized patients to focus more clearly on both their own body movements and those of others. These warm-up movements can be done either in a seated position or standing, based on the needs and abilities of the group or individual.

Body Boundaries　Prior to the process of differentiation, young children have no clear definition of their *body boundaries*—where their bodies end and Mothers' begin. With many regressed patients a similar merging of body boundaries (often with the therapist) can occur due to faulty body image and perception. Fragmented and fluctuating body boundaries are also common occurrences in psychiatric patients. As a case example of the need for psychiatric patients to confirm body boundaries: "A," a young male patient, must reach out and make subtle tactile contact with a person before he can speak with them, in a sense "bridging the gap," or merging the boundaries to allow communication to occur.

Many persecutory or paranoid delusions are related to invasion of the body boundaries (i.e., being followed, poisoned food, being spied on, feelings of other "beings" inside the body). As Fisher (1973) writes, each person has to develop confidence that the walls of his or her body (the most fundamental "home base") are adequate enough to shield and protect him or her from outside forces that can do potential harm.

A case example of building delusional body boundaries is "S," a young schizophrenic woman who created an imagined "shield" in front of her body that kept her from being harmed or feeling ill. Techniques available to the dance/movement therapist to help patients become aware of body boundaries, strengthen or adjust them into a necessary and functional protective system include tactile stimulation of the body periphery and other surfaces in the environment such as the floor and by holding hands with others. Work with body weight (i.e., grounding, shifting); use of advance and retreat movements; and pushing and pulling motions can help patients re-confirm body boundaries. Specific exercises that are particularly useful are coming together as a group leading with a specific body part and then separating; closing eyes and meeting someone by touching tops of heads; and rolling the body along the floor, arms and legs held together and outstretched.

Use of the "imagined hoop" exercise developed by Dr. Alma Hawkins (1987) has proven successful in facilitating movement range expansion experiences and understanding of joint rotation, dimensionality, and use of force. Preliminary work in chairs is optimal for severely fragmented individuals as a method of further "grounding" them. Being grounded or having the sensation of feeling stable and secure while connected to the earth provides patients with a safe place to begin their movement exploration.

Kinesthetic Awareness   Having an image of the body and knowing body boundaries are both fundamental sources for body attitude. A further basis for movement discovery is the *kinesthetic awareness* of the body as both a static and mobile structure. The sense of body position and movement of joints, or kinesthesia, is another aspect integral to knowledge of "self." Kinesthesia can be considered the "sixth sense" (Feldenkrais, 1977). Todd (1937) described the process by which the brain uses the information regarding position and direction of motion in space received by the otoliths and semicircular canals of the ear:

> (These impressions) are combined in the brain with the kinesthetic sensations of movement, weight pressure, and relative position, coming from other parts of the body, to give us our minute-to-minute information as to the movements of our limbs, neck, and trunk, where we are at a given moment, and how we can get somewhere else. (p. 28)

Feldenkrais (1977) associated "inefficient moving" to a low kinesthetic sense and believed that unskillful use of the body structure uses up more energy than proper utilization. Apparent in the majority of hospitalized patients is their inefficient use of the body: either moving in a tension-ridden, limited range or often in a frozen, immobile body posture lacking the necessary cycle of relaxing and tensing the muscles. While Feldenkrais (1977) believes that those who have a fine kinesthetic sense continue to improve the efficiency and fluidness of their movement and that those who haven't continue deteriorating, he claims that this cycle can be broken through practice of more productive use of the body and awareness of this "sixth sense."

DMT, in making use of the body as the vehicle leading to health and healthful action, offers individuals the opportunity to become aware of and re-attune their kinesthetic sense. Some techniques might include internal, personal sensing of the body followed by a verbalized description of where the body is in space and the manner and range in which the limbs, trunk, and head are moving. Articulation of joints, including hips, ankles, shoulders, and exploration of range of movement (including high, medium, and low levels of space; forward and backward motion; near and far, etc.) and efficient use of weight and gravity are further techniques that build awareness kinesthetically.

Sensitization

As an action-oriented form of psychotherapy, DMT puts the body senses into motion. Full sensitization includes visual, auditory, olfactory, tactile, taste, thermal, pain, synthetic, (itch, tickle, vibration), and kinesthesis. The healthy body selectively censors and screens perception of many of these senses to avoid overstimulation and subsequent chaos. For example, if we were constantly aware of the contact and textures of our clothing on our bodies it would be quite difficult to tolerate being clothed.

Many times, due to conditions of their pathology (i.e., visual or auditory hallucinations) and flooding of sensations and emotions, patients may attempt to block external (and often internal) stimulation. They may selectively attend to visual stimulation (specifically, avoidance of direct eye contact) and auditory stimulation (not responding to questions). The dance/movement therapist, in an attempt to focus the patient on more appropriate, reality-oriented processes, might direct the dance/movement activity in sessions toward a heightening of awareness of simple, non-threatening stimuli—sensing temperature, color, tactile stimulation, texture, etc. Throughout the session, patients can be reminded to stay aware of how their bodies are feeling both physiologically (body temperature and heart rate changes), and psychologically (emotional and feeling state changes). The therapist needs to be attuned to the appropriate time to introduce sensitivity experiences and only when the patient is sufficiently capable of processing it. Overstimulation may lead to a flooding of sensations and cause confusion or further disorganization in a psychotic or manic patient.

Spatial Awareness   As we move through the environment that surrounds us, a further awareness, *spatial awareness*, becomes apparent. Few of us know, in a literal sense, how much space our body takes up; our "body volume" is something we rarely calculate. For the layman, the how and why of using space seldom exists. The dance/movement therapist is a keen observer of the individual's use of space: choice of location, amount, direction, dimension, and size. Studies have shown that personal distance, social distance, and intimate distance, as well as the effects of crowding and poorly planned space, are all connected to and influence the way we behave (Hall, 1969).

Attention to the details of how we use space, such as where one sits in a crowded room, how one claims a "personal space" and what one's *Interactional* distance might be, are all useful elements of sensitization. A patient's use of space elements, as observed by a dance/movement therapist, may give heretofore unknown insight, understanding, and clarity about that patient and his or her behavior. For example, an isolative patient might begin to verbalize a wish to live in a house with many people or enjoy moving with a partner or as a member of a large group. This might signal an underlying wish to be with people and establish contacts, thereby ending his or her isolation. DMT can uncover another psychological dimension of that patient and provide material for processing in both movement and verbal modes. Specific exercises using space elements can include choosing a place in the room where it is most comfortable, then least comfortable, and then sharing verbally; or building a "personal house" describing its size, shape, location, furnishings, etc.

Motility   As the body moves through space creating ever-expanding patterns, our perceptions also change. Boas (1978) believed that even moving one's head into a different position in space can alter the world that individual perceives. *Motility*, moving the body with force through space and time, shapes our perceptions of who we are and the world we live in. Boas writes: "Through motility the individual learns to establish and expand concepts of his body image, thereby gaining confidence in his reality and control of his body" (p. 116).

Developmentally, neonates first become aware of their bodies because they move: they wriggle, push, slide, open their mouths to feed and communicate, lift their heads, and eventually pull themselves up to crawl and then finally walk. The concept that man moves to survive recognizes the anatomical and physiological nature of man. Furthermore, motility is essential so that humans can explore and understand their environments. Once the recognition of the self as a moving entity is established and the environment is understood, humans move to control and adjust to their environments (Allenbaugh, 1970).

As dance/movement therapists we base our belief in the success of our work on the knowledge that as we move we learn more about ourselves; as we understand and gain personal insight we feel prepared to reach out to others; as we make contacts with others, they, in turn, provide us with new information about ourselves. This is how we grow and develop. As unique as fingerprints, each person possesses a movement style that distinguishes him or her from others (Hunt, 1964). DMT, as opposed to more structured dance training or sports activity, deals directly with the dynamic, individual quality of movement ability inherent in each person. As we encourage and exercise expansion of range and exploration of the environment, patients are literally "moved" to another level of behavior and interaction. Dance forms involving mirroring, circle formations, partner work, and varying musical rhythms can motivate the reluctant mover. Expanding the spatial formations of the group to include moving in lines, snaking serpent-like through the space, and encouraging individual patients to explore moving in the center of a circle, have proven to be valuable techniques.

A common problem in many urban psychiatric facilities is the lack of space. Patients sleep in multibed rooms and spend most of their time in crowded day areas. Compounding the effects of minimal space on movement opportunities are the side effects of many psychotropic medications, which can result in stiffness, lethargy, and drowsiness. The result is an individual who minimizes overt and extraneous movement, shrinks into a near-reach kinesphere, and retreats into a self-involved, self-centered sphere of intra-action. The modality of DMT is ideally suited to these conditions, as it offers the patient the freedom and opportunity within the structured session to dissolve those barriers to movement and proceed from isolative *intra-action* to healthy, socialized *interaction*.

Selfhood

As we move within the *Intra-Actional System* of the BASCICS model from Body Attitude to Selfhood, we begin to observe the true reciprocal quality of both categories. Building from the foundations of the body, our "home base," through awareness of body image, we begin to formulate the idea of self-concept—the "me." As it will be apparent in the following, this is a notion that has different definitions.

Self-Concept The concept of "self" occurs when young children begin to differentiate themselves from the environment and from others within their environment. Once differentiation occurs and children are no longer completely self-oriented, the role of mother, father, and similar "significant others" begin to play the most important part in the development of the child's self-concept. The formation of the self-concept is never accomplished in isolation; rather, it is the result of interpersonal relationships.

Fundamentally, the self-concept is learned; it is basic to individuals' personality structure. The self-concept is a person's feeling, knowledge, and reaction toward their bodies—physical, emotional, social and intellectual (Jervis, 1959). McDonald (1965) defines self-concept as being the way one sees oneself—the set of inferences, drawn from self-observation in many different situations that describe one's characteristic behavior patterns. William H. Fitts claims that when we speak about an individual's self-concept we refer to "the image, the picture, the set of perceptions and feelings which he has of himself" (1967, p. 1).

According to personality theorists, an individual's self-concept is the result of the reflected appraisals of significant others (Sullivan, 1947) and the give and take of interactions with people (Commins & Fagin, 1957). It is acceptable to infer then, that no one is born with a fully formed self-concept. The development of the self-concept begins in infancy and goes through a series of stages into adulthood. It develops as children experience approval and criticism, success and failure; it grows with children's perception of the world around them—their families, friends, and their places in society. It matures as their bodies mature and they begin to evaluate themselves according to characteristics of their physical, social, and emotion being (Capello, 1979).

In DMT we are constantly providing answers to the patient's question, "Who am I?" Depression and regression reinforce the feelings of depersonalization, the fragmented and confused identities, and the decisive loss of sense of self that characterizes psychosis. Using techniques intrinsic to DMT, patients are encouraged to reacquaint themelves with their moving bodies, to redefine and clarify their body images and body boundaries, and become sensitized to the world (and its inhabitants) around them. Supported by a receptive therapist and a non-threatening environment, patients in DMT can focus on the search for self through their exploration of the range of movement, expansion of that range, and physical investigation of their surroundings. Being mirrored by others (validation) and taking center stage (perhaps in the middle of a circle) can concretize and reconfirm his own identity and experience of the moving self.

Self-Esteem   The feeling state that accompanies perception of self is defined as *self-esteem*. The "normal" person has a healthy love for him or herself and depends on others only partially for attention, affection, and praise (Buss, 1966). Individuals with mental illness are observed to have a considerable loss of self-esteem and often seek the affection of someone else to maintain their sense of self-worth. Contingent with feelings of low self-esteem are inadequacy, inferiority, and lack of self-confidence.

Developmentally, when the ego is starting to form, the child's self-esteem is entirely dependent on the affection of the parents (Buss, 1966).

Psychoanalytic theory maintains that the loss of self-esteem occurs in schizophrenics as patients regress back into an early oral stage in which they cannot test reality adequately and, unlike the infant, reject reality. In the here and now realm of a DMT session, with physical boundaries clearly set (i.e., the room) and within the structure of the session itself (from warm-up to closure), there is the potential for the patient to "test" his selfhood against that of others. In reflecting others' movements, by permitting and accepting physical contact, and through the integrating quality of activating the muscles and joints, patients can move toward an acceptance of both reality and themselves within that reality.

As dance/movement therapists accept the movement of individuals and "tries them out" on their own bodies, and as they provide an open, consenting environment for personal movement opportunity, untrained "dancers" can feel new confidence in themselves as worthwhile, esteemed individuals. A sense of pride and accomplishment can only add to the good feelings of "self" as the patient in a DMT session offers the group a personal movement that is received, duplicated, and expanded upon. Specific dance activities that foster positive self-esteem can include patients' taking turns in the center of the circle ("spotlight dance") and two members' changing places in the circle by dancing across the middle and over to the opposite side ("change partners dance"). Increased self-esteem is illustrated by brighter affect and smiling, sustained eye contact, as well as spontaneous applause from group members for each other's accomplishments.

Authentic Movements   While structured education of the body (i.e., through exercise and technical practice) and more formal, social dance opportunities are part of the realm of recognized dance activities, the principle of accepting the unstylized movement of the group member is unique and specific to DMT. DMT recognizes and accepts this basic movement offered by group members as important to the process of change and growth. More importantly, the dance is not judged by codes of good or bad; all movement expression is deemed acceptable within the realm of safety for both the individual and the group. Diem (1970) writes that *authentic movements* (or what she calls "self-movement") are a naturally learned expression of man. An individual's personal movement repertoire is acquired, not through formal dance/movement training, but by sensing, by feeling, by watching, by trying, by experimenting and creating. Diem writes:

> Self-movement leads to a greater self-expression, to increased self-control, to better self-understanding, to progressive self-responsibility, to more independence, and to greater self-realization in becoming a whole person. (p. 4)

Dosamantes-Alperson (1974) states that it is through authentic movement that it is possible to discover the meaning of the felt experience. Using the term "spontaneous dance," Bender and Boas (1941) saw authentically improvised dance/movement as a method of creative liberation and expression. The role of the dance/movement therapist is to search among this authentic thematic material for relationships and symbolic associations. Once this information is revealed, the dance/movement therapist can make interventions and interpretations when appropriate and necessary.

By working with the "flow" of the group, the dance/movement therapist permits an atmosphere of creative freedom and consent. She accepts the movements of her clients (barring physical abuse) for their intrinsic value and symbolic material. Unlike the dance educator or choreographer, dance/movement therapists are not product-oriented, they do not criticize the movements, or, as Maslow (1971) says:

> Edit, pick and choose, correct, improve, doubt, reject, judge or evaluate. They merely accept the patients' movements and let it flow upon them; they let it have its say; they let it be itself. (p. 32)

Therefore, there are no failures in a DMT session. The simple beauty of the moving body and its relationship to other moving bodies in space offers success in each session. Often, the most regressed and ill patients or those with dual diagnosis of both mental illness and developmental delay will spontaneously applaud each other when a dance has ended to signal their delight in the process. Use of imagery and developing movement patterns sparked from an inner cue or impulse are techniques that inspire authentic movements. Often, use of pedestrian or work-related movement sequences (i.e., walking or task-oriented patterns) can provide basic material for un-stylized movement. From these simple and recognizable steps, the patient and therapist are able to design a more fully experienced aesthetic and creative dance.

Creativity   *Creativity* is a force that can be fostered and sensitively nurtured by the dance/movement therapist. While educators and artists have long sought to explain and duplicate the creative act in measurable terms, the fact that creativity is not reproducible remains apparent. Dance is a creative act; it springs from the depths of creative wells immersed within each carefully trained body. As dance/movement therapists we should not shrink from the history of the performing art from which the therapeutic function of dance was recognized and extricated (Capello, 1980).

In the belief that DMT is both a therapeutic and creative event, the benefits of creativity must be considered. Maslow (1971) wrote that creative people are comfortable with change, enjoy change, and can handle a new situation with confidence, strength, and courage. Translated into a life situation, the creative person can make adaptations and function adequately in the face of change (including economical, social, environmental, and role changes). Within a DMT session is the opportunity to face change (shifting levels, varying rhythms, negotiating personal space) and to react to it. In the secure atmosphere of a session, coupled with a firm therapeutic alliance of mutual trust and respect, patients might be inclined to be more flexible in their choices and decision-making and seek alternatives to situations presented.

A case example of alternate choice was observed in a session in which we created a "human fence" with the task being to "get to the other side." The majority of the patients sought to use aggressive movements to force their way through without success. Finally, "D" utilized the option of asking politely in a quiet voice while moving with small gestures. She alone succeeded in solving the problem.

If we view the movement of the body in DMT as a vehicle for creative, expressive release, and accept the fact that body movement is basic to life, the experience of dance furthers our creativeness in everything we do (Mettler, 1960). A DMT session can provide an arena for experiencing characteristics important to creative functioning—courage (accepting limits and structure), independent thinking (choice and responsibility), intuitiveness, and absorption and persistence in the activity (Torrance, 1965). All of these elements are also characteristics of healthy adaptive functioning throughout one's life.

Leadership   We have traced the meaning of "selfhood" as incorporating properties of self-conceptualization, self-esteem, authenticity of movement, and how the creative process enhances the search for self. A further potential of selfhood, the capacity for *leadership*, is a quality of personality that embraces all these properties. A common technique used in a DMT session is the changing and sharing of leadership. An individual may be provided with the opportunity to create a movement, share it with the group, and then pass the leadership on. Although a "simple" process and one that patients who are veterans in DMT come to accept and anticipate, taking the leadership furnishes a circumstance in which, perhaps only on a primary level, the drives for self-determination and self-mastery are satisfied. As leader, patients learn to take responsibility for the choices they make—the direction and dimension in which to move, the pattern and shape of the movement, and the rhythm or time element in which it is done. The positive validation that occurs when therapist and peers alike are focused on and execute the patient's personal movement choice can promote a true sense of pride and accomplishment. The "reflective" experience of observing others in your posture and movement qualities can confirm a realistic image of the body and present another awareness for understanding of "self."

As the leadership changes in the group, visual and tactile contact can be heightened as the perception of self and others becomes more acute. The dance/movement therapist may help guide the leadership experience for the patient who is unsure about his own capacities thereby reducing feelings of failure or ineptitude. It has been observed that hospitalized patients are extremely supportive and tolerant of their peers and their leadership attempts and often offer both verbal and nonverbal encouragement and acknowledgment.

For hospitalized psychiatric patients, the DMT session may well be the only occasion for them to "present" themselves and develop skills as leaders in an appropriate, productive manner and receive immediate feedback about their behavior.

As therapists and patients work in partnership and take responsibility for the success of the session, patients can help choose music they believe will guide the group to a creative expression. Music plays an essential role in DMT sessions, helping to evoke an emotional and aesthetic response. Often patients choose music that has personal meaning to them and want to share these memories with the group. Music helps to foster relationships among generations of dancers (helping both older and younger patients learn new tunes and dance forms) and works to prolong involvement and interest in the session. Music and lyric can both support and sustain the dance and promote success in the group experience. By supporting the dance, music aids in synchronizing the movement, unifies the voices with a shared lyric, promotes reminiscence and communal memory, and establishes an environment of familiarity. Music works to sustain the dance, allowing it to reach its fullest potential.

Through the musical foundations of rhythm, melody, verse, and chorus, the choreography of the dance is created. The specific time limitation of each song condenses the group experience by creating an opportunity for a brief choreographic creation that has a beginning, middle, and end. Within this time frame, every song can offer a special moment that people can claim for themselves. For one, it can be a chance to dance with full energy and vibrancy; for another, a time to reflect on a special time from the past; for others, an opportunity to master a new form or style of dance. Finally, singing and vocalizing to the lyrics will encourage fuller use of breath and sound.

The Interactional System

Communication

Movement Dialogue　In her book *The thinking body*, Mabel Elsworth Todd (1937) writes of the language of the body, or nonverbal communication, by stating, "often the body speaks clearly that which the tongue refuses to utter" (p. 295). In DMT we tap into the nonverbal mode by creating *movement dialogues*. Over the years, dance/movement therapists have catalogued their experiences in using the dynamics of a nonverbal approach. Working with patients who may have adapted to the outside world by establishing an effective system of protective verbal defenses, dance/movement therapists can effectively evaluate and understand the individual's symbolic gestures, postures, movement quality, rhythms, and patterns.

Verbal language is a complex process. As with all complex, multi-systemic procedures, true, accurate meaning can be distorted and often lost completely. One is reminded of the party game of "telephone" in which a verbal message is sent through a network of people receiving and transmitting and is ultimately altered to the point when the original message is not comprehensible. A dance/movement therapist writes:

> Movement responses, which involve a lower brain level are less a part of conscious awareness, are more reliable expressions of feelings than words. (Burton, 1974, p. 21)

In utilizing movement dialogues for communication between patient and therapist, and patient and peers, DMT becomes the optimal treatment alternative for the preverbal developmentally delayed child, the mute autistic youngster, and the silent or intellectualizing mentally ill adult. Samuels (1972) writes that because a patient's reaction to other people is often so defended, initial contact established by a nonverbal mode of expression is often easiest to achieve. From his studies on kinesics, Birdwhistell (1970) claims that the communication behavior of a schizophrenic is actually not disordered or chaotic, but *appears* so because it has a different pattern, a different system of communication. At the primary level of communication, the body level, the "pictures" or forms created by both the static and moving body are "worth a thousand words." In DMT our movements speak resoundingly louder than words.

In DMT sessions, movement dialogues are facilitated through techniques that include the mirroring, reflecting, expanding, and diminishment of movement expressions. In group work, giving each patient an opportunity to present a movement to the group and then observe their response is a method of back-and-forth dialogue. Asking members to take on a posture or explore a gesture that is related to their feeling state at the moment is another form of nonverbal exchange. Alternately leading and following group movements is a further occasion for expressing and reacting to information offered by other group members. While communicating through movement in a DMT session, members become aware of the need to find and take on the group rhythm, adjust to the quality of each movement, and adapt to the spatial configuration of the group.

The movement dialogue expands as emotional content is brought to the surface through the experience of moving the body. Patients can explore the increasing exposure of moving alone, with a partner, or as part of a larger group. Often they are observed smiling to one another, making better eye contact, and permitting more intimate contact through hand-holding and support of each other's body weight as they both lead and are led in the dance.

Symbolic Expression   In her writings on DMT, Marian Chace (1975), a pioneer dance/movement therapist, observed that although people may remain silent verbally, they never stop communicating on the non-verbal level. When emotions are strongly felt and important to a person, communication of those emotions may be expressed in the less-threatening nonverbal mode. For Chace, this mode was the *symbolic expression* of the moving body:

> One aspect of people with emotional problems is the fact that they use physical action to express feelings more readily than the majority of people in our culture who are so restricted in this direct expression. (p. 210)

As the dance/movement therapist works toward enabling patients to experience themselves on the level of bodily sensations and impulses, thereby allowing communication to occur, it is based on the belief that "movement is an honest reflection of the self, one that cannot be hidden by words" (Chaiklin, 1975, p. 707). While words can be consciously disguised and self-censored to suppress the expression of emotional states, body movement is a more basic form of emotional disclosure (Berger, 1972). In addition, if patients feel inadequate to describe feeling states verbally, "body actions can be used to convey emotions which are factual or symbolic expressions" (Samuels, 1972, p. 66).

Symbolic gestures and postures come to the surface as the moving body promotes a level of felt expression. Aggressive expressions, which may have been successfully blocked on a verbal level, come through in DMT with symbols of hostility (facial expression, clenched fists). The dance/movement therapist can redirect aggressive impulses by initiating percussive, full-bodied moves such as stamping, swinging fists, and jumps with impactive phrasing. Cathartic discharge of aggression can be redirected to an imagined "symbolic foe."

As a case example, one group of inpatients shaped a large, heavy "imaginary" boulder, then ritualistically shattered it with axes and fists, and finally ended by jointly throwing it out of the window. Verbal reactions afterward included expressions such as "cleansed," "relieved," and "satisfied." The imagined *enemy* took on varying characteristics for each patient; one saw it as the hospital; another as mother; another as spouse.

Similarly, expressions of hopelessness and despondency, perhaps symbolized by repetitive self-rocking or a limp, collapsed posture, can be shared on a movement level and explored through mutual trust and support experiences such as back-to-back stretches, leans, or pushes and pulls. As the dance/movement therapist provides experiences to enlarge the repertoire of body movements, patients are better equipped to express their own impulses and emotions, and can more accurately interpret the nonverbal signals of others (Feder and Feder, 1977). Symbolic sharing, through postures and gestures and feeling tones, are methods that can elicit expressive movement responses.

Rhythm   *Rhythm* is a definitive element in the human interactive behavior of communication. According to Kendon (1970) two people engaged in a conversation are, on one level, rhythmically linked:

> The listener dances with the speaker to show he is "with" him, receiving him; he then gets the speaker to dance with him as a way of heightening the synchronization between them, so they can both reach the point of disengagement at precisely the same moment. (p. 67)

In her article "Some aspects of the nature of the rhythmic experience and its possible therapeutic value," Allegra Fuller Snyder (1972) traces the history of research on the implications of rhythm as a tool in DMT and as a fundamental part of the human experience. The rhythms of our heartbeat and the flow of blood through the body, along with the rhythm of our walking gait and conversational patterns, are just a few elements of the body's rhythmic expression.

In DMT, rhythm is utilized as a communicative force between therapist and patient and among patients themselves. There is some undefined sense of satisfaction that is felt when a group of discordant and isolative patients becomes unified through synchronized rhythmic movement. Often, psychiatric patients exhibit arrhythmic movement patterns, the element of rhythm being impaired, undeveloped, or inhibited. Movement patterns within the DMT session provide rhythmic experiences that foster communication and relationship:

> Psychologically, rhythm integrates the individual with himself by centering his thoughts on the rhythm he feels within his body at the same time integrating him with the group. (Keen, 1972, p. 132)

Rhythm, as an expressive, communicative mode, is a viable part of the DMT session. Techniques vary as some dance/movement therapists use external rhythms (recorded music and instruments) and others use internal rhythms (breath patterns, heartbeat, voice). By combining methods using both externally and internally produced rhythms, the dance/movement therapist offers a fuller, more inclusive opportunity for independent choice and expression.

Emotions are often brought into awareness and communicated in shared symbolic rhythmic action (Chace, 1975). In addition to its communicative element, the healing aspect of rhythm is described in the following:

> In the healing rites of the Kung of the Kalahari Desert, the Vedda of Ceylon, and the Ute of North America, for example, participants are led by a shaman through rhythmic, repetitive movements which lead to altered states of consciousness. These are aimed at exorcising illness and relieving physical and mental suffering. (Dosamantes-Alperson, 1979, p. 114)

While working with psychiatric patients who display disorganized thinking and altered perceptions of reality, the dance/movement therapist relies on the use of the properties of rhythm to organize and structure the experience. Through moving in unison in a particular rhythmic relationship, patients can find both comfort and success being in the "here and now" of the session. Dance as a therapy, based on its use of rhythmic patterning of force/space/flow, is a communicative and healing energy. In an outpatient DMT group in which the rhythmic action of the flow of water (waves, tide, surf, whirlpool) was explored, members expressed feelings of being "cleansed," "purified," "purged," "blessed," and "refreshed."

The rhythmic component is a unifying, integrating, and powerful force that can release tension and serve to "center" the individual and group. Rhythmic activity (whether projected by a musical selection or an inner beat) can provide themes for movement exploration. Often certain musical selections (particularly ethnic and folk songs) can evoke emotional memory release and provide the group with thematic material to explore and process through dancing, singing, and verbal interchanges.

The picking-up and sharing of personal and group rhythms can promote a sense of group cohesiveness; it can energize a lethargic group; and when necessary, provide a satisfactory closure and resolution to the movement experience.

Verbalization   Although DMT is described as a non-verbal form of psychotherapy it is certainly not mute. *Verbalization* before, during, and after a DMT group can be an effective, necessary component of the therapeutic process. The dance/movement therapist might begin a group by greeting the patients individually and welcoming them to the session. During the group he or she may ask a patient to describe an image or compose a story in reference to a particular movement pattern. At the conclusion of the session, verbal sharing of any insights gained or feelings evoked by the movement experience may provide a further opportunity for communication and interaction. Chaiklin (1975) writes:

> While movement is the prime tool, verbalization should not be ignored. There is a need to develop cognitive and thought processes in relation to movement in order to maximize its potential. Imagery and verbalization in response to movement patterns involve the individuals further. (p. 710)

Chaiklin augments her ideas about verbalization by qualifying the depth of discussion as dependent upon the abilities of the particular group to process and deal with insight and language.

W. S. Condon (1968), a proponent of linguistic–kinesic research, states that "both speech and body motion share in the on-going, rhythmic waves of ordered change (at many levels) which constitute the flowing stream of behavior" (p. 22). Language, then, can be seen as another dimension of the movement experience; it can give crucial, in-depth meaning to symbolic gestures and postures; it can further "link" the patient and therapist into an alliance of trusting candor; and it can enrich the movement experience by connecting past memories, present situations, and future goals.

Another method that encourages use of language and verbalization is to utilize the lyrics of songs during a session. Singing out loud and along to music while dancing fosters integration of the music, movement, and words. Groups become more cohesive and their members intimately related to one another as they share in the expression of rhythmic and patterned sound. Activating the voice deepens breathing and further improves the mind–body connection. Often the lyrics themselves evoke emotional response and help the group create a "spoken/sung dialogue" that raises their awareness and often leads to meaningful discussions and revelations. A clear example of the power of the lyric is seen when the song entitled "I'm Alive" (performed by Celine Dion) offers the group members a chance to both sing the title words and gesture (hands to heart and then lifting upward toward the sky in exaltation) in an empowering *symbolic and verbal* illustration of hope and survival.

For high-functioning groups, verbal sharing at the conclusion of a session can prolong the impact of mutually experienced emotional states uncovered by the movement. Feelings of relief experienced by the knowledge of the commonality of feelings, as well as the acceptance and tolerance of contrary feeling states among group members, is a process of social learning. In lower-functioning groups, verbalizations in the form of greetings, introductions, and saying "goodbye," promote appropriate conversational exchanges in the reality of the here and now.

As group members attend DMT, it seems that the quality and quantity of conversation among patients increase significantly over the course of a session and over a series of sessions. While the group members may come into the session in silence and in an "intra-active state," they invariably leave in a flurry of conversation, commenting on the activity and acknowledging one another verbally. Clearly, they have moved into an "inter-active state." Finally, thanking the group participants for their work and effort acknowledges each person's contribution to the process. The group members may then express their gratefulness to the leader as well, building appropriate social skills and anticipation of the next session.

Interpersonal Dynamics

As part of the *Interactional System*, communication on a movement, rhythmic, and verbal level is a prerequisite to the development of the *therapeutic alliance*, a foundation for *group experience*, and a forerunner to *socialization*. These are the essential components of Interpersonal Dynamics.

Therapeutic Alliance　One form of relationship necessary to the process of therapy is the *therapeutic alliance*. According to Berger (1977) it is based on mutual trust and respect. Belief in the sincerity of the therapist as an empathetic listener and guide, and a feeling of positive regard or acceptance of the patient's total being are foundations of the therapeutic alliance. Once the therapist–patient relationship is established in an atmosphere of frankness and concern, the patient can face the risks of change, trying new ways of seeing, understanding, and behaving both when alone and with others (Berger, 1977).

Any therapeutic relationship is characterized by similar components:

1. Validation of the individual as an important, worthwhile person
2. Setting of realistic goals
3. Respecting the rights and wishes of others
4. Realizing one's potential
5. Encouragement and support in growing toward health

Kopp (1972) adds the element of "self-disclosure" or "transparency" as an aspect of the therapeutic alliance. His belief is that if I, as the therapist (or guide), can be firmly centered in my own inner feelings and can be "transparent" to myself (and reveal myself to others) in a non-selective, accepting way, my commitment

> … invites a like commitment to my patients, we can offer each other courage to go on, joining each other along the pilgrim's way, foregoing semblance for openness, and solitude for community. (p. 26)

The relationship between dance/movement therapist and client is built on both verbal and non-verbal exchanges and interactions. Because the dance/movement therapist uses movement and rhythm as communication, verbal barriers and deceptions are set aside (Keen, 1971). In developing a therapeutic alliance, the therapist uses methods specific (and unique) to the dance/movement experience—the mutual sharing and exploring of physical space; flow and force elements, and time fluctuations; conversing in movement dialogues of rhythmic harmony; establishing appropriate physical contact and eye contact; and the setting of limits and boundaries. A provocative conjecture regarding the dance/movement therapist–client relationship is the suggestion that this alliance (as compared with those of traditional psychotherapies) is formed in less time and with a higher degree of empathy. A cursory explanation can be based on the contention that the nonverbal mode of DMT simulates the preverbal, primitive communication system, thereby setting up an "unspoken" network of mutual understanding and intuitive interaction.

Group Experience The relationship between therapist and patient can serve as a foundation for relationships and interactions that develop as part of the *group experience*. Berger (1977) describes the group experience as one in which the patient can communicate, relate, and work with others ..."in a corrective, interactional, re-educative, emotional, and attitudinal experience focusing on individual and group dynamics in a spirit of trust, mutuality, and confidentiality" (p. 88).

The group DMT experience provides a supportive basis for both group and individual expression (Samuels, 1972). The group works as a "sounding board," an opportunity for the individual to receive realistic feedback or validation for his actions from other group members. In the face of the group response (to personal movements or verbalizations), the patient learns how to cope with rejection as well as acceptance and approval. Rejection becomes a less threatening, less self-defeating experience. Defense mechanisms can be lowered as the individual's movements, and thereby self, is accepted and understood by the moving group; fear of contact is reduced as the experience continues without threat; movement goals become group goals and seem more attainable and less overwhelming.

Mettler (1960) described the group as a living organism made up of differentiated parts that must work as a whole to function effectively. For the self-centered, disoriented, retreating psychiatric patient, the group is a "connective" device connecting the patient to the environment, to the session, to other group members, and to the therapist. The circular structure is useful as it provides tactile contact on either side and inclusive group eye contact and visibility. The circle is also a relatively easy and familiar shape to create and is a stabilizing, centering position for both warm-up and closure. Chaiklin (1975) saw group rhythmic movement to musical accompaniment as an alternate means of relating for the mentally ill patient who finds it difficult to interact. The activity becomes a method of responding "first to the structure of the music, then to the therapist and each other" (p. 709).

Within the group context, an individual has a chance to express, reflect, and respond to emotional material. The symbolic expression of anger, without retribution from the therapist or group members, can provide an opportunity to examine and understand the source of that anger (Berger, 1977). The "collective" feeling of the group as they share in the emotions of an individual, gives that person a sense of belonging and recognition. Emotional maturity is developed as the patient learns that members of the group may have both similar feelings, and yet very different needs, desires, and wants. This knowledge becomes valuable when a patient uncovers painful material and seeks consolation and understanding from the group.

Although the group may be moving in unison, the fact that each individual is making a personal movement statement is not overlooked. At times, the synchrony of repetitive unison movement may prove restricting or suffocating. The dance/movement therapist can then use techniques that encourage alternately moving away from the group individually or with a partner, and then returning to the group structure. This process of separating and regrouping challenges the patient to individuate from the group, provides an opportunity to practice self-control and develop listening skills, and demands concentration and focus. Random regrouping at various points in the session allows new contacts to be made and can facilitate increased quality and quantity of interaction.

At all times within the group, patients are simultaneously moving on their own ("doing their own thing") and acting as a part of a group. Mettler (1960) writes:

> A group movement is not a sum of individual movements. It is something quite different: a different *kind* of movement. In group movement expression, each separate member of the group must be aware of the movement which he himself is making, but this awareness is subordinate to an awareness of the group as a whole. (p. 404)

During the dance experience, as the patients respond and interact with one another's movement, "we then see a reorganization of the emotional responses and very often greater organization of the cognitive response" (Dyrad, 1968, p. 1).

Along with the development of learning skills, tolerance of others, reduction of isolation, alternately separating and merging, and creation and processing of group themes, the simple *joy* of moving harmoniously in a group is one of the most important and satisfying elements of the group DMT process. Patients return to DMT groups throughout their hospital admission, seeking the emotional and physical pleasure of dancing with their peers. The cumulative experience of the simple act of each human connection (including handholding and direct eye contact) encountered in the session, contributes to both psychological healing and physiological recuperation.

Socialization   In addition to "activating" the individual toward understanding of body and self, allowing communication of ideas and emotions, and dealing with the dynamics of the group, DMT is an experience in *socialization*. Even prior to the session, the act of being invited to join, making a choice about attending, and expressing that choice, are all opportunities to practice social skills. As the group begins, each person introduces him or herself or in some way acknowledges his or her presence and the presence of others.

Many times it has been observed that patients come into a DMT session (particularly inpatients) and don't know each other's names. Often these patients have been living close to each other for a period of days or weeks as "anonymous" beings. Time spent within the session learning and memorizing others' names is an important socializing process and builds relationships and camaraderie. On a movement level, social interaction is practiced through turn-taking—learning to wait and delaying gratification; anticipating one's turn and preparing a response (as in conversation); and attending to the movements of others using visual, auditory, and kinesthetic cues.

As social beings we learn to accept limits and guidelines that are necessary to maintain reasonable order. Within a DMT session there are also boundaries and structures. Foremost, there is the structure of the session itself from warm-up through closure. While fantasy material may be developed and imagery is utilized, the moving body can be experienced only within the boundaries of the here-and-now reality—in the particular facility, the room, the hour, the day, etc. Other limits such as no phone calls, eating, or drinking during the session are restrictions that the patient comes to accept and tolerate as being a part of the social sphere. Contracts regarding time limitations, expectations, and acceptable behavior characterize the DMT session as a socializing event.

A more intimate construct of interpersonal dynamics is that between partners. Partner work in DMT furnishes the patient with one-on-one interaction. This coupling requires the patient to make spontaneous, self-initiated decisions and responses: the therapist is no longer the direct guide. Patients focus in on one another seeking other leadership figures and assuming leadership positions themselves. While working in dyads, patients become sensitive to contrasts and similarities in movement style and may find it necessary to adjust and adapt to a new partner at any given time. Social liaisons form and relationships grow out of the give-and-take of moving with a partner.

At the conclusion of a session another socializing experience takes place. Each individual is acknowledged by name and thanked for participating. Personal issues may be addressed either privately or by the group. Making some kind of direct, physical contact—such as shaking hands or reaching out to touch arms or shoulders along with focused eye contact—completes the event and encourages future participation. Closing rituals help to ground and center the members, preparing them to move on to other hospital activities and anticipate the next DMT session. Deep breathing in unison, passing "energy" and thanks from hand to hand with a squeeze, serve to balance and focus the group. Rituals can vary from group to group but usually incorporate a symbolic sharing or gift giving, with the leader requesting that the members offer each other something they believe the group needs or desires. Often, gifts of "going home," "good health," "peace," and "love" are commonly heard. Another aspect of closure that is important to sustain is the group's acknowledgment of the leader and his or her efforts in guiding the group and providing the experience. Usually, the group members show their gratitude spontaneously as part of the ritualized sharing and offer smiles and thanks. It is important for the dance/movement therapist to then accept the group's appreciation with grace and humility. Thus, both a strong social and therapeutic interpersonal connection has been established, confirming the validity of the session.

Conclusion

In the BASCICS system we have traced the theory and methodology of DMT from the re-education and awareness of the *body attitude*, to the concept of *selfhood*, to the notion of *communication* through expressive, *authentic movements* and rhythmic dance, and finally to the realm of *interpersonal dynamics*. The relationship among all four categories is clear; each grows and develops and is reciprocal to the other, each one is affected by changes or blocks within any one category, the potential of each one is both limited and expanded by the others, the capacity for health is determined by the health of each part.

Although the BASCICS system is organized where body attitude is followed by selfhood, then communication, etc., the succession of categories is interchangeable. While it is true that, as Chaiklin (1975) writes, "One must first have a perception of oneself, some sense of control and choice before one is able to perceive clearly and relate to others" (p. 709), exposure to group process and interactions can lead to a more authentic awareness and clarification of self.

Each section of this system with its descriptive elements (i.e., body attitude, body image, boundaries, etc.) does not stand alone or exist as a separate entity from the entire model. Rather, the double-arrowed lines that connect each category as diagrammed in Figure 5.1 indicate the inter-related dynamics of this system. As a flexible system, these fundamental concepts and theories can be put into practice, and then further modified and expanded by the individual therapist. In originating, developing, and substantiating the BASCICS model, I have come to recognize a personal identity and belief system and its relationship to the fundamental constructs of DMT as a viable, joyful, and potent form of psychotherapy.

References

Allenbaugh, N. (1970). Learning about movement. *Selected readings in movement education*, R.T. Sweeney (Ed.). Reading, MA: Addison-Wesley.

Bender, L., & Boas, F. (1941). Creative dance in therapy. *American Journal of Orthopsychiatry 2*, 235–241.

Berger, M. M. (1977). *Working with people called patients*. New York: Brunner-Mazel.

Berger, M. Roskin (1972) Bodily experiences and expression of emotion. *ADTA Monograph No. 2*, 191–230.

Birdwhistell, R. L. (1970). *Kinesics and context: Essays on body motion communication* Philadelphia: University of Philadelphia Press.

Boas, F. (1978). Creative dance. In M. N. Costonis (Ed.), *Therapy in motion*. Chicago: University of Illinois Press.

Burton, C. L. (1974). Movement as a group therapy in a psychiatric hospital. In K.C. Mason (Ed.) *Focus on dance VII. Dance therapy Journal of AAHPERD*.

Buss, A. H. (1966). *Psychopathology*. New York: John Wiley & Sons.

Capello, P. P. (1979). The role of parental attitudes in the development of self-concept in blind children. Unpublished paper.

Capello, P. P. (1980) Dance therapy as a creative event. Unpublished paper.

Chace, M. (1975). *Marian Chace: Her papers*. H. Chaiklin (Ed.), ADTA.

Chaiklin, S. (1975). Dance therapy. In S. Arieti (Ed.) *American handbook of psychiatry* (2nd ed.) Vol. 5, pp. 701–720. New York: Basic Books.

Commins, W. D., & Fagin, B. (1957). *Principles of educational psychology*. New York: Ronald Press.

Condon, W. S. (1968–69) Linguistic–kinesic research and dance therapy. *Combined Proceedings of the ADTA 3rd and 4th Annual Conferences*.

Davis, C. J. (1964). Development of the self-concept. *New outlook for the blind 58* February.

Diem, L. (1970). Basic movement education with simple elements in primary schools. In R. T. Sweeney (Ed.), *Selected readings in movement education*. Reading, MA: Addison-Wesley.

Dosamantes-Alperson, E. (1974). Movement therapy: A treatment framework. *ADTA Monograph No. 3* 1973–1974, 87–99.

Dosamantes-Alperson, E. (1979). Dance/movement therapy: An emerging profession. *Journal of Energy Medicine 1*, 114–119.

Dyrad, J. E. (1968–69). The meaning of movement: As human expression and as artistic communication. In S. Chaiklin (Ed.). *Combined Proceedings of the ADTA 3rd and 4th Annual Conferences*, Madison, WI.

Feder, E., & Feder, B. (1977). Dance therapy. *Psychology Today,* February, 76–80.

Feldenkrais, M. (1977). *Body and mature behavior.* New York: International Universities Press.

Fisher, S. (1973). *Body consciousness.* Englewood Cliffs, NJ: Prentice Hall.

Fisher S., & Cleveland, S. (1968). *Body image and personality.* New York: Dover.

Fitts, W. H. (1967). The self-concept as a variable in vocational rehabilitation. Nashville Mental Health Center Project No. RD2419-668cl.

Freud, S. (1927). *The ego and the id.* London: Hogarth.

Hall, E. T. (1969). *The hidden dimension.* New York: Doubleday.

Hawkins, A. (1987). *Creating through dance.* East Windsor, NJ: Princeton Book Co.

Hunt, V. (1964). *Movement behavior: A model for action.* Quest, Monograph #2, 69–91.

Jervis, F. M. (1959). A comparison of self-concept of blind and sighted children. *Guidance Program for Blind Children, 20,* Watertown, MA: Perkins.

Keen, H. (1971). Dancing toward wholeness. F. Donelan (Ed.). ADTA, *Monograph No. 1, Combined proceedings of the ADTA 2nd Annual Conference,* Washington, D.C.

Kendon, A. (1970). A movement coordination in dance therapy and conversation. *Workshop in dance therapy: Its research potentials.* New York, CORD, 64–69.

Kopp, S. B. (1972). *If you meet the Buddha on the road, kill him!* Palo Alto, CA: Science and Behavior Books.

Leventhal, M. B. (1974). Dance therapy with MBD children. In K. C. Mason (Ed.), *Focus on Dance VII: Dance Therapy.* Washington, DC: AAHPERD.

Maslow, A. H. (1971). *The farther reaches of human nature.* New York: Penguin.

McDonald, F. J. (1965). Journal of, *Educational Psychology.* 2, 1–16.

Mettler, B. (1967). *Materials of dance as a creative art activity.* Tucson, AZ: Mettler Studios.

Samuels, A. (1972). Movement change through dance therapy: A study. ADTA, *Monograph No. 2.*

Schilder, P. (1950). *The image and appearance of the human body: Studies in the constructive energies of the psyche.* New York: International Universities Press.

Snyder, A. F (1972). *Some aspects of the nature of the rhythmic experience and its possible therapeutic value.* Monograph 2. In F. Donelan (Ed.), Writings on Body Movement and Communication, Monograph 2 (pp. 128–150). Columbia: ADTA.

Sullivan, H.S. (1947). *Conceptions of modern psychiatry.* Washington D.C.: William Alanson White Psychiatric Foundation.

Todd, M. E. (1937). *The thinking body.* New York: Dance Horizons.

Torrance, E. P. (1965). *Rewarding creative behavior: Experiments in classroom creativity.* Englewood Cliffs, NJ: Prentice Hall.

CHAPTER **6**

Body, Style, and Psychotherapy

VARDA DASCAL

Contents

Introduction

In his book *Neurotic styles*, David Shapiro employs the term "style" in the sense of "a form or mode of functioning—the way or a manner of a given area of behavior—that is identifiable in an individual through a range of

103

his specific acts" (Shapiro, 1965, p. 1). I believe that this notion, originally from literary and arts studies, is extremely pertinent to the topic. I will therefore develop and apply it in this chapter and consider some of the results of my own clinical practice and research in relation to this broad concept of style.

By "neurotic styles," Shapiro means "those modes of functioning that seem characteristic, respectively, of the various neurotic conditions" (Shapiro, 1965, p. 1). By "modes of functioning," he subsumes ways of thinking and perceiving, ways of experiencing emotion, and modes of activity under various conditions, including pathological conditions—in other words, a whole gamut of phenomena associated with the cognitive, emotional, behavioral, and physical spheres. In cases that require psychotherapy, these factors are present in the patient's symptoms and are part of their etiology; at the same time, these factors also point to the kind of therapeutical intervention that might be most adequate for each particular case and patient.

The notion of style as applied to psychotherapy by Shapiro is, in my opinion, both valuable and helpful inasmuch as it relates directly to the psychotherapeutic effectiveness. I had the opportunity of experiencing this when applying a *figure of style*—in the rhetorical sense—namely, metaphor. One of the reasons for this effectiveness is precisely the fact that the metaphor, by its own nature, brings together the various spheres mentioned earlier. As is well known, what characterizes the metaphor is that it operates by linking distinct and often distant domains as in, for instance, "John is a lion," or "the roots of Peter's thoughts come from far." John is not literally a feline, nor do Peter's thoughts grow on trees. And yet, the metaphor creates a new relationship between the distinct domains it connects, providing us thereby with a new way of looking at them and giving them a new meaning. Consequently, it can be argued that metaphors connect the various spheres through which the style of the individual manifests itself. What the dance/movement therapist does is call attention to these spheres and thus create the conditions for the patient to elaborate the metaphors following his or her inclinations.

For a dance/movement therapist, the relation between body and mind, between action and intention, between feeling/thinking and experiencing is, to be sure, of particular interest. In effect, many authors from different disciplines agree nowadays that it is impossible to separate (as it was once rather common) mental activity from its embodiment.[1] Moreover, many of the most often used metaphors are actually based on bodily activities and experiences[2]; thus, states of mind, emotions, and ideational contents are frequently conceptualized in terms of bodily terms. Insofar as the therapeutic work consists of creating the conditions that will, if necessary, produce some sort of change—e.g., reframing—it is evident that interventions at the "style" level can only be beneficial. This style level furthermore includes (although not exclusively) the bodily metaphors, which in turn provide access to the various layers of internal and external phenomena— both past and present—that may eventually lead the individual to seek therapeutic help. The clinical examples analyzed in this chapter will serve, then, to illustrate these processes and stress the role played by body and movement in them.

After presenting and analyzing in the next section the clinical examples alluded to, I will proceed to discuss the theoretical significance of the psychotherapeutic implications of a theory such as Shapiro's, which conceives of neurosis as a style and its variants as stylistic modalities. In particular, I will emphasize the possibilities of reframing, which this new approach seems to provide, especially with reference to the bodily dimension.

The Ball and the Balloon

During one of her therapeutic sessions, N—a successful academic, a persistent and serious woman aged 32, the only daughter of holocaust survivors and recently divorced, who had sought therapy as a way of overcoming her emotional limitations—described her problem in establishing a fulfilling relationship with men in the following terms:[3] "I meet somebody. I tell him everything straight away. I throw everything at him.[4] I don't know what I should tell and what I should keep to myself, what to give and what to keep."

The Ball

"To throw," literally, refers to some kind of movement, and this leads me to propose to N that we play at throwing and passing the ball between us. After a while, I ask her to keep on throwing the ball at the wall by herself. I notice that while the distance between her and the wall is small enough to barely require the thrust of her arms, N actually flings her entire body: she pushes extensively forward with her head and shoulders, and she bends her trunk toward the wall as she steps forth. The wall, of course, remains static and non-elastic, thus causing the ball to bounce back with greater force every time, since N's position is closer to the wall and her thrusts become harder. Consequently, the increasing difficulty in catching the ball seemed to surprise N as she was forced to adjust her position continuously.

I pointed out to N that she should pay attention to her performance (in particular, to the solution she had forged in order to tackle the specific motor problem she was facing) as well as to her feelings and sensations. In addition, I asked her to examine whether these emotions might be familiar to her and, if so, whether she could specify in which contexts. Eventually, N's performance and responses revealed that her relational problem could not simply be reduced to a lack of self-control, as she had initially assumed. In effect, N's performance vis-à-vis the wall—which functions here as a metaphor of "the other"—exposed a certain lack of sensitivity regarding the needs, feelings, and capabilities of this other, namely of this other's "position" as opposed to her. She had been unable to anticipate correctly her recipient's reactions and had thus failed to make the necessary adjustments and adaptations of her own actions so as to fit the dynamics of the exchange. By "throwing everything at him," by telling and disclosing indiscriminately everything to her partner, she transfers to the other the entire responsibility of adapting and readjusting, she places upon him the onus of controlling and shaping the relationship.

We observe in N, therefore, a problem involving limits, lack of flexibility, and a certain bodily, behavioral, and cognitive rigidity: she performs the activity of "throwing and passing the ball" with the utmost seriousness and concentration, without—so it seems—being aware of the problem. To be sure, this same serious and rigid behavior may, in a different context or point in time, constitute an advantage and even a necessity of a sort, as for instance when she is required to be persistent and uncompromising in the performance of a research task. Yet in other circumstances, as in her relationships with men, a rather more flexible attitude would be advantageous. Indeed, as we will see below, even extremely rigid people may, under the right conditions, learn to be more flexible.

The Balloon

In the following session with N, I concentrated on a kind of movement not unrelated to our previous one. I asked N to blow up a balloon in various different ways: for instance, by blowing slowly and carefully so as to have full control of the amount of air being introduced, by inhaling and exhaling only once, etc. The balloon's flexibility allows us to have some control over its shape. When I asked her to blow into the balloon with as much air as she could, she stopped and declared: "I won't go on blowing because otherwise the balloon will explode." In other words, she realized that the recipient's capacity has a limit and took upon herself the responsibility of adjusting her behavior according to the observed limitations. Later on in the course of this same session, N—throwing the balloon up and down, exploring its qualities and creating a sort of dance with it—expanded her own repertoire of movements, a process that continued in subsequent sessions. As a result, her potential capacity to take the other into account and act with more flexibility came to light, thus revealing additional possibilities of reaction in interpersonal relationships.

It is important to stress the role played by the therapeutic space, as well as the specific bond with the therapist, as necessary conditions that enable the original spark of change to kindle in due time. I will return to this later on when I deal with reframing.

Going back to N and the balloon, however, this particular activity with the balloon also yielded unexpected dividends. In her diary (I normally request my patients to record their therapeutic experiences in a diary),[5] N wrote down that, to her surprise, she had associated inflating the balloon with the act of sucking her mother's breast. Her surprise stemmed from the fact that the act of sucking is a way of "receiving" whereas inflating a balloon implies "giving." N connected this, moreover, with her constant concern to "fill her mother with life."[6] And the latter, in turn, was linked, on another occasion, to her perception of her parents as cold, emotionless, strictly rational beings, whom she pictured as automata. At home, she recalls, the only mode of communication was verbal; only words existed, and everything had to be literal and explicit. There was no room for hesitations, doubts, feelings, or flexibility. "I was not surprised," she said, that the world was grasped as "rigid, unchanging, non-breathing." In such a world, to have strong emotions was threatening; what is more, these emotions could not be expressed. If the world was so predictable and rigid, it meant that all actions and reactions not only follow fixed rules but likewise there was no need to learn to adjust to changing circumstances.

Between the Ball and the Balloon

We see, therefore, that the issues that had emerged initially through the ball-throwing metaphor have reappeared yet again—this time within a different conceptual structure introduced by a new metaphor: rigidity or flexibility, to be concerned or not with the other, to take responsibility or not. At the same time, the images elaborated within the therapeutic process, all part of the same "family" of movement metaphors, offer N the possibility of articulating a new attitude toward her problems that takes shape in the course of the process. Let N say it in her own words:

> I enjoy writing, giving expression now to what fills me and changes in me. Like the balloon, no matter how much air I blow into it and how much air gets locked up inside, there will always be more air to keep on blowing, and the balloon will fly up high, and the air will come out, and a new balloon might be filled up.

As we activate the movement underlying a certain verbal expression, we are in effect putting into action the "experiential basis" of the metaphorical expression being used. If it is true that "no metaphor can ever be comprehended or even adequately represented independently of its experiential basis" (Lakoff & Johnson, 1980, p. 19), then the movement metaphor constitutes a crucial tool not just for verifying the descriptions and tenets at the basis of the theory, but it similarly serves to explore the details of the experience through the movement's subtle qualitative variations. By focusing on what it triggers in the individual, it broadens significantly the experiential understanding of the initial metaphor.

We are thereby recovering the full range of meaningful and creative possibilities encapsulated in a metaphorical concept and the frozen metaphors through which it is conveyed. It is as if the frozen or petrified metaphor was melted down and came back to life again, flaunting its full associative force and revealing thereby unexpected paths that might be pursued in exploring its hidden metaphorical network. It is the specific path chosen by the patient in this physical and verbal exploratory adventure, this new dimension of freedom, that unmasks or forges for himself or herself and the therapist the ultimate "meaning" of the patient's metaphor.

The acts of turning the metaphor into movement, of feeling the vividness of the experience, of acquiring knowledge by doing something, all constitute the type of knowledge that Ryle (1979) called "knowing how" as opposed to "knowing that."[7] We may read an entire encyclopedia on the laws of gravity, on the various component parts of a bicycle, on human anatomy, but we only learn the ability of throwing a ball, walking on the tightrope, riding a bicycle, or dancing by engaging in the action. Indeed, we learn and master these activities without knowing anything or hardly anything about what the encyclopedia tells us about them. Our psychomotor development is essentially a "knowhow."[8]

The Tightrope

Pale, hanging onto her handbag rather than letting the bag hang from her shoulders, and walking over a narrow band as if encased in an invisible membrane confining her personal space, D enters the therapeutic space. She says: "I feel I am on a tightrope."

Feet on the Ground

I ask D to imagine that in our therapeutic space there is a tightrope such as the one she has just mentioned and to imagine herself walking on it. D is a short, lightweight woman around her 40s. She walks as if hovering over the ground. On closer inspection, her feet seem to hardly touch the ground; she seems to be lacking proper support. She displays stiffness along the spine, up to the neck, as if she was suspended from above, hung by vertebrae three to five. We therefore devote several sessions to working on posture and grounding.[9]

D: "What does it mean to walk on a rope?"

She provides the answer herself: "It means to keep balance." And she proceeds to walk like an acrobat on the tightrope. As she does so, the rope acquires a concrete existence: it has color, texture, tightness, height, etc. Similarly, the walking activity itself is now more definite, as walking on *this* particular rope, in a specific context. Although object, action, and context here constitute imaginary constructs, the fact of being confronted by the body lends them a degree of reality that the mere fiction or the conceptual construction does not have.[10]

D: The rope is slightly broad, the breadth of my foot, not more than that. It is tied to two trees and is high up.
V: How high?
D: Half a meter.

Throughout our verbal exchange, she keeps walking back and forth on the rope. Her posture is upright, her arms straight open at shoulder height, in a crosslike position. At about the middle of the rope, D recurrently loses balance. Nonetheless, she does not bend her arms or knees in order to regain balance; rather, she stops and keeps rigid.

V: What do you feel?
D: Afraid! When I reach the middle of the rope, I realize I'm scared. My ankles are not stable, I have no balance.
V: Is there any danger?
D: Yes, of falling. If I fall down I will hurt myself, I may get injured and even have something broken. This scares me.
V: Is this feeling familiar to you from other contexts? Have you had this feeling before?
D: Yes. It is a fear of falling. I often dream about this. I see myself falling from a great height and wake up with the heart pounding, horrified while I'm still falling.
　　When I'm falling, there is no ground under my feet. The foundation disappears. Sometimes in my dreams I have to go down, but then there are no stairs or anything of the sort to do that. I have this other dream where I run toward something and once I get there it is an abyss.
V: What are you feeling now?
D: I absolutely have to get to the other side. There is an abyss below. I start up at the lower side, the easier end, and walk toward the higher side. In the middle of the way it is high enough to fall. The lower side is also the safer, it is like my home. The working place is here, at the higher side—more dangerous and threatening. There are many fights and tensions.

We might observe that in her narrative the rope no longer connects two trees, as it did in the beginning, but rather two meaningful "places" for D. The notions of conflict and tension between home and work, as well as the struggle at work, have emerged. The experience of danger is reaching its peak; it is probably the right time to start dispelling it. I first of all let her know she has been walking on the tightrope with her eyes closed; thereupon she proceeds with her eyes open.

D: I don't know why I have been walking with my eyes closed. Now I can actually see the danger in front of me and organize myself better.

As she walks with her eyes open, her hands and knees become more flexible. I suggest that she might play somewhat with the rope, by pressing upon it with her weight, or bending the knees, for example. She begins to feel more comfortable, and even bends down to touch the rope with her hands. Contrary to her original belief regarding the rope as rigid and unchanging, D has found out now that she can acquire control over the situation, provided that she changes her attitude.

V: When you go to work, what do you say to yourself?
D: I'm all tense. The way is full of obstacles.
V: Maybe you could tell yourself: "Whether I feel more or less tense inside my car, the conditions outside will be the same." Do you like music?
D: Yes, I do.
V: Tomorrow then you could choose some music that you like and play it on your way to work.
D: I never thought of that.

By the end of this session, D dances on the rope to the sound of drums. She then steps off the rope and continues dancing on the floor, her arms moving freely and harmoniously, her whole being more fluid. She finally says:

D: Now I realize to what extent my father has his both feet on the ground in whatever he does.[11]

Balance, Effort, and Tension

The experience of walking the tightrope certainly elicits the paradigmatic schema that characterizes *balance*: "a symmetrical (or proportional) arrangement of forces around a point or axis" (Johnson, 1987, p. 85). The Hebrew expression for balance is *shivuy mishkal*, literally "equalization of weight," which is intrinsically linked to the schema and its static aspect. In Spanish, the words "balance" and "balanceo" refer to the dynamic aspect of the schema, namely to the backward and forward movements that result in the balance or imbalance situation. In effect, to keep one's posture—an ability closely related to balance—involves the activation of a number of muscles.[12] The schema of equilibrium, as pointed out by Johnson, is therefore preconceptual (and hence preverbal) because (a) it goes back to the child's early experiences such as standing or falling, and (b) its use and full mastery have to do with "knowing-how" rather than "knowing-that."[13]

The acquisition of these balance-related abilities does not actually involve knowing and applying any system of rules; it is a rather automatic effortless skill. Consequently, any conscious interfering in the action may lead to a momentary imbalance, as when we stop to reflect on each and every one of the sequenced movements one usually performs automatically when riding a bike, driving, walking or breathing. To reflect on one's movements introduces an unnecessary cognitive effort in the action, because its automatic aspect consists precisely in the elimination of the cognitive element and the sparing of mental energy. To be conscious of an automatic behavior as a result of external restrictions or learning produces a self-representation of ourselves performing these actions. It was precisely this phenomenon that we observed in N's case discussed earlier. When she paid attention to her breathing on one occasion, or to her walking on another, there was some disturbing change in what before had been automatic and spontaneous.[14]

In D's case, the situation of walking on the tightrope produces a sudden de-automatization of the balance mechanism, which then requires putting some effort into actually not losing balance. The latter brings about an array of metaphorical extensions centered on the scheme of *effort*. D expressed this metaphorical turn by remarking on the extra effort required to push up the inclined rope. She furthermore associated the effort with *tension*, the latter reflected in her body's disposition and the nature of her movements. Metonymically, it was no longer the tension of the rope—as in the beginning, during the space construction—but rather the tension of the individual walking along the path traced by the rope. Metaphorically, the tension refers to the tension involved in other conflict situations.

An additional aspect of this same effort-based metaphorical extension employed by D concerns the way in which effort-laden situations are perceived as unstable, uncomfortable and unwanted. In other words, situations that one wishes to get over with as quickly as possible. The rope, in this case, is a path that ought to be traversed headlong. There seems to be no attempt to make the experience more bearable (as, for instance, listening to music while driving to work in the example mentioned above), for in reality it is not the path or its crossing that are unpleasant, but the actual goal, the final destination. The rope had the function of connecting two points assumed to be stable (fixed, roots)—and yet, we might ask, what happens if the tension of the pathway extends also to its end points? This exercise revealed to D that *work* (one of the two presumed fixed end points to which the rope is tied) was not a balanced, stable, cherished place where she wants to be. Instead, it was a place riddled with tensions and conflicts that she wishes to avoid. This place obviously did not provide security or stability to D. In one of the dreams associated with the rope experience she recalled that the final goal was pictured as a void, an abyss. Going back home—the other end of the rope—was easier, according to her, but not entirely free of tensions either, because, once at home, she had to face a series of unfinished tasks and the consequent tough decision regarding what to tackle first. This clearly relates to her constant difficulty in making decisions, which is a characteristic of her "psychological style."

At the same time, the danger motive is inextricably linked to the rope's instability. Here it is important to distinguish between two levels of this relation. The first, more directly dependent on motor activity, has to do with a certain difficulty in making the necessary postural adjustment: "If we cannot maintain our relationship to the center of gravity and our relationship to the earth's surface, we are not in a position to move or to respond quickly and efficiently, and therefore we are in danger of harm from external sources." (Kephart, 1971, p. 82).

At the second level, it is the ultimate dangerous outcome of walking on the rope, rather than the walking itself, that is feared. In D's case, it means specifically to fall and get hurt or injure herself. Our childhood is replete with falls that are part of our learning, that teach us how to learn to fall, how to get up again and reorganize ourselves so as to avoid new falls. To learn all of this is to acquire a new know-how that turns the eventual future fall into a less threatening event—the same is true of course about learning to keep one's balance on the rope or to play in general (Winnicott, 1974, pp. 44, 48). The fear and insecurity might be thus dispelled, at least in part. As for learning to deal with conflicts, I believe that learning to respond adequately to the variations in tension of the imaginary concrete rope may produce a reframing of the entire way of dealing with dilemmas in general. It means acquiring a know-how that allows one to tackle metaphorically identical situations in a more balanced way, namely by achieving the goal while expending less energy.

The enactment of the tight-rope metaphor can be seen as having provided D with a "corrective experience," inasmuch as it enhanced the above-mentioned learning. By the end of the experience, D was able to remain longer on the rope, to walk more smoothly, and be more confident about maintaining her balance without too much tension and effort, either muscular or emotional. The danger of falling became less threatening. The situation is accordingly no longer dominated by irrational, indiscriminate fear. These new attitudes and perceptions, achieved by the metaphor enactment at the physical, emotive and cognitive spheres, are ripe enough now to be applied in the reframing of further situations.

Style and Psychotherapy

Psychic Style: Nature or Nurture

Working with emotional or behavioral disorders, and with neurotic manifestations in particular, raises the crucial question regarding determinism: is the organic level, for genetic or other reasons, the determining cause of the observed disorder? And if it is the cause, is there any room for therapeutic interventions that operate on this level? We are faced here with yet another battle in the long fight that has nature and nurture as the two opposite poles of the inescapable dichotomy: physical–chemical–biological causality on the one side, cultural–mental–historical causality on the other. But is it really the case that we have to accept the dichotomous terms of this opposition? Or maybe we can, more sensibly, admit the organic foundation of these mental and behavioral disorders without necessarily endowing the former with the entire causal monopoly. Moreover, by doing so, we might be able to recognize the role played by other factors—e.g., social, educational, and psychotherapeutic factors—in the treatment of these disorders. From a theoretical point of view, this more moderate option would allow us to account for the nature and effect of the various factors that, within a theory such as Shapiro's, make up the individual "style."

According to Shapiro (1965, p. 178), we are born with an "initial organizing configuration" that consists of an

> … innate psychological equipment [that] imposes some form of organization, however little differentiated it may be initially, on drives and external stimuli and, in general, on all psychological tensions. More exactly [...] such innate apparatus imposes some form of organization on the *subjective experience* of internal tensions and external stimuli from the beginning.

In this sense, the infant is not merely a passive agent vis-à-vis both the biological drives as well as the external stimuli that shape him or her, but rather "he may be said to exist psychologically and his psychology to constitute an autonomous factor in the determination of his behavior" (Shapiro, 1965, p. 179). In other words, for Shapiro—as opposed to behaviorism—we are equipped with an innate active component which from the beginning shapes our psychic life or "subjective experience' and structures the latter, albeit in a rudimentary form. It is within the individual variations of this innate psychological equipment that Shapiro identifies "the beginnings of psychological style" of each individual. He adds, however, that these rudimentary and diffuse beginnings are enriched, differentiated, and specified, both in their form and content, through maturation and the interaction with the external world, resulting eventually in the crystallization of "highly differentiated adult styles" (p. 180).

For instance,

The baby cries initially not for its mother, nor with an expectation of satisfaction, nor even with a sense of its need, but only, we may imagine, from discomfort. The mother responds, and the baby is satisfied. In the course of such experience, the initially diffuse tension becomes organized into a more directed tension, into an experience of need eventually directed clearly toward the mother. Along with this directedness, anticipations of satisfaction appear, perhaps a sense of expectancy and trust, and, with these, a greater capacity to endure delays in satisfaction (Shapiro, 1965, p. 183); [...] a tension finds an external object, and gradually, the baby comes not only to anticipate or expect satisfaction, but also to experience the tension in a more directed way and ultimately to learn to cry *for* the mother. (pp. 188–89)

Thus, where there was diffuse tension, there is now a specific tension and a new mode of organization: tension is converted into intention; one is replaced by the other.

This process not only results in more complex and richer mental operations, but also in a higher level of style differentiation, and consequently in the decrease, yet not disappearance, of the weight attributed to the innate component in this structure. Shapiro's formulation of his position regarding the nature/nurture factors and their subtle relation ought to be a cautious one: "The more specific the style feature, the less the innate responsibility for it. On the other hand, however, much innate determination of exceedingly general style tendencies seems quite likely" (1965, p. 180).

The psychic style of an individual is therefore the point of intersection of both innate and maturational factors with a wide array of environmental elements—physical, social, and cultural—that "make up the climate in which innate potentialities develop" (Shapiro, 1965, p. 196). By referring to neurotic *styles*, it is clear that Shapiro is trying to emphasize precisely the fact that the former cannot be reduced either to instinctual origins or to environmental sources, as both factors are at play in the crystallization of style.

Take, for instance, a typical mode of functioning of the neurotic style: the intensified use of defensive mechanisms that exclude from consciousness certain classes of subjective experience in order to eliminate the anxiety this experience provokes. We observe that, in the neurotic style, it is not just the motivational source of the anxiety that is excluded but this exclusion is extended to a whole *group* of contents, affects, modes of communication, interpersonal relationships, etc. This extension takes place, apparently, through mostly unconscious associative inferences, undoubtedly derived nonetheless from interaction with the environment. The neurotic style, as it involves an entire defensive *mode of functioning* vis-à-vis the tensions and thus extends far beyond its immediate internal cause, clearly illustrates the double nature of every style. The latter, as we will see, has important implications for psychotherapy. The following example offers a more concrete picture of the mode of functioning of one of the neurotic styles.

In my clinic I experienced an episode very similar to the one discussed in Shapiro (1965, p. 192) with reference to the obsessive-compulsive style. It involved N, whom we have met before. N, a very serious scholar, had, as we have already mentioned, difficulties in establishing satisfactory relationships with men and came from a family where affection was not expressed. During one of our sessions, while she was talking about the possibility of being successful in a new relationship, her voice suddenly went up, she smiled, and her whole body seemed to bloom with the anticipated emotion. For some time she went on like this, already making plans for the future. A few minutes later, she lowered her voice and said gloomily, "Well, of course nothing is for sure"; for sure "this relationship won't work out." The situation of expecting success seems to have raised the tension and anxiety, which in its turn triggered her defensive system and made her withdraw to her usual controlled position. In body movement terms this would be analogous to allowing yourself *free flow* at a point when momentarily the expansion overrides the confidence to *bound flow*, which provides her with more confidence through shrinking back to a more controlled mode.

Style, Reversal, and Mastery

Although developed to account for neurosis, Shapiro's concept of psychological style based on the interaction of both innate and acquired factors might be very helpful for conceptualizing and treating of a variety of conditions.[15] Let us take an example.

The phenomenological theory of motivation, better known as Reversal Theory (see Apter, 1982, 1989; Kerr et al., 1993), starts off from the experience many have of quick and multiple mood alternations. The consequent instability brought about by this series of successive shifting is, according to the theory, the norm. It is nonetheless directed by at least four pairs of meta-motivational states (Potocky & Murgatroyd, 1993, p. 22). For each individual it is possible to identify, for each pair, the dominant state, namely the type of meta-motivation that rules most of his or her experience and behavior. This does not mean that the nondominant, opposite states do not occur; in fact, they do occur in the alternations series, albeit with shorter duration and intensity.

Consider, for example, the pair telic/paratelic (from the Greek *telos*— "end"). A dominantly telic subject is characterized by being oriented toward the future: by being goal-oriented, he plans ahead in order to achieve the goal and to effectively apply his plan; he is focused and has the capacity to avoid arousing and distracting stimuli. The subject with paratelic dominance, on the other hand, is characterized by being oriented toward the present, looking for stimuli and sensations as well as responding to them, by being spontaneous and playful, happy to be distracted and entertained with activities not directly relevant to the goal, and enjoying humor. An individual may be predominantly telic or paratelic, but is able to experience both moods. The state of an individual at a given point in time is the result not only of his or her predominant telic or paratelic characterization, but also of the interplay of internal forces and motivations that, combined with the external forces, produce the mood reversal. A very serious boss, for instance, may be concentrated and demanding at work, where his telic aspect predominates, and yet in a party he may easily revert to a paratelic state, being funny and playful. A sportsman in a formal competition must deploy all his telicity to win, but when playing football with friends or jogging he may revert to a paratelic mood.

Mood alternations, then, include moving out from or reversing back to the dominant meta-motivation. Furthermore, it is important to note that there are various levels of dominance, and there is always the option of getting away from it. Meta-motivational mood dominance, it might be argued, is thus an important component of style, inasmuch as it is a mode of functioning and of organizing experience that directs and dominates, but neither excludes nor determines.

Movement and bodily expression, in fact, manifest this mode of functioning. Furthermore, in my ongoing research I have observed a clear influence of the body and movement in mood reversals, in particular when the telic/paratelic pair of states is involved. Thus, for instance, different positions and rhythms affect differently the mood and its alternations between telic and paratelic. For example, the same relaxing technique may not be equally appropriate for both groups; whereas a certain position of low arousal, like lying still, may be experienced by one group as pleasurable, it may be felt as threatening by the other, for whom keeping still in one position is likely to increase tension. I have furthermore observed a correlation between the use of space and the basic meta-motivational dominance; the telic, for instance, shows a more direct use of space and movement style, while the paratelic is more indirect, i.e., he uses more space and more mannerisms. Shapiro, it is worth recalling, describes the obsessive-compulsive style (1965, pp. 23–25) as showing a dominant rigidity related not only to a style of thinking (dogmatic, stubborn, unable to have a true dialogue), but also to body rigidity (posture, the features that characterize his or her movements). He notes that it is as if the obsessive-compulsive were constantly making some effort, without relaxing for a minute, affecting also the muscular system, body, and form of expression, and thus constantly putting pressure on himself or herself.

The anti-dualist conception of the mind's *embodiment* mentioned earlier stresses the fact that the mind works in close interaction with the body. Hence, the body is no longer viewed as a mere external wrapping of the mental dimension. What we have presented so far indeed justifies this perspective. We may nevertheless advance further with this partial justification, and in fact, the psychotherapies based on dance/movement have done precisely that. Besides, we possess nowadays a theoretical basis for this justification.

Marcelo Dascal, who in his philosophical and linguistic work has emphasized the relation between the use of language and thought, proposed the term "psychopragmatics" for the investigation of this phenomenon (1983, 1987, 1995). The psycholinguist David McNeill made a significant contribution to this field by showing that gestures do not simply accompany speech but are rather a constitutive part of it (1979, 1992). In his most recent work, moreover, he has established the direct relation between gestures and thought (McNeill, 2005) by developing a new theory whereby gestures are an integral part of thinking. He argues that gestures initiate and are part of emerging psychological states, producing images and linguistic enunciations. Accordingly, speech, gestures, and thought are components of the same complex process, inextricably linked to one another.

In my opinion, McNeill's research supports the hypothesis that the work done *from* the body and *with* the body—including gestures and movement with the latter's basic components of space, time, rhythm, weight, etc. (Laban, 1971)—reaches the essence of the human experience. Dance/movement therapy comprises parameters for the observation of movement that grant it precision and subtlety. Thanks to these methods, the body style is thus revealed to the psychotherapist, as well as to the patient, through a variety of perspectives.[16] Furthermore, as shown by McNeill's findings, the bodily experience cannot be approached any longer as *purely* corporal; the work *from* the body, *with* the body, *in* the body and *on* the body unfolds necessarily additional aspects of the *integral* individual, both at the intra-psychic and the interpersonal levels (2005, pp. 35, 231). Dance/movement therapy, which has never accepted the body–mind dichotomy, may be rightly considered the pioneer of the *embodied mind* concept.

Style and Reframing

The therapeutic space is a privileged one. On the one hand, its intimacy is protected from outside. It allows working with the particular rhythm of the individual, forgetting external pressures. This is a secure space with its own internal rules, which, as in a laboratory, permits experimenting with new, different, and at times dangerous things. What is crucial is that being a laboratory-like space, it is nonetheless a space of living experience, in which the same real and concrete experiences are lived out as in the person's daily life. This specificity is what makes it possible to transfer what has been learned in this space to the life beyond this space. But the question is how?

The key to an adequate answer resides in recognizing the crucial value of *reframing* in the therapeutic process. I have dealt with this subject elsewhere (Dascal & Dascal, 2004). Here I will make a few brief comments.

Let us start from the assumption that all human beings need to hold on to some sort of system of beliefs, be it justified or not. When, for some reason or other, this aforementioned system causes problems that lead to dissonance (Smith, 1997, pp. xiv–xv) and eventually anxiety, some leeway or flexibility is needed for adjusting or replacing it. Reframing consists precisely in providing the means for finding, when necessary, one or more alternatives for a problematic system of beliefs. The first step is to try to unravel, to shake, its rooted character. One of the reasons for the tenacity of these kinds of systems lies in the fact that our beliefs are not purely internal mental states; rather, they actually reflect in a direct way the public image we project, our *ethos*, our reputation. This image includes, moreover, what is known as the self-image and body-image of the individual, an entity that is holistic and multidimensional, simultaneously a socio-psychological construction and a physical structure.[17]

Our beliefs are connected, among other things, as much to our personal identity as to our group identity, and thus, to try to change them might be felt as threatening, as questioning our sense of belonging and self-determination, as putting in danger our sense of control. The difficulties in modifying a belief are also related to the filter effect these factors have vis-à-vis the credibility of our sources of information, the kinds of innovation we will accept, the patterns of criticism, and the whole class of arguments and actions that we will accept as possible and reasonable.

The concept of reframing is used in various psychotherapeutic approaches and refers to a specific type of intervention strategy. Furthermore, there is a sense in which reframing extends over a whole gamut of means that help eliminate or decrease the above-mentioned filter effect. These means offer a way of overcoming the crucial obstacle whereby the individual is confined to one single point of view, one single exclusive mood. Reframing involves multiple processes and levels—both intra- and inter-psychic—in the cognitive, behavioral, interactional, emotive, corporeal, and experiential spheres through distinct channels of perception, expression, and communication.

Certain conditions must be satisfied if reframing is to materialize:

(a) The suspension of judgment during the therapeutic course
(b) The legitimization of possible innovations

(c) The emergence of options that can co-occur with the existing system of beliefs

(d) The reduction of the potential threat of new alternatives

(e) A change of attitude toward the other, be it external or internal

The task of the therapist is to create the above conditions within the therapeutic space. It is crucial to take into account the psychic style of both the patient and the therapist in order to achieve reframing. For, as we have seen, the style is characterized precisely by not being a determining or exclusive factor. Accordingly, by stressing in our sessions the fact that each individual's psychic life is not entirely determined, even when it has a dominant style, but is rather open to dynamism and change, we are creating the most essential condition of all to achieve reframing.

Conclusion

This chapter examines specific theoretical issues that have practical implications for psychotherapy, in particular for dance/movement therapy. I first showed the use of a figure of speech, the metaphor, within the therapeutic space and two cases were analyzed in which movement metaphors had been employed. Several basic aspects of David Shapiro's concept of style within his analysis of neurosis were described. I argued that this concept serves to explain further psychological phenomena and supports the efficiency of body psychotherapy praxis, wherein human action is perceived as essentially integrated and interactive, simultaneously mental, physical, and social. It is a praxis that thus rejects dichotomies and dualisms. Finally, I outlined the ways in which an elaborated concept of style may justify the most important postulate of all therapeutic practice: the fact that in the therapist–patient encounter it is possible to create the conditions for reframing, which, in its turn, may lead to a significant change in the patients' lives.

Acknowledgment

I am grateful to Tal Goldfein for her excellent translation of the Spanish version of this chapter, and to Adam Marcus for his expert proofreading.

Endnotes

1. See, for instance, Gallagher (1998, 2005), Johnson (1987), Lakoff & Johnson (1999), McNeill (1992, 2005), Shanon (2002).
2. In fact, according to a number of theories, *all* common metaphors are bodily based, as argued for instance by G. Lakoff. See Lakoff (1987) as well as Lakoff & Johnson (1999).
3. This case has been partially presented in Dascal (1992).

4. The sessions are in Hebrew and sometimes in English.

5. To write a diary recording the experiences of the therapy's sessions allows a further active elaboration of the therapeutic process beyond the actual sessions. Thus the here-and-now of the session acquires thereby a temporal dimension that significantly enriches the awareness of the bodily experiences.

6. The Hebrew expression involved here is "*lehafiah bah ruah haim* and it literally means to "infuse/fill her up with the wind/spirit of life." This expression is particularly significant given that N's mother is a holocaust survivor.

7. This subject has been dealt with extensively in Dascal, V. and Dascal, M. (1985) as well as in Dascal, V. (1985).

8. In my opinion, the "know-how" and the "know-that" are, not a dichotomy, but the two poles of a continuum that starts off with birth and its accompanying sensorial, proprioceptive, motor (possibly a pure know-how), and psychomotor development, goes on to the acquisition of language and reaches abstract thought (a possibly pure know-that). In dance/movement therapy, as I practice it, work is done on this continuum exploring both kinds of knowledge, either alternately or simultaneously.

9. Schilder (1970) is still a fundamental source for a proper understanding of the importance, meaning, and consequences of posture and grounding for human development and, therefore, is a basic tool for dance/movement therapy.

10. It is important to note that this exercise involving the construction of an imaginary object, itself part of an actor's training, is not based exclusively on conceptual imagination, but is also related to the sensorial and preconceptual memory. The imagined object *activates* those bodily mechanisms that allow relating to this sensory and preconception element. It is thanks to the latter that one may experience or re-experience the imagined situation, and participate entirely in it. The exercise's main strength resides here. Within the therapeutic space this is particularly valuable because experiencing or re-experiencing a situation serves not only to enhance dramatic effects, but is effectively part of the therapeutic process. There is empirical evidence showing that motor alterations induced by the imagining of the motor action are very often equivalent to the movement itself (Feldenkreis, 1972, p. 130; Bijeljac-Babic, 1978; Frith, 2007).

11. Schilder (1970, p. 16): "The postural model of our own body is connected with the postural model of the bodies of others." On the connection between posture and the primary sensation of security, see Kephart (1971, pp. 81–83).

12. "Posture is a positive neuro-muscular act in which a series of muscle groups is innervated in pattern so that the position of the body with reference to its center of gravity is maintained. These postural adjustments are very basic and are among the most rigid in the organism." (Kephart, 1971, p 81, referring to Dusser de Barenne, 1934).

13. See notes 6 and 7.

14. For further discussion and analysis of the implications of this phenomenon, see Gallagher, 1998 (pp. 229, 238–239).

15. This is not surprising given the evolution of the concept of neurosis itself. Since it was first introduced by Freud in 1895, the definition of neurosis has evolved, and by the turn of the 21st century it is not employed by the *DSM-IV* as a basic category in its taxonomy of psychopathology. At the same time, it

has been argued that neurosis is now a general mode of being within western culture, whereby one can speak of a "normal neurotic" who does not require "cure," but rather "adaptation" or "good integration" (Shapiro, 1975, p. 195; Sodré Dória, 1974).

16. See Laban (1963, 1971), Bartenieff et al. (1965), Dell (1970), Preston (1963). These authors as well as other sources allowed me to envisage a movement observation scale that I apply in my clinic.

17. "The image of the body is not a static phenomenon from the physiological point of view. It is acquired, built up, and gets its structure by a continual contact with the world. It is not a structure but a structuralization in which continual changes take place, and all these changes have relations to motility and to actions in the outside world" (Schilder, 1970, pp. 173–174). For Gallagher (1998, p. 226), on the other hand, the body-image is "a mental construct or representation, or a set of beliefs about the body [that] can include at least three aspects: the subject's *perceptual* experience of his body; the subject's *conceptual* understanding of the body in general [...]; the subject's *emotional* attitude toward her own body." Neisser (1988), in turn, when dealing with both physical and social self-knowledge, identifies no less than five different kinds of self: the *ecological, interpersonal, extended, private* and *self concept.*

References

Apter, M. J. 1982. *The experience of motivation: The theory of psychological reversals.* London: Academic Press.

Apter, M. J. 1989. *Reversal theory: Motivation, emotion, and personality.* London: Routledge.

Bartenieff, I., Davis, M., & Paulay, F. 1973. *Four adaptations of effort theory in research and teaching.* New York: Dance Notation Bureau.

Bijeljac-Babic, R. 1978. Langage et activité tonique posturale: Aspects psychophysiologique et psycholinguistique, Thèse de 3ème Cycle, Université de Paris 6.

Bermúdez, J.L., Marcel, A., & Eilan, N. (Eds.). 1998. *The body and the self.* Cambridge, MA: The MIT Press.

Dascal, M. 1983. *Pragmatics and the philosophy of mind,* vol. I. Amsterdam: John Benjamins.

Dascal, M. 1987. Language and reasoning: sorting out sociopragmatic and psychopragmatic factors. In J.C. Boudreaux, B.W. Hamil, and R. Jernigan (Eds.), *The role of language in problem solving* 2. Dordrecht: Elsevier, pp. 183–97.

Dascal, M. 1995. The dispute on the primacy of thinking or speaking. In M. Dascal, D. Gerhardus, G. Meggle, & K. Lorenz (Eds.), *Philosophy of language: An international handbook of contemporary research,* vol. 2. Berlin: De Gruyter, pp. 1024–41.

Dascal, M., & Dascal, V. 2004. A des-fixação da crença. In F. Gil, P. Livet, & J. Pina Cabral (Eds.), *O processo da Crença.* Lisboa: Gradiva, pp. 321–53.

Dascal, V. 1985. A case for art in therapy. Assaph—Studies in the Arts, Section C, 2: 142–52.

Dascal, V. 1991. Walking the tight rope: The psychotherapeutic potential of a movement metaphor. *Assaph—Studies in the Arts,* Section C, 7: 103–12.

Dascal, V. 1992. Movement metaphors: Linking theory and therapeutic practice. In M. Stamenov (Ed.), *Current advances in semantics*. Amsterdam: John Benjamins, pp. 151–57.

Dascal, V. 1995. Art as therapy. *Mahanaim* 11: 322–29 [In Hebrew].

Dascal, V., & Dascal, M. 1985. Understanding art is knowing how. In A. Ballis et al. (Eds.), *Art in culture*, vol. 2. Ghent: Communication and Cognition, pp. 271–98.

Dell, C. 1970. *A primer for movement description using effort-shape and supplementary concepts*. New York: Dance Notation Bureau.

Dusser de Barenne, J. G. 1934. The labyrinthine and postural mechanisms. In C. Murchison (Ed.), *Handbook of general experimental psychology*. Worcester, MA: Clark University Press, pp. 204–46.

Feldenkrais, M. 1972. *Awareness through movement*. New York: Harper & Row.

Frith, C. 2007. *The making of the mind*. Oxford: Blackwell.

Gallagher, S. 1998. Body schema and intentionality. In Bermúdez, J.L., Marcel, A., and Eilan, N. (Eds.). *The body and the self*. Cambridge, MA: MIT Press, pp. 225–244.

Gallagher, S. 2005. *How the body shapes the mind*. Oxford: Clarendon Press.

Granger, G. 1968. *Essai d'une philosophie du style*. Paris: Armand Collin.

Gross, A.G., & Dascal, M. 2001. The conceptual unity of Aristotle's rhetoric. *Philosophy and Rhetoric* 34(4): 275–291.

Johnson, M. 1987. *The body in the mind: The bodily basis of meaning, imagination, and reason*. Chicago: University of Chicago Press.

Kephart, N.C. 1971. *The slow learner in the classroom*, 2nd ed. Columbus, OH: Charles E. Merrill.

Kerr, J. H., Murgatroyd, S., & Apter, M. J. (Eds.). 1993. *Advances in reversal theory*. Amsterdam: Swets & Zeitlinger.

Laban, R. 1963. *Modern educational dance*. London: MacDonald & Evans.

Laban, R. 1971. *The mastery of movement*. London: MacDonald & Evans.

Lakoff, G. 1987. *Women, fire, and dangerous things*. Chicago: University of Chicago Press.

Lakoff, G., & Johnson, M. 1980. *Metaphors we live by*. Chicago: University of Chicago Press.

Lakoff, G., & Johnson, M. 1999. *Philosophy in the flesh: The embodied mind and its challenge to Western thought*. New York: Basic Books.

McNeill, D. 1979. *The conceptual basis of language*. Hillsdale, NJ: Lawrence Erlbaum.

McNeill, D. 1992. *Hand and mind: What gestures reveal about thought*. Chicago: University of Chicago Press.

McNeill, D. 2005. *Gesture and thought*. Chicago: University of Chicago Press.

Neisser, U. 1988. Five kinds of self-knowledge. *Philosophical psychology* 1: 35–59.

Potocky, M., & Murgatroyd, S. 1993. What is reversal theory? In Kerr et al. (Eds.). *Advances in reversal theory*. London: Taylor & Francis, pp. 9–26.

Preston, V. 1963. *A handbook for modern educational dance*. London: Macdonald & Evans.

Ryle, G. 1979. *The concept of mind*. Harmondsworth: Penguin.

Schilder, P. 1970. *The image and appearance of the human body in everyday life*, 2nd ed. New York: International Universities Press.

Shanon, B. 2002. The embodiment of mind. *Manuscrito* 25(2): 531–72.

Shapiro, D. 1965. *Neurotic styles*. New York: Basic Books.

Smith, B.H. 1997. *Belief & resistance: Dynamics of contemporary intellectual controversy*. Cambridge: Harvard University Press.

Sodré Dória, C. 1983. *Psicologia do ajustamento neurótico*, 5th ed. Rio de Janeiro: Vozes.

Winnicott, D.W. 1974. *Playing and reality*. Harmondsworth: Pelican Books.

CHAPTER 7

Becoming Whole Again

Dance/Movement Therapy for Those Who Suffer from Eating Disorders

SUSAN KLEINMAN

Contents

Introduction

Sufferers of eating disorders have difficulty tolerating and containing feelings. They often describe the experience of being in their bodies as disembodied, as if living with a stranger or an enemy (Kleinman & Hall, 2006). Helping these individuals reawaken their life force by connecting with their feelings is critical to their recovery. Martha Graham (1952) said:

> There is a vitality, a life-force, an energy, a quickening that is translated through you into action. And because there is only one of you in all of time, this expression is unique. And if you block it, it will never exist through any other medium and be lost. (p. 335)

Because an eating disorder is such a bodily-focused experience, dance/movement therapy is uniquely suited to address related issues. In short, dance/movement therapy allows sufferers to become more embodied, by experiencing themselves more fully and identifying connections between their eating disorders and the issues that underlie them (Kleinman & Hall, 2005). The sufferers' way of being in their bodies and willingness to access their own unconscious material is part of their sense of self, and plays an important role in the degree to which they will be able to heal.

The writings that follow are intended to provide a context in which to delve into understanding why and how dance/movement therapy with those who suffer from an eating disorder is integral to their recovery. Although dance/movement therapy for boys and men would be the same, language used in this chapter reflects treatment in the context of women and girls, as this has been almost exclusively the author's working experience. Names and identifying information of all patients have been changed to protect their privacy.

What Is an Eating Disorder?

It is speculated that a complex interplay among biological, environmental, and cultural factors contribute to this destructive condition that is referred to as an eating disorder (Kleinman & Hall, 2005). Although the percentage of people whose eating disorder may have a biological base is unclear, it is believed that a built-in component may exist and research is currently in progress (National Eating Disorder Association, 2008). An eating disorder can be developed at any age. It is often triggered by events in people's lives that leave them feeling vulnerable. These may be transitions connected to growing up or maturing, such as graduating from college, or marrying; or losses, such as divorce or the death of a loved one. Markers for people with eating disorder tendencies include obsessive thinking and ritualistic behaviors, never feeling good enough, a constant striving to be perfect, and difficulty tolerating emotional situations. Someone who is a survivor of verbal, emotional, or sexual trauma has a tendency to turn toward an eating disorder in an attempt to avoid an otherwise too painful connection with reality. Also, individuals from cultures that are steeped in high, or very specific, expectations for their children, are especially vulnerable to developing a climate for eating disorders. When external structure is perceived as too controlling, an eating disorder may provide an illusion of control, as well as a safer focus.

Women make up at least 90% of diagnosed cases of both anorexia nervosa and bulimia nervosa. These disorders appear to be most common in industrialized countries. This could be in part due to pressure to compete and excel in the world as well as to the influence of the media in promoting and influencing certain physical standards (APA *DSM-IV*, 2000, pp. 583–595). It is possible that the stress in these cultures could trigger someone with a propensity for an eating disorder to act on these behaviors. The largest numbers of people with eating disorders are reflected in the category referred to as binge eating, which includes compulsive overeating or emotional eating. A provisional diagnosis in the DSM-IV also recognizes binge eating disorder (BED) as a discrete eating disorder. According to current research, BED is the most common form of an eating disorder, affecting 3% of the adult population and approximately 8% of the obese population (Grillo, 2002). There are dire medical consequences for sufferers of eating disorders, including loss of life. For females between 15 and 24 years old who suffer from anorexia nervosa, the mortality rate associated with this illness is 12 times higher than the death rate of all other causes of death, and has the highest premature fatality rate of any mental illness (Sullivan, 1995).

Although the term eating disorders implies that these disorders are about food, they really should be called emotional disorders, because the individual turns toward food as a substitute for dealing with larger emotional issues. An eating disorder is considered an adaptive disorder because people are not born with this problem, but acquire it as they grow and develop. Schwimmer (2003) says:

> In normal development individuals learn how to maintain an appropriate level of self-awareness, affect regulation, impulse regulation and emotional self-protection. When these capacities are missing or inadequate due to a variety of pathological [or invalidating] experiences, other maladaptive coping patterns are likely to develop. The inner experience of an eating disorder and the proliferation of eating disordered symptoms are sometimes best understood as expressions of these alternative and maladaptive patterns. (p. 7)

Living in a Body Inhabited by an Eating Disorder

Movement defines us from the moment we are born to the day we die. From the first kick in our mother's womb, until our dying breath, we participate in the dance of life and experience the power of movement" (Kleinman, 1994, p. 70). For individuals with an eating disorder, their experience of embodiment and sense of being in their bodies has become distorted and their primary relationship has shifted to their eating disorder, which they often refer to as "ED." In essence, their body image has become distorted. Body image is defined by Ressler (2000) as "the picture in our mind's eye of how we look to ourselves. It reflects our beliefs about how we think others perceive us and captures how we experience the feeling of "living" in our bodies" (p. 35). Individuals with eating disorders make their life about food, weight, the size of their bodies and, at all costs, they avoid a *dance* that is full of life and expressive movement.

A hallmark of people with eating disorders is their tendency to try to control or numb feelings and instead, worry obsessively, engage in black-and-white thinking, and fix their attention on a distorted perception of themselves. As one patient explained to me, "It is much easier to focus on how many calories I have consumed in a day than it is to deal with day-to-day events such as arguments with my parents, getting good grades, or feeling accepted by others." Two examples follow that describe how these sufferers attempted to deal with life by using eating disordered behaviors.

> Carol, an outpatient, suffered from anorexia as well as exercise bulimia. Her body image was severely distorted. Sexually abused from at least the age of five, she targeted her body as her enemy and devoted herself to trying to disconnect from all her feelings. She slept little because it was too scary for her to relax. She spent a great deal of time planning and ruminating, which caused her to feel tense, burdened, and alienated from herself. She explained to me what happened one morning that reflected her daily experiences. She said:
>
> "This morning I woke up, stepped on the scale and of course I weigh exactly the same as I did yesterday, and the day before, and the day before that. I pretty much "lost it" this morning. I cried the entire time I was in the shower and was still in tears by the time I got to work. So, I made myself get to the gym by 4:30 this afternoon and I didn't leave there until 8:30 tonight. I took two classes, ran on the treadmill, rode the lifecycle, and did a few of the machines. I don't know what I am going to do if I get on that scale tomorrow and my weight hasn't changed."
>
> If Carol is to recover, she will need to build on her strengths and rebalance her body image more equally so that her negative thoughts are no longer dominant. In short, she will need to expand her ability to

resolve her body image issues by examining how her image of herself impacts on her life. This includes an emphasis on living in rather than attempting to control the experience of living in her body.

Jane, who was diagnosed as bulimic, also developed her eating disorder as a way of coping with early childhood sexual abuse. Her behaviors fluctuated between restricting food so she wouldn't have to taste it or binge eating and then purging as a way of emptying herself of the uncomfortable feeling of containing the food in her body. One evening, during a support dinner I was leading, she acknowledged that she couldn't tolerate the sensation of tasting the food and wanted to get rid of it by eating more. She acknowledged her discomfort and need to get a dessert to take the taste away. I encouraged her to explore what her discomfort with taste was about as an emotional need rather than a physical hunger, and as Jane's eating experience was followed by dance/movement therapy, she was able to feel safe enough to move in her body and to speak freely about her discomfort. Both examples represent a slice of the anguish and torment sufferers of eating disorders experience on a daily basis.

Methods Used to Treat Eating Disorders

The effect of an eating disorder impacts on a person's whole being. Therefore, treatment methods need to reflect the magnitude of the disorder. The *APA Practice guidelines for the treatment of patients with eating disorders* (2006) recognizes the value of using a multidisciplinary approach. Disciplines that are suggested for treatment of this tenacious disorder include a medical manager, or physician to access, diagnose and treat the devastating physical consequences; a medication manager, or psychiatrist to alleviate symptoms of underlying emotional conditions; a nutritionist specifically skilled in treating eating disorders, an individual psychotherapist who uses approaches such as cognitive behavioral therapy, interpersonal therapy, and psychodynamic therapy, and family or couples therapy. Dance/movement therapy is also mentioned as a potentially helpful therapeutic modality (p. 17).

Alexithymia, a personality trait, having to do with difficulty expressing feelings and thoughts, is a prevalent symptom of eating disorders. Helping the patient express feelings on both a verbal and nonverbal level is key to eating disorder recovery. Individuals with eating disorders have shifted their life focus to make it about food, weight, and the physical body, and the challenge of therapists is to shift the focus back to the more natural way of living that includes experiencing feelings. Kleinman and Hall (2006) state that "Ignoring internal states amounts to burying feelings and the burial site exists in the body itself. Since feelings may fester underneath the body's surface and erupt when they become intolerable, it behooves us to help our patients develop a stronger relationship with this vital part of themselves" (p. 3).

Dance/Movement Therapy in the Treatment of Eating Disorders

Although readers will no doubt recognize various psychotherapeutic influences such as Sullivanian, Jungian, and Feminist theories, this particular approach to dance/movement therapy is built on the opportunities I have had to first explore and understand how to work expressively on a body level and later articulate the creative process that unfolded for me over time. This process is as follows:

- Building on the foundation that bodily felt experiences spark cognitive understanding, dance/movement therapy can transform idiosyncratic behaviors into expressive behaviors, and cause disconnected experiences to ignite into meaningful expression and understanding of one's experience that can contribute to lasting change (Kleinman, 2003).
- Because women with eating disorders have difficulty tolerating as well as expressing feelings, they often turn to these alternative behaviors as a way of attempting to feel more in control. Dance/movement therapy provides a means for patients with eating disorders to begin again to experience feelings, to express these feelings through their body language, and to articulate what their experience means to them in terms of larger emotional issues and coping patterns.

The Role of the Dance/Movement Therapist

Because human beings communicate through their bodies long before they learn to talk, the language of the body is, in essence, our native language (Kleinman & Hall, 2006, p. 2). Dance/movement therapists work directly with feelings using their whole bodies as empathic receptors and responders to the patients (Harris, 2008). Honing their native language into therapeutic skills frees the dance/movement therapist to spontaneously develop the body language of those they are working with into meaningful interactions. Essentially, they devote themselves to trusting their innate ability to "attend" empathically, respond authentically, and translate nonverbal experiences into cognitive insights. Responding to the patient's nonverbal signals, including tone of voice, facial expressions, eye gaze, and bodily motion, can reveal the otherwise hidden shifts in states of mind and body. According to Siegel (1999), "Resonating with these expressions of primary emotions requires that the therapist feel the feelings, not merely understand them conceptually" (p. 290).

The therapists' own experience of embodiment, ability to access unconscious material, and way of being in their bodies, is part of their sense of self, and plays an important role in the healing process (Kleinman, 2004). Supporting this premise, Virginia Satir (1987) eloquently states:

> When I am in touch with myself, my feelings, my thoughts, with what I see and hear, I am growing toward becoming a more integrated self. I am more congruent, I am more "whole," and I am able to make greater contact with the other person. (p. 27)

The dance/movement therapist facilitates expression by inviting patients to begin to notice their otherwise deadened, or overly controlled sensations, impulses, and natural movements, and to consciously embody these movements. This may occur as part of a group, individual, family, or couples experience. Often frightened to connect with feelings as well as to move in their bodies expressively rather than through exercise or stylized movements, they are more easily engaged when they cognitively understand why this therapy is important to their recovery, what will be expected of them, and that their input is important to the process. The therapist therefore provides a brief orientation or, in a group or family session, may invite identified patients to share from their own experiences.

All behavior is considered relevant, and communication is always present. Patients are encouraged to set aside their tendency to focus on food and physical weight issues in order to explore larger underlying emotional issues. Issues such as loss, fear of success, failure, change, losing control, lack of awareness of body boundaries, and being seen, to name a few, quickly become visible in the experience that unfolds. Patients are quick to recognize their own quintessential experiences and seem to take solace when others commiserate and give voice to this recognition.

Because dance/movement therapy begins with permission to bring these experiences to the foreground, the patients are able to explore their emerging awareness and to risk identifying how and why it takes form in their lives through the actions they choose, either consciously or habitually. This acceptance of self lends itself to exploring challenges in which to incorporate change.

Concepts of Practice

Three interrelated concepts represent the underpinnings of this therapeutic process: rhythmic synchrony, kinesthetic awareness, and kinesthetic empathy. These concepts blend together to promote the development of meaningful relationships that foster collaboration, empowerment, and mutuality (Kleinman & Hall, 2006, p. 4).

Rhythmic synchrony is the ability to be in tune with ourselves and our patients. This could occur by moving in rhythm with another person (e.g., walking with them, breathing in the same rhythm or even speaking at a pace that duplicates their rhythm). When dance/movement therapists are not in rhythm with their patients they may move too fast or too slowly, give directions that are too complex, or even speak too quickly. This can cause patients to detach if they become overwhelmed. However, when they are able to share a rhythm with the patient by consciously attuning to the patient's rhythms, they then may be able to also share emotions later in the process.

Kinesthetic awareness is the ability to sense one's self physically on both an internal and external level. For example, dance/movement therapists might make an intervention and simultaneously focus on their own inner feeling states. If they rely on the language of their cognitive mind only and are detached from the language of the body, their interventions may reflect their lack of connection to themselves. Therefore, it is likely that their patients will respond with the same degree of detachment. To facilitate experiences that help their patients experience and "move" their feelings, they need to not only be able to move their own feelings, but to understand how to do this without losing their therapeutic balance. Essentially, maintaining appropriate boundaries is necessary to balance attuning to our patients while simultaneously attuning to ourselves (Bloomgarden, Mennuti, & Cohen, 2003, pp. 9–10).

The third concept, called kinesthetic empathy, represents the therapist's ability to foster shared expression. Gerstein, Botwin, and Kleinman (2004) state that,

> Exquisite attunement to one's self (kinesthetic awareness) can permit therapists to sift through and discard feelings which indicate that they may be over-identifying with patients, while still allowing for the possibility that they may also be tapping into the patient's issues in an embodied, less conscious, fashion. (p. 16)

The dance/movement therapists' responses include conscious awareness of their own sense of the patient based on the feelings they experience. Pallaro (2007) says that, "The recent discovery of mirror neurons may indicate that the ability to respond to another's feeling states and understand them is, in fact, a result of bodily based kinesthetic empathy" (p. 183).

Focusing on facilitating experiences that access the language of the body, and expressing feelings and thoughts that underlie the presented problems, is critical to challenging patients with eating disorders to explore how they feel living in their bodies, a central ingredient for genuine change. This, in turn, affects how they live their lives, the real sign that recovery has occurred and that the patient is on a pathway into fuller, more meaningful, and productive life experiences (Ressler & Kleinman, 2006, p. 17). In contrast, when they try to be *in control,* they initiate planned, forced actions, causing them to feel tense, burdened, and alienated from themselves. When we are able to help them to be *in charge,* they may be able to begin to yield to their authentic life forces, creating a natural flow from within that is empowering.

One patient, Mary, explained to me what this meant to her. She said:

> Being in control means that we spend so much of our energy trying to attain perfection in every sense of the word that we miss out on day-to-day life. The unfortunate thing is that attempting to be in control usually leads to more things being out of control. Life then becomes stressful, and all of our attention becomes focused on controlling the stress in our lives. I want to eventually be able to feel as if I don't need to be in control of everything. I want to be in a place where I am okay with allowing life to happen as it should. When you are in charge, you trust your authentic, true self. You know that your true self is okay and you know that you can trust that inner part of you in every aspect of your life. How wonderful that must feel. That is something I strive for: to be able to trust myself enough to want to be in charge.

Clinical Application

The therapist's ability to facilitate meaningful expression leads to patients being able to experience a stronger connection with their bodies, trust their feelings, explore what they are communicating through their body language, and discover the metaphorical connection between how they move through life and problems they are facing. The session that follows describes how a group of seven patients were engaged in a process that facilitated all of the above-named goals.

I began the group by asking each patient to make a statement about what she was feeling. This allowed me to get a sense of how they communicated as well as to hear anything they wanted known in the group, such as if they felt anxious, had a headache, or were worried about a family session. I absorbed what they shared, and together, we chose music and prepared to move through the room as a way of beginning to explore and get our bearings. Next, I asked them to each choose a space to settle into. Because so many individuals with eating disorders tend to be good followers, I was looking for the emergence of spontaneous or authentic expression. I was also looking for signs of leadership that I could build on. How they had shaped themselves as a group looked interesting to me as a possible thread

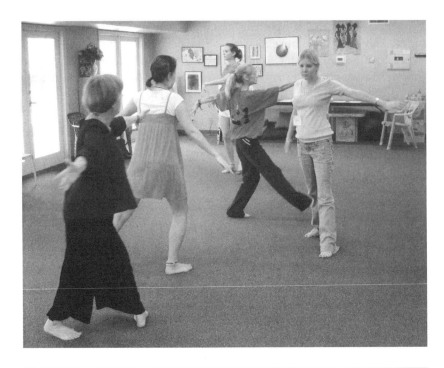

Figure 7.1 Exploring feeling free. (Photo courtesy of the Renfrew Center of Florida.)

to follow. Thus, I asked each patient to describe how they saw the shape of the group as if it were a dot-to-dot drawing. Each of them identified descriptive words like birds, free form, or expansive, and this led to associations with freedom and taking flight. Wondering what that might mean to them, I decided to explore these associations in movement to further understand. I asked each patient to initiate a free, expansive movement (Figure 7.1).

We all joined in, trying on each movement that was initiated to see what it felt like in our own bodies. Each movement was therefore validated nonverbally, as well as verbally though supportive comments from me and various group members. The last to go, Tess, initiated a movement like a swimmer's breast stroke. Sensing that it offered a potential focus because of the clarity of the movement, I decided to develop it further by asking everyone to work with a partner and to identify their own creative way to move across the space (Figure 7.2).

I knew that by doing this, we would be problem solving experientially and that in following this line of thinking, we would also be working metaphorically on patterned ways each patient problem-solved issues related to change. I realized this would lead us, both as a group and as individuals, to bring to light issues of significance; issues that related to each patient's relationship with herself and others, and caused her to

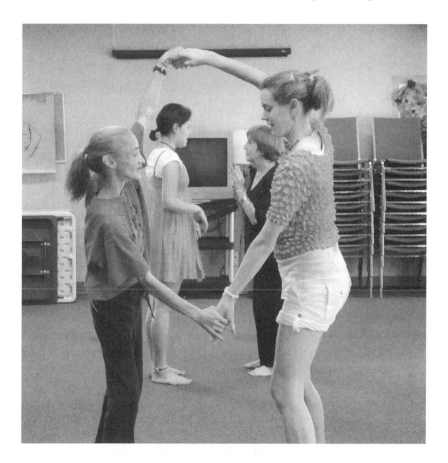

Figure 7.2 Collaborating with a partner. (Photo courtesy of the Renfrew Center of Florida.)

retreat to eating disorder behaviors instead of dealing with the inherent larger emotional issues.

Once the dyads had time to identify and practice the movements they had chosen, I asked each to perform them. As a group, we observed as each pair moved across the space, then the pairs shared their observations. We added our own comments based on our individual perspectives. Each pair repeated the experience again one by one, but with their eyes closed so that their experience could be intensified.

Observations and Insights

1. Ann and Marge leapfrogged, using one another as stepping stones. Ann identified a fear of getting too close, both to herself and to another person, while Marge, a professional dancer, recognized her tendency to become so involved in the experience that

she detached from being in her body. This led her to recognize a familiar pattern of ignoring inner cues that often resulted in serious physical injuries. She also recognized that this estrangement from herself caused her to numb herself to her ability to experience emotional cues.

2. Tess and Addie turned and twirled over and under each other's arms, spinning wildly until they reached their destination. Both recognized their tendency to create chaos in their lives. They discovered that when they slowed down, they were able to go farther as well as to listen to each other. They related this to listening to their bodies.

3. Allie and Rebecca stood sideways to the direction they planned to move in, standing back to back. Allie placed her hand on Rebecca's shoulder, making Rebecca the lead person. Both sashayed down to their goal but never faced it. Rebecca discovered that she moved smoothly and related it to her tendency to demand perfection of herself in every aspect of her life. She connected this with times when she performed as a singer and worried about what others thought, and then feeling judged, panicked. She also acknowledged that she felt as if she were always screaming on the inside, but on the outside trying to appear calm. This caused her to almost always experience anxiety in an attempt to control her uncontrollable inner feelings. Allie recognized that she often let others take the lead and that this provided her with direction because she was scared to make mistakes and be seen as imperfect.

4. I partnered with Ari. We sidestepped toward our destination, facing one another, hands in our pockets. Once we had gone a short way, we turned with our backs to the destination, took our hands out of our pockets, and moved backwards toward our goal. Ari recognized that she was often dependent on her parents or others for directions and was looking to me for cues. Therefore, when we moved parallel to each other, she felt more pressure because she couldn't see exactly what I was doing.

The simplicity of this process left room for us to collaborate as a group in the creation of a space where we could be free and spontaneous. This lent itself to discovering insights that validated and confirmed the patients' abilities to understand and move toward taking charge of their lives.

Getting Creative with Resistance

The following vignette illustrates a group of five teenage girls in a residential program.

Most of the girls were new to the group. As they walked into the room I noted that a few seemed very uncomfortable. I knew that I would need to create a sense of safety to encourage their involvement. I reasoned that providing a concrete task might help to ease the tension, increase safety, and provide a springboard for exploring and expressing feelings.

I asked the group to go outside and choose an object they were attracted to such as a leaf, a twig, or a piece of grass. Once they were back inside, I asked everyone to briefly describe their object in writing; to describe three things they thought were strong about their object, and then three things that were a problem for their object. Once this was accomplished, I asked each to read her description, identifying both the strengths and the problems related to the object.

Anna described her object as a very small leaf that was shaped like a heart. She said it was lonely. Betty shared her piece of driftwood with the group, noticing aloud that the outside was rotting away layer by layer even though it looked tough and sturdy on the inside. Cindy noted that her delicate leaf was becoming frayed around the edges. Dana showed the others her strong twig that supported a tiny sharp and pointed limb. "It could hurt someone," she added.

I was learning something about each girl through the descriptions they provided in relation to their objects. I knew it would be important to simply engage them in this process and not move them too far into self disclosure that could overwhelm them and affect their willingness to return for more sessions. After each girl had read her description and processed it briefly, I asked her to choose a safe place in the room for her object. I asked each to represent her object by choosing a body position from which to let the object come to life. By identifying a safe space and then embodying the object, I thought it might be possible to eventually lead them into moving for themselves. Anna chose a space along a far wall, curled up tightly, then rolled over onto her back; Betty sat by an open door, half in, half out, facing away from everyone; Cindy sat by another door holding herself together; Dana lay by my office door with her head inside her tee shirt, like a turtle. She eventually began to bring her head out and said that, for her, that was progress.

Because the group members seemed frozen in their safe spaces, I approached each individually, discovering a common theme related to fear of losing control. Eve entered the room at this time. She had been in the group many times before and was comfortable with the modality. I quickly explained the task. Following my instructions, Eve went outside and returned with a leaf that she identified as becoming frayed. She acknowledged her safe space as under a table, lying flat on her back and holding on to the table legs. The others watched as I engaged Eve in a playful interaction where she held onto the table and I moved as if trying to take it away from her. I asked Eve to take the same position away from her table, leaving her lying flat on her back with no cover. Eve acknowledged how exposed she felt. Taking cues from Eve, the "barometer" for the group, I intuited that allowing them to "move the therapist" would be more successful than the reverse. Therefore, I invited group members to give me movement directions, and I dutifully complied. Eve began first and others quickly followed suit. This intervention seemed to empower them and a playful movement interaction ensued. Much to my surprise, all of the girls moved from their safe spaces and joined in. Afterward, they spoke briefly about their fears and ambivalence about giving up their eating disorder.

Cognitive Markers of the Therapeutic Process

The *Cognitive Markers* represent five stages of the therapeutic process, namely, exploration, discovery, acknowledgment, connection, and integration (see chapter appendix). These markers give form to the therapeutic process and represent a frame of reference for what is occurring (Kleinman, 1977; Stark & Lohn, 1993, pp. 130–131; Kleinman & Hall, 2006, pp. 14–15). They can be used to assist therapists in tracking the process of therapy and not become lost in the experience of attending. They can also be used by patients to help them process on a body level both in the therapy room and with everyday experiences. Patients report that using the *Cognitive Markers* provides them with a focus that helps them understand and explain themselves more clearly.

From the therapist's perspective, it means recognizing that facilitating an experience guides the patient in exploring herself inter- and intrapersonally. This includes making discoveries regarding what she has explored, acknowledging that this discovery holds truths, connecting its meaning with a familiar pattern or experience, and integrating the meaning of the discovery with the connection so that insights can develop and be examined further. Integration also entails providing some kind of closure. Although the markers are nonlinear, a definable path is followed (Kleinman & Hall, 2005, p. 224; Kleinman & Hall, 2006, pp. 14–15).

The example that follows describes an individual dance/movement therapy session with Tracy, a 24-year-old anorexic who was preparing to leave residential treatment within the week. The *Cognitive Markers* are used to explain the experience occurring within the relationship. Tracy *acknowledged* that she was extremely anxious and frustrated. She said that it was difficult to "be in" her body. Her obsessions were relentless. I knew I needed to help her feel more comfortable before she would be able to focus on problem solving. I *explored,* probing a bit, to identify, through her verbal and non-verbal communication, what was happening. Once I intuited that I had enough information, I devised a plan to attempt to quickly get behind the obsessions, so we could address underlying issues. First, I had her identify her frustration level (between 1 and 10) and vent by hitting a soft foam bat on a chair to help her release enough tension to reduce her discomfort. She related her frustration to her distorted body image, complaining that she was fat and ugly. I knew that this focus on her body was her way of attempting to gain control, so I asked her to close her eyes and create a snapshot in her mind so that she might be able to identify deeper issues that she was not consciously aware of. She *acknowledged* more body obsessions and eating disordered thoughts, so I continued to ask her to symbolically move the snapshots until, eventually, she *discovered* one that was about something else. In this picture, she saw herself as a child of 8, trying to hold onto her father's leg. He traveled frequently and was preparing to leave on another trip. We processed this *connection* only enough for both of us to understand the impact her father's departures left on her as a child. Remembering she once shared that she liked to ride horses, I introduced this topic to provide a safe way to address her painful acknowledgment of insecurity and abandonment. Given her continued difficulty with anxiety, I decided to focus on trying to re-create Tracy's feelings of satiety and comfort derived from her relationship with her horses. I thought that this could help her experience a sense of wholeness and feel more in charge.

We explored our relationship with each other through a piece of elastic we both held (Figure 7.3), verbally processing and making connections regarding our experiences as they occurred. For example, Tracy was aware of moving fast. I *acknowledged* that I could feel that, and we *explored* the conflict she experiences with her horses when she speeds, *acknowledging* that she repeats this same pattern in other aspects of her life also. She understood how, when she tried to control her horses, they would resist because she automatically aims for outcomes rather than experiences. We *explored* how she needs to apply this same kind of bodily felt awareness in her relationship with herself, in order to *integrate* it. She *discovered* and *acknowledged* that in using her senses to increase awareness, in contrast to running from them, her anxiety had diminished. I gave Tracy a *Cognitive Markers* worksheet so she could process further in writing, as a way to *integrate* this experience. Later, she gave it back to me for feedback. What she wrote on the form indicated that she'd understood both cognitively and on a body level. In the Integration section, she said: "I need to work through family issues; issues of abandonment; conquering fears instead of running from them; and trust myself more." In closing, she *acknowledged,* "What I enjoyed most [when we worked together] is when I was most in touch with my body and let go and worked with another being." I told her

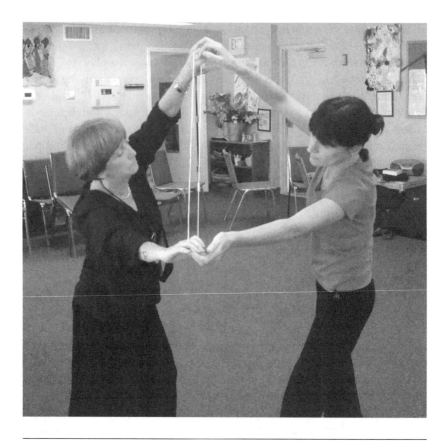

Figure 7.3 Relationship through an elastic. (Photo courtesy of the Renfrew Center of Florida.)

that she had identified her goals, as well as her objective in life. In our last session, she asked if she could keep the elastic. She said winding it around her wrist or in her hair would help her remember what was really important to her (Kleinman, 2004).

Summary

Human beings communicate through their bodies long before they learn to talk. Individuals with eating disorders, however, detach from listening and responding to their bodies as much as they possibly can. They attempt to control the anxiety caused by shutting down emotionally through a variety of behaviors aimed at distracting them from themselves. These behaviors, all body based, range from leg shaking to cuticle picking, hair pulling, and even overworking. In attempting to create an illusion of control, they often find themselves withdrawing from life, alone with their thoughts, disordered behaviors, and the part of themselves they have come to call "ED." Dance/movement therapy helps individuals with eating disorders learn how to reconnect with themselves, enabling authentic change in both actions and words to occur and to recognize their whole self to be a necessary part of their life force.

Appendix: Cognitive Markers: A Guide to Process Experiences

Copyright Susan Kleinman, 1977, 2001

The Cognitive Markers give form to the process of living and represent a therapeutic frame of reference for what is occurring. These markers provide a guide to:

1. Explore an experience.
2. Make discoveries regarding what has been explored.
3. Acknowledge a discovery that seems important.
4. Connect the meaning of the discovery with a familiar pattern or experience.
5. Integrate the meaning of the discovery with the connection so that insights can develop and be explored further at another time. Integration also includes closure to end the current experience.

Use these markers as a guide to process your experiences. Keep your descriptions simple and remember that these are YOUR feelings and thoughts and you cannot make a mistake. Imagine that you are a detective, collecting clues to solve a mystery—the mystery of your experiences (one at a time). Good luck.

Exploration

Write about your experience by exploring and noting feelings, sensations, and subsequent thoughts that are emerging from it.

Discovery

Write about your awareness of your feelings and sensations as well as any observations you've noticed regarding what you have just explored. What did you discover? Be as specific as possible.

Acknowledgment

Acknowledge that your discovery has meaning in your life—or if not, why you think you made this discovery and it is NOT relevant in your life.

Connection

Recognize HOW the feelings, sensations, and thoughts you've discovered and acknowledged are important in relation to your present experiences, how they fit into your life and parallel past similar experiences.

Integration

Sum up this experience, noting any issues you think are important that you want to note for further exploration, including questions or things that you found interesting. Also, identify actions you might take, or strategies you might use to further help you deal with these issues.

Remember to give yourself permission to explore and discover new ways to cope with these old problems and patterns as well as to begin to include these new tools as part of your growing repertoire of skills. Then, you'll begin to have new connections to add to your experiences.

References

American Psychiatric Association. (2006). Treatment of patients with eating disorders, third edition. *American Journal of Psychiatry 163* (7 Suppl) pp. 8–57.

American Psychiatric Association. (2000). *Diagnostic manual and statistical manual of mental disorders, DSM-IV-TR* (4th ed.). Washington, DC.

Bloomgarden, A., Mennuti, R., & Cohen, E. (2003).Therapist self-disclosure: Implications for the therapeutic connection. *The Renfrew Center Working Papers.* Volume 1, Fall. (pp. 9–10). Philadelphia, PA.

Gerstein, F., Botwin, S. & Kleinman, S. (2004). Developing connections in group therapy. *The Renfrew Center Working Papers.* Volume 2, Fall, (p. 16). Philadelphia, PA.

Graham, M. (1952). Beautiful morning. In DeMille, A. *Dance to the piper.* Boston: Little, Brown (p. 335).

Grillo, C.M. (2002). Binge eating disorder. In C.G. Fairburn & K.D. Brownell (Eds.), *Comprehensive textbook of obesity and eating disorders* (2nd ed.). New York: Guilford Press. pp. 178–182.

Harris, R. (April, 2008). Personal communication.

Kleinman, S. (1977). A circle of motion. Unpublished master's thesis, Lone Mountain College, San Francisco, CA.

Kleinman, S., & Hall, T. (2006). Dance/Movement therapy: A method for embodying emotions. *The Renfrew Center Foundation Healing Through Relationship Series: Contributions to Eating Disorder Theory and Treatment Volume 1: Fostering Body-Mind Integration.* Philadelphia, PA (pp. 2–19).

Kleinman, S. (October, 2004). Use of self as a dance/movement therapist: Our greatest therapeutic tool. *Proceedings of the American Dance Therapy Association 39th Annual Conference.* Columbia, Maryland: American Dance Therapy Association.

Kleinman, S., & Hall, T. (2005). Dance movement therapy with women with eating disorders. In F. J. Levy (Ed.) *Dance/movement therapy, A healing art.* Revised ed. (pp. 221–227). Reston, VA: The American Alliance for Health, Physical Education, Recreation, and Dance.

Kleinman, S. (2003). Body talk: Giving form to feelings. *Proceedings of the American Dance Therapy Association 38th Annual Conference.* Columbia, Maryland: American Dance Therapy Association.

Kleinman, S. (February, 1994). Submission for the Record, Statement of The American Dance Therapy Association to the Sub-committee on Ways and Means, House of Representatives Hearing on The Congressional Budget Office's Analysis of the President's Health Care Reform Proposal, Volume X11, President's Health Care Reform Proposals: Impact on Providers and Consumers, Part 3 of 3 (pp. 70–74). Serial 103–91, US Government Printing Office, Washington, 1994.

National Eating Disorders Association (2008). Research Committee. Retrieved on July 10, 2008 from.http://www.nationaleatingdisorders.org/research-efforts/research-committee.php.

Pallaro, P. (2007). Somatic countertransference: The therapist in relationship. *Authentic Movement: Moving the body, moving the self, being moved* (pp. 176–193). London: Jessica Kingsley.

Ressler, A. (2000). A body to die for: Rethinking weight, wellness and body image. *The Official Publication of the International Spa Industry*. (p. 35). September–October. Lexington, KY.

Ressler, A., & Kleinman, S. (2006). Reframing body image identity in the treatment of eating disorders. *The Renfrew Center Foundation Healing Through Relationship Series: Contributions to Eating Disorder Theory and Treatment Volume 1: Fostering Body-Mind Integration*. Philadelphia, PA.

Satir, V. (1987). The therapist story. In M. Baldwin & V. Satir (Eds.), *The use of self in therapy*. (p.23). New York: The Haworth Press.

Schwimmer, C. (2003). Psychoeducation and skills development. *The Renfrew Center Working Papers*, Volume 1, Summer. (p. 7). Philadelphia, PA.

Siegel, D. J. (1999). *The developing mind* (p. 290). New York: The Guilford Press.

Stark, A., & Lohn, A. (1993). The use of verbalization in dance/movement therapy. In *Foundations of dance/movement therapy: The life and work of Marian Chace*, edited by S. Sandel, S. Chaiklin, and A. Lohn. Columbia, MD. The Marian Chace Memorial Fund of the American Dance Therapy Association. p.130–131.

Sullivan, P. (1995). *American Journal of Psychiatry*, 152 (7), 1073–1074. Retrieved on June 2, 2008 from http//www.nationaleatingdisorders.org/p.asp?WebPage_ID=286&Profile_ID=41138.

CHAPTER **8**

Family Dance/Movement Therapy
A Systems Model

DIANNE DULICAI

Contents

Introduction

This chapter describes the use of dance/movement therapy (DMT) as used in families and the theoretical basis that underpins the intervention. Historical development of the author's synthesis includes aspects of family therapy theory, DMT theory, movement observation, and developmental movement. Practical use of family DMT therapy is described accompanied by the clinical implications of nonverbal movement assessment and the skills necessary to move easily between verbal and nonverbal streams of communication. Examples of sessions that highlight theory and research projects testing this model under a variety of settings and populations are cited.

Family as a System

The American Dance Therapy Association defines DMT as, "the psycho-therapeutic use of movement as a process which furthers the emotional, social, cognitive, and physical integration of the individual." Integration, the concluding element and for me the salient quality in therapy, provides the bedrock of this kind of intervention as well. To integrate the whole-ness of any person, it is necessary to conceive of that person as a part of a family system embedded within a community, involved within a nation that is a part of the world. Even when working with an individual alone, integration is achieved best when the therapist considers the client within a context of family and culture.

Families most commonly come or are referred to therapists with a view of their difficulty and frequently know within whom the problem lies. Use the first one or two sessions to get to really know the immediate family as well as the nuclear families of both parents. For example, the family may tell you the younger of two children has always been sickly and anxious, unlike the older sibling. A family therapist would use the term "identified patient" for that child. However, the situation is different as other factors are considered. The child may have a genetic disposition for asthma living near a polluting industry in a very poor country with scarce health care resources.

Assessment of the situation and the resulting treatment plan might be very different if the family lived in a less polluted area and where health care was available. The family's stress in dealing with an illness differs in different circumstances and their ability to access resources may vary. Mature stable parents most probably will have less stress and more ability to cope with illness in the family and therefore have less conflict. At times, an individual is overwhelmed with factors that cause severe strain on the family system. We must consider whoever comes to us within the con-text of micro and macro aspects of their lives in order to develop appro-priate goals for therapy. Consider how each family member describes the difficulty he or she faces. Some cultures believe an illness may be a sign of weakness—they may not understand anxiety as a signal rather than a problem. The wholeness of your evaluation will enhance your potential for assisting the family that comes to you.

Very early in my professional development I was dissuaded from the idea of treating an individual in isolation. While at my first DMT job and still a beginner, I participated in a fairly new discipline, family therapy. Training required assessing not a patient but a family system of which the patient was a part. Albert Scheflen (1972), director of research and clinical development, had previously published articles, some conjointly with Ray Birdwhistell, defining the indices of movement behavior to be considered while interviewing families (Birdwhistell, 1963). A thorough understanding of Scheflen, Birdwhistell, and Beels and Ferber (1969) is outside the scope of this chapter, but I will summarize those theoretical components important to this work throughout the following pages.

While watching other colleagues in training, I began to note movement characteristics in interaction and trained my eye to observe patterns of a number of participants. The skill for observing families is quite a different ability from what I had been taught in movement observation studies where we were required to observe a single person. It was only later that I had the opportunity to study Kestenberg's mother and child interactions (Kestenberg, 1975).

Scheflen and Birdwhistell defined nonverbal units of communication—kinesic factors regulating and expanding verbal interactions, particularly in families. These movement behaviors, such as a posture shift or a gesture toward another member, when seen synchronized with the spoken components, yield more information than the verbal channel of communication alone. Patterns of movement behaviors help monitor or negate an oral statement. Examination of the patterns of nonverbal expression yields the characteristic rules of exchange in communication of the family. My experience suggested that the elements of the Laban analysis of movement qualities* were also important to family communication and I was excited about testing that hypothesis under such ideal circumstances. For example, when a mother reaches across the table to place a finger on the shoulder of her young son, she may do so with a delicate touch or a forceful pressure—each communicating quite different information. Scheflen would note what was done (gesture toward child, i.e., M–g > c). Combining the kinesthetic movement with Laban's effort elements yielded a more nuanced evaluation (M–g > c with lightness or strength), which became the beginnings of the "Nonverbal assessment of family systems" (Dulicai, 1977). I continued seeing families over the next decade.

Important Observational Skills

In an early publication, Schmais stated the major hypotheses upon which DMT is based (Schmais, 1974). She states:

> (1) Movement reflects personality, (2) The relationship established between the therapist and patient through movement supports and enables behavioral change, and (3) Significant changes occur on the movement level that can affect total functioning. (p. 10)

---

* For information about Laban's system of movement observation and analysis, see Chapter 12.

This is equally true for movement behavior within a family system where their relationships are displayed in the interactional movement behavior. The family dance/movement therapist (dmt) enters the system and therapeutic interventions begin. When changes occur in the way the system deals with each other, the movement interplay changes and then the outward display of behavior changes. For the observation skills required, one begins by observing a number of persons at once—say a dialogue of two persons, the first doing several seconds of a phrase of movement answered by the second person. Though normal interaction doesn't follow a stimulus/response format, it is the best way to work up to more complex observation. The onlooker should view this from a distance, as you want to use your choreographer's eye to see the relational dance. The observer is recording what happens (kinesic movement) as well as how it happens (effort elements). I often begin practice with only the kinesic movement and add the effort qualities with more practice. Readers interested can refer to the Scheflen (1972) text for the full range of movement interaction characteristics and/or to the Dulicai assessment (1977) for those included in the 1974 study.

The narrative of the data sheet may look something like this:

Seated #1 leans toward his right side slowly with lightness slightly retreated backward and reaches right arm to side with a great deal of restraint, returning to center with upper torso still retreated.

Seated #2 responds from a posture slightly leaning to left, legs crossed, moves to her center quickly and with strength with a small circular gesture of right lower arm matching the slow light gesture of #1.

Obviously, this is far too much writing for an observation without videotape. Displayed below is a look at the data sheet. I have found the shorthand described in the original article shown below quite helpful and with practice the therapist can do the observation live (Dulicai, 1977). For those unfamiliar with Laban notation I have used words for the qualitative description rather than symbols. T indicates the therapist.

Nonverbal channel: Person #1 -seated M > r (moves to right), PB < T (posture/gesture away from therapist). Use Laban symbols for slow/light gesture—torso held and retreated

Verbal channel: When she left I knew she wouldn't come back.

Nonverbal channel: Person #2 (therapist) T-P < #1, (therapist postures away from client) x-lower (crosses lower torso), use Laban symbols for, strong and quick, acc #1 G (therapist accommodates #1 gesture)

Verbal channel: Leaving the room after a tense moment means what to you?

In this example, the words are recorded on the video and the movement is described with its quality. The effort language used consists of terms used in previous studies by Marion North (1972). You see person #1 (the client) display a posture and gesture away from his center containing his use of lightness with an ability to take his time—all the while using a retreated posture. The verbal channel indicates they were discussing when his fiancée left the room after harsh words. Before he completes his sentence, the therapist is aligning her posture with his and echoing the quality of the gesture displaying what Scheflen called "quasi-courting behavior." The therapist accommodated the client's gesture—a gesture of affiliation—while challenging the verbal component (Scheflen, 1965). For this example I used a small phrase shown on video though these skills can be practiced with peers role-playing any short movement phrase. If you find the verbal distracting, try moving outside hearing distance from the interaction. From this point there is need for practice and gradually increasing the length of observation.

Television interviews are quite good for practice, though it is better to turn off the sound in the beginning. In the example above, you saw the observation of movement, with the verbal section added, and finally the interpretation of what you saw. This is only an example of a few seconds, unlike a therapeutic session of an hour in which pages of data are collected and analyzed, informed by knowledge of research. It takes a great deal of experience to accomplish this skill but it is important in deciding the appropriate intervention with the family. Again, remember to be careful; a short sequence happened at that moment in time in a certain situation in this particular relationship. You need far more information under various circumstances to compare a movement profile with that same person's abilities at interaction over time. It is, however, a skill that is necessary for this kind of work. Working with a family is like playing cards with a group of people who know the rules and you do not. You need to first find out the rules of this system and the family cannot or will not tell you in words alone.

Data can be arranged and analyzed in several ways, depending on how one wishes to use it. One way may be by finding the number of incidences of a kinesic event of each individual in the family, often the most helpful method in research. It is equally useful in building norms for a particular population or group. For example, it can be used in comparing normal with disturbed families or changes in families over time. For clinical use of the data, it is far more useful to begin by identifying repeated sequences or patterns in the session in a vertical form and the verbal content that accompanies them. For example, you will see sequences of movement appear among a long string of data and if you examine the discussed theme each time the pattern appears, you have identified a characteristic mode of coping for this family. In one case, each time the subject of intimacy arose, a characteristic movement pattern accompanied it, demonstrating the family's way of coping with the subject.

Your data sheet is vertical, one event following another such as this example:

M-P/G > F (Mother, Posture/Gesture, toward Father)

F-acc M (Father accommodates Mother's action)

PP-dis.r ft (Presenting patient discharges right foot) with strength and quickness

M-P/G < F (Mother, Posture/Gesture away from Father) (Dulicai, 1977)

Helpful DMT Skills

While achieving proficiency in family observation, let's review a skill that has been learned in DMT training—the ability to move from movement to speech and vice versa. First and foremost, trust the movement; it has meaning and it is up to you to discover the meaning.

Bartenieff quoted Laban, who wrote, "The source whence perfection and final mastery of movement must flow is the understanding of that part of the inner life of man where movement and action originate." (Bartenieff & Lewis, 1980). In a DMT session, after you have completed the warm-up, you may begin a simple movement, say shifting weight from side to side, and soon enough one member of your group will somehow modify it. If you follow those small changes you may see that personality imposed on the movement, just as in conversation a person takes a theme and person-alizes it from a particular perspective. You are observing the process of the group just as you would if you were a verbal therapist listening to an initial opening as described by Yalom (1985). However, while watching, you are also asking yourself questions. Why is that person the one who changes a side-to-side rocking motion to one forward toward the group with great strength and rocking back with great restraint of strength? Is he speaking for himself or the group's process? By waiting to watch how the group deals with this initiation, you find it has accepted the stronger, differently directed movement. You may ask several questions about the new action, hoping to move from expressive movement to expressive verbalization. Or the opposite may be the case, as you may have a person who always wants to talk as a defense to interrupt the movement. I often ask this kind of person to "move it" rather than talking about it. Shifting from feeling to thinking or the reverse, as your clinical judgment guides you, is an impor-tant skill. A dmt may learn to beautifully continue movement through a whole session, but often with families as with individuals, we need to crys-tallize the moment into movement and talk. It is also a way we teach clients to recognize movement behavior as a tool in therapy and one they can take with them to make use of.

A simple example from a group movement session demonstrates both. While running a session with long-term-hospitalized in-patients, a gentleman who would shuffle into the room, his head bent down, always without interacting unless conversation was directed to him by name, participated in a group action similar to holding a shovel and digging a ditch. My concern about continuing this theme was that the (primary) process would likely lead to digging a grave.

In this instance, I determined that they were not sufficiently defended to explore this theme and so took the lead by moving the downward shoveling to a slower movement of the tool forward at waist height and asking what tool was used this way (secondary process). My shuffling participant changed his body to upright and looking directly at his fellow group members said, "I was a baker once." He told them about the job he really once enjoyed. It allowed him to enter into interaction with his peers. At times, you ask a group what the movement feels like and you get a response at the secondary process level when you are looking for primary process or the reverse. However, in circumstances in which the typically well defended and insightful client wants to continually explain, obfuscate, deny any meaning to the movement, you need the skill to move the session to a feeling level. It's necessary to be comfortable moving back and forth, as you will need to do so in working with families.

Case Study

Here is an example from a family session in which I missed the obvious clues that unconscious contents and specific dynamics would appear. This family came in with the "presenting patient" being the youngest of five children. The parents explained that the 5-year-old boy had numerous problems such as bedwetting, thumb sucking, tantrums when stressed, and cruelty to the family pet. While I obtained information about the family structure including the parents' families of origin, the first 10–15 minutes occurred between the parents and myself. They had separated several times, the mother in each case leaving the house. While the parents discussed this briefly, the presenting patient began banging his feet on the rungs of his chair and poking his brother. I incorrectly thought that he was getting bored and instituted a family genogram in which all could participate.

As the family drew their genealogy in three generations and discussed how each related to the other, again the subject of "leaving" rose, this time about a grandmother's dying. Suddenly, the room became dark, chaos occurred, with great laughter from some of the children. The "identified patient" had found the light switch in a one-way screened room without windows. Fortunately for my learning, a colleague had been notating the session and I could review her notes to see how I had missed the first clue. This family was not going to talk about their conflict as long as the youngest provided disruptions. There was an understood agreement—though not conscious—that the child could deflect difficult issues by acting out to his own detriment. Later, I understood that themes of loss or abandonment were issues that both parents had not been able to resolve in themselves and which negatively interacted within their family. Neither parent could see that this issue was affecting their son or influencing his behavior. To the contrary, they cared deeply for their son but thought his "problem" rested with him.

Upon checking my colleague's notation we found the pattern had emerged early in the session. When the mother and father would speak about any issue in which they disagreed, mother would block the father by crossing her leg away from him, gesture across her body to close the upper away from the father, all accompanied by a nervous discharge with her foot. The child would pick up the rhythm of the discharge in his feet or sometimes in the rhythm of his fingers on the chair. The boy picked up on the anxiety of the parents, particularly the mother, and "acted it out" for them. One or both of the parents would stop the conversation, address the boy's "bad" behavior and work would begin again. In fact, it happened three times before the lights went out.

Having identified the pattern, the therapist needs to consider what function this serves for the family homeostasis. Consider what we know from this sequence. Unresolved conflict exists between the parents, though at this point the source of the conflict is unknown to the therapist.

We also know that the youngest child tunes into the nonverbal behavior of the mother, sometimes escalating into misbehavior. At age 5, he is beginning important work such as entering kindergarten and moving toward independence. Separation is present in the family system and each member is being affected. Why is he reacting to his mother's anxiety?

System purists such as Beels and Ferber (1969), mentioned earlier, as well as Boszormenty-Nagy and Spark (1973) and Bowen (1976) are interested in the relationship between the current interaction patterns in the family and the interpersonal patterns of the past. Learning the interaction style of this particular family gives a chance for the youngest member to be free of that kind of responsibility and the parents to begin to talk about their own conflict. Looking at their genogram revealed another clue. The therapist asked the family members to join their closest members with a red line and join difficult members with a green line. Our presenting patient joined his parents in bright red marking, and remarking it, formed a triangle of red with his parents and himself and excluding his siblings.

Further discussion of the genogram revealed that this family lives in a middle class area of a large city within a multicultural section. Both parents have some education above high school and both have good-paying and interesting jobs. The children's public school has a good reputation and the older children have done well. The youngest child's teacher states he would do well in academics if he were not diverted by behavior problems. I learned that the mother's father had been in the military service and moved numerous times during her childhood and finally, when she was an adolescent, he left the family. The grandmother is particularly close to the youngest child. On the paternal side, both grandparents live across the country and visit infrequently though the father, an only child, states his relationship with both is good. If you watched the videotape of the genogram activity, the distance between all members would be seen as the few accommodations of postures or gestures and very little touch, though the space was rather small.

Our presenting energetic and attractive patient has an age-appropriate movement repertoire. Readers should familiarize themselves with works of Kestenberg (Amighi et al., 1999) and North (1972) as well as being able to use child assessment instruments such as the Peabody Developmental Motor Scales (Folio & Fewell, 1983). It is equally important to survey cognitive development as a part of the integration of the individual (Rosen, 1977). Izard's work is useful to our understanding as he sees motor, neurological, emotional, perceptual and cognitive systems as interrelated systems, allowing the human to develop as the organized holistic set that we identify as the autonomous person (Izard et al., 1984).

With this family, finding no evidence of cognitive deficit or movement characteristics that would suggest a neurological problem, we need to consider more complex movement patterns.

All the qualities Laban referred to as efforts are present, so let us consider combinations seen and how they are used in phrases. The boy uses two elements more frequently than combinations of three during the interview time, which would be expected, but moves into action during activity and when his parents get close to a conflictual subject. Most commonly, he uses two elements of strength and suddenness, suggesting his energetic forcefulness, and also bound and sudden movement displaying his restlessness and withholding propensity. When he picks up the emotional discharge of his mother, he moves to three elements of strong, direct, and quick quality that accelerates from the normal swing phrase to an impactive phrase. Occasionally, another three-element pattern appears, particularly when his father uses a postural shift away from his mother. Wringing motions appear at this time, usually beginning with a small object that becomes larger and more disruptive.

Reviewing all the information, my verbal interview, the genogram, and the movement information with my supervisor, we planned my next session with the following goals and objectives:

1. Strengthen the generation boundaries
2. Increase the sibling relationship independent of the parents
3. Expand the presenting patient's ability to move from high action without exaggeration and acceleration

Boszormenyi-Nagy and Spark (1973) stress the importance of secure and firm boundaries between the generation of parents and children and possible forms of acting out when such boundaries are not clear. In this case, it is seen that the youngest child is "acting out" when he sees unresolved conflict appear in the parents. His role is to become distruptive when the subject of his parent's relationship is discussed in the session. They have a stake in his activity as well, as it serves the function of preventing the conflict from being resolved and thereby maintaining the homeostasis.

Lewis and colleagues developed an assessment of family functioning based on their research project of functioning and nonfunctioning families. First on the list of items assessed is the structure of the family's use of power, ranging from overt power to egalitarian. Parental coalition is the next in importance that ranges from parent–child coalition to weak parental coalition, and strong parental coalition (Lewis et al., 1976).

Looking at the possibilities of what the DMT session might look like, it should be kept in mind that there are a variety of ways to approach these goals. Another thought deserves consideration—a cotherapist—either another dmt or another mental health practitioner familiar with movement and if possible a female/male combination to work with families. Fortunately for me I could, in this instance, call on one of my peers, a social worker who became familiar with DMT during his training. These ideal situations are not often replicated and I have worked alone on many occasions, although it is much more difficult.

We started the next session with an explanation of how we use nonverbal as much as the verbal expression to understand how the family works and we would follow the warm-up with an avoidance game with the whole family. During the warm-up, Mom placed herself next to the presenting patient while Dad took a position directly across from Mom next to the oldest daughter. After a few minutes, we suggested that we have two circles, one for the children and one for the parents. My co-therapist took the youngsters into a larger room while I stayed with the adults. He continued the game but worked on changing places around the circle as the center person changed and ending with talking about what it was like playing in each position. My task was to use the stretch cloth while working with the parents to try to get a triangle with them and to play the most distant position, more commonly myself in that spot. Theoretically, this would be bringing to awareness a triangle position concretely in the game. Afterward, I could bring that concept of a triangle between people to a conversational level applying it to their family system. We reviewed the genogram and talked about the triangles there.

The following session began by reviewing the previous session and the week in between. My co-therapist and I placed ourselves together and opposite the parents with the children to the right and left of us with the presenting patient closest to my co-therapist. During the warm-up I took the family through a range of effort modulations ending with time possibilities. I assigned the oldest daughter to be the referee first to call "losing it" when it was getting close to being dangerously fast and assigned the presenting patient to be the referee to call "too boring" when it got too slow. Numerous times the parents wanted to intervene, though both therapists kept the game proceeding and allowing the children to regulate it. We were able to talk about who gets to regulate whom and what makes good leaders, starting with revealing how therapists plan treatment plans, but must accommodate to changes that occur. Without examining the following sessions step by step, you can see where we were going, how we were getting there using both movement and talking guided by goals and objectives but taking into consideration life changes. After 8 months we had witnessed the parents jointly increase their ability to assume their roles and develop new coping mechanisms for their anxiety and conflict, without allowing the children to be scapegoated. The presenting patient finished kindergarten, gradually containing his need to act on his anxiety and talking more when he felt anxious.

Summary and Conclusions

In addition to these examples, one may be asked to work with couples only or in combination with a family session. Kluft's thesis (1981) outlined the movement aspects of nonverbal behavior in marital partners and she has continued to use them as guideposts for guiding DMT interventions. Loman (1998) proposes a developmental model working with children and their parents. Meekums and Sbiglio focused their work on children who are in families where abuse is present (Meekums, 1991; Sbiglio, 1999). This presents particular problems such as understanding the laws under which a therapist must work with reference to violence to children. This kind of work calls for especially close supervision and co-therapy if at all possible.

In the late 1960s, researchers began investigating the nonverbal channel of communication and its importance in family relationships. Davis examined sequences of movement and the accompanying speech and illustrated both channels in words and effort notation (Davis, 1966). During the same period, Kestenberg (1965) began her long history of movement publications relevant to children and their families and integrating concepts and theories of Laban with psychoanalytic thinking. A decade later, influenced by these pioneers, I built on their research to develop "Nonverbal assessment of family systems" (1977) and in a later study (1995), the cognitive deficits in children with lead exposure. The interaction of the family proved to be an intervening variable as a high level of family interaction seemed to compensate for cognitive skills with these children. Peterson (1991) chose to use the assessment instrument to study distributional features of nonverbal behavior in families. Goodill (1980) chose to use the Action Profile Movement Analysis (Ramsden, 1973) normally used in management studies to apply to movement characteristics of normal and dysfunctional families.

This collection demonstrates only the highlights of continuous research examining families in various circumstances, cultures, and configurations. I would like to close with a fine example of family therapy clinical teamwork culminating in the thesis of a former graduate, Casey Slayton. Her research examined children with pervasive developmental disorder and their parents under stress circumstances. She participated in a mobile team from a mental health center in a collaborative project within a larger urban city police department. When the police received a report of domestic violence in a home with children, the mental health team was alerted and joined the response. It was hypothesized that the children's trauma could be addressed more quickly and would reduce the long-term emotional damage to the child with immediate intervention. Director Bert Ruttenberg thought the dmt should be placed on the team, citing their ability to use movement intervention as immediate soothing intervention with children. This was Slayton's job—similar to the emergency room clinician and she did it well. Her thesis would make important reading for those interested in this work (Slayton, 2000).

References

Theses from Hahnemann's Creative Arts Therapy Department, Drexel University discussed in this chapter are marked with asterisk in the reference list. They can be obtained through interlibrary loan by contacting the director, Sherry Goodill, Ph.D., ADTR, at Drexel University at sg35@drexel.edu.

Amighi, J. K. L, Loman, S., Lewis, P., & Sossin, K.M. (1999). *The meaning of movement*. London: Brunner-Routledge; Amsterdam: Gordon and Breach.

Bartenieff, I., & Lewis, D. (1980). *Body movement: Coping with the environment*. New York: Gordon and Breach.

Beels, C.C. & Ferber, A. (1969). Family therapy: A view. *Family Process*, 8, 280–318.

Birdwhistell, R. L. (1963). The kinesic level in the investigation of the emotions, in P. H. Knapp (Ed.). *Expressions of the emotions in man*, New York: International Universities Press. p. 396.

Boszormenyi-Nagy, I., & Spark, G. (1973). *Invisible loyalties: Reciprocity in intergenerational family therapy*. Hagerston: Harper & Row.

Bowen, M. (1976). *Theory in the practice of psychotherapy*. New York: Gardner.

Davis, M. (1966). *An effort-shape movement analysis of a family therapy session*. New York: Dance Notation Bureau, 21.

Dulicai, D. (1977). Nonverbal assessment of family systems: A preliminary study. *International Journal of Art Psychotherapy*, 4(2), 55–62.

Dulicai, D. (1995). *Movement indicators of attention and their role as identifiers of lead exposure*. Unpublished research, The Union Institute, Cincinnati.

Folio, M. R., & Fewell, R. R. (1983). *Peabody developmental motor scales and activity cards*. Chicago: Riverside Publishing Co.

*Goodill, S. W. (1980). *A comparison of normal and dysfunctional families using the action profile movement analysis*. Philadelphia: Hahnemann University.

Izard, C. E., Kagan, J., & Zajonc, R. B. (1984). *Emotions, cognition, and behavior*. Cambridge: Cambridge University Press.

Kestenberg, J. (1965). The role of movement patterns in development: *International Psychoanalytic Quarterly*, 34, 1–36.

Kestenberg, J. S. (1975). *Children and parents: Psychoanalytic studies in development*. New York: Aronson.

*Kluft, E. (1981). *Nonverbal communication and marriage: An investigation of the movement aspects of nonverbal communication between marital partners.*, Philadelphia, Hahnemann University.

Lewis, J. M., Beavers, W. R., Gossett, J. T., & Phillips, V. A. (1976). *No single thread: Psychological health in family systems*. New York: Brunner/Mazel.

Loman, S. (1998). Employing a developmental model of movement patterns in dmt with young children and their families. *American Journal of Dance Therapy*, 20(2), 101–114.

Meekums, B. (1991). Dance/movement therapy with mothers and young children at risk of abuse. *The Arts in Psychotherapy Journal*, 18(#1), 223–230.

North, M. (1972). *Personality assessment through movement*. London: Macdonald and Evans.

Peterson, D. (1991). *The kinesics of family systems: Distributional features of nonverbal interaction*. Unpublished research, Minneapolis: Minnesota School of Professional Psychology.

Ramsden, P. (1973). *Top team planning: A study of the power of individual motivation in management*. New York: John Wiley and Sons.

Rosen, H. (1977). *Pathway to Piaget: A guide for clinicians, educators and developmentalists* (1st ed.). Cherry Hill: Postgraduate International, Inc.

*Sbiglio, M. G. (1999). *A pilot comparative study of nonverbal interactions in Puerto Rican families with and without a history of family violence*. Unpublished research, Philadelphia: Hahnemann University.

Scheflen, A. E. (1965). Quasi-courtship behavior in psychotherapy. *Psychiatry*, 28, 245–257.

Scheflen, A. E. (1972). *Body language and social order.* Englewood Cliffs, N.J.: Prentice Hall.

Schmais, C. (1974). Dance therapy in perspective. In K. Mason (Ed.) *Focus on dance VII.* Reston, VA: American Alliance for Health, Physical Education and Recreation), pp.7–12.

*Slayton, C. (2000). *Mobile family dance/movement therapy for children with pervasive developmental disorder: A multiple case study.* Unpublished case study, Philadelphia: Drexel University.

Yalom, I. D. (1985). *The theory and practice of group psychotherapy* (3rd ed.). New York: Basic Books.

CHAPTER 9

Dance/Movement Psychotherapy in Early Childhood Treatment[*]

SUZI TORTORA

Contents

---

[*] Parts of this chapter were adapted with permission from Tortora, S. (2006). *The dancing dialogue: Using the communicative power of movement with young children.* Baltimore, MD: Paul H. Brookes Publ.

> I want to go in. ... I want to go in, I want to go in. ... I want to go in.
> Is the door opened yet? Is the door open yet? Is Suzi inside? Is Suzi
> inside? I want to go in. I want to go in. I want to go in.

Through the closed door of my studio office I hear the rapid, punctuated yet "singsong" voice of my new patient, Timothy, age 6, diagnosed with pervasive developmental disorder, not otherwise specified (PDD.NOS). As I open the door, I am met by a small thin boy with sparkling blue eyes. He looks at me fleetingly as his glance shifts to scan the interior of the room behind me. His head rocks side to side as his body appears to be stepping forward and backward at almost the same time. His arms are intertwined, as he grasps his hands with a quick short pulsing rhythm, tightly woven together at the wrists. The force of this rhythmic hold causes Timothy to almost jump, up and down. Is this a dance of welcome or hesitation, I immediately wonder? Watch the movements, follow his actions, and soon I will know, I remind myself. Everything will be revealed if I stay attuned to the quality of his actions.

Pause, forward, pause, tighten the grasp, look around, prance a step or two—Timothy enters the room on his own. Forward, then a step back. "Dancing? Hi Suzi. Dancing." Is this a question or a statement, I wonder? I notice my body is very alert, ready to respond to his words or his actions. I'm not sure where he will take me as we begin our dancing dialogue, but I notice an awakened sensation in my every limb; my thoughts are filled with questions and my emotional reaction is one of excitement, with a hint of concern. I am intrigued, yet sensing I must proceed with caution. I note these reactions and wonder how they may relate to how Timothy is feeling at this moment.

Thus begin Timothy's dance movement psychotherapy sessions. During weekly visits, I, as Timothy's dance therapist, will use my observations and experiential sense of Timothy as tools to gain insight into how Timothy experiences and expresses himself in his surroundings. Through a very eclectic yet specific method I will get to know Timothy on his own terms, creating a safe "holding environment" (Winnicott, 1982) that will enable him to express himself while developing his ability to cope in his emotional, social, and communicative world. Because this method is very physically oriented, Timothy will also make many advances on a physical and cognitive level. This chapter will provide an overview of the method that I have created, using case studies to demonstrate how it is used both in private practice and in medical and hospital settings.

Basic Methods

This program utilizes nonverbal movement observation, dance, music, and play for the assessment, intervention, and educational programming of children and their families. It is a multisensory approach based on the principles of Laban Movement Analysis (LMA), the discipline of authentic movement, dance movement therapy practice, early childhood development research, play, creativity, mindfulness mediation, and hypnosis. The term *ways of seeing* was chosen to describe this program to emphasize that there are many ways to look, to assess, to receive information about self and other. In this method, the therapist is asked to become aware through observation and interaction of how nonverbal and multisensory-based experiences may be influencing an individual's experience. These individuals include oneself, children, and other family members involved in the child's intervention or educational program. Observing personal experiences as the therapist or parent is as essential a component of the treatment as the observations of the designated patient. Ways of seeing emphasizes that observation of nonverbal and personal "felt-sense" experiences are key techniques that facilitate the understanding of self and others.

A basic principle is that every individual creates a nonverbal movement style or profile composed of a unique combination of movement qualities that are observable to the trained eye. These movement styles reveal aspects of the mover's experience with his or her surroundings. The therapist and parent are encouraged to look beyond their initial impression of a child's behavior and ask, "If this action is a communication, what might this child be saying?" In turn, the therapist and parent are asked to pay attention to their own reactions and responses to the child's behaviors—through a particular self-observation system that will be discussed later in this chapter—to become aware of how these personal internal and external behaviors may be contributing to the interaction, known as the dancing dialogue.

It is relationship based, with the strength of the emotional bond being paramount, supporting all other areas of development. Parental involvement is encouraged both within the sessions and in separate individual sessions. This treatment is helpful with a wide range of children, including those with autism, pervasive developmental disorder (PDD), developmental delays, communication and language disorders, sensory integration disorder, attention deficit hyperactivity disorder (ADHD), Tourette's Syndrome, issues associated with dysfunctional relational skills, adoption, trauma, and parent–child attachment issues. This program has also been adapted to work in integrative-medicine hospital settings, with a particular protocol to support painful medical procedures. Each of these applications of the program will be discussed in this chapter through discussion and case study presentation.

A Dance/Movement Psychotherapy Theoretical Approach

The term psychotherapy is added to the dance movement therapy description to highlight that the foundation of this program is psychotherapeutic. The primary focus of this form of treatment is psychological. The first task is to create a socially, emotionally, and neurologically safe environment that enables the child to express feelings, issues, concerns, and past and current experiences that are affecting optimum psychological functioning. Dance movement psychotherapy utilizes the mediums of music and dance as modalities to support mental and emotional growth. Because body movement is a salient element of the treatment, this form of therapy also supports growth and integration of motoric, perceptual-motor, verbal processing, and social skills, cognition, and communication. The multifunctional aspects of this treatment modality frequently cause observers to mislabel it as a form of physical therapy or occupational therapy.

Psychotherapy is emphasized to distinguish dance/movement therapy from other body-based therapies that are frequently used with children. These methods are typically skill-based, setting goals that specifically target functional skills such as improved hand grasp, muscle strengthening, muscle relaxation, or improved coordination. Although such improvements will also be evident in a dance movement psychotherapy treatment, the primary focus is emotional expression, building relationships, and improving social skills. The body, movement, and dance serve as added tools within the psychological therapy process used to support the unfolding of the child's social and emotional current and historical experience. Using such nonverbal means of expression enables preverbal, unconscious, or traumatic experiences to be revealed.

Core Principles of the Program

The core principles of this program state:

- Every individual creates a nonverbal movement style based on multisensory experiences composed of a unique combination of movement qualities.
- These qualities are the child's expressive/communicative style regardless of how conventional or atypical that style may be.
- Skill and developmental levels are looked at within the context of the quality of the child's nonverbal behaviors.

- Even severe movement limitations have a qualitative element to them; it may be in the level of tension in their musculature, the position the body habitually takes, or the frequency of eye contact.
- How these qualities are expressed create a sensation, an attitude, a response from the "mover" to those in the environment.
- In return, the observer of these behaviors has a reaction, based on his or her own experiences.
- It is this action–reaction that influences the developing social/emotional relationship, and impacts therapeutic and educational interventions.

Based on authentic movement practice (Adler, 1987, 2002), therapists are asked to monitor personal multisensory and nonverbal reactions through a specific self-observation process involving objectively mapping the details of the mover's actions (witnessing); becoming aware of and reflecting upon their own sensorially based reactions (kinesthetic seeing); and becoming aware of and reflecting upon their emotional reactions derived from experiencing these interactions, which include actually "trying on" the mover's actions (kinesthetic empathy). In this way of working, therapists take a very active role during engagement with the child.

Becoming aware and attuned to one's own multisensory reactions and responses has two functions. First, it enables therapists to become more open to the possible multisensory ways children may be experiencing their surroundings. Young children initially explore, discover, and express themselves in their world primarily thorough their multisensory and nonverbal experiences. Second, the therapists' self-monitoring of multisensory and nonverbal reactions enable them to become aware of the role they are playing in the developing relationship on a more subtle experiential level. Though nonverbal actions and reactions occur simultaneously with verbal and cognitive processing during communications and engagements with others, we tend to not register these reactions and modes of expression. Much of the detail of sensorial and nonverbal communication is unconsciously recorded. It is essential to emphasize that therapists must be careful to view their observations as their own, not assume they represent the child's experience, for one cannot truly know another's experience. The self-observation process expands the therapists' attentiveness to this way of seeing, providing an added perspective in which to support the growing relationship and the intervention.

The opening vignette exemplifies how I used this self-observation process to attune to Timothy. I carefully describe his actions and my first thoughts as I hear him outside my office door, and he enters the room (witnessing). I pay close attention to alert sensations of my body (kinesthetic seeing) as I take in his questioning; and I notice my emotional excitement, laced with caution, as I begin to engage with him more deeply (kinesthetic empathy).

Sense of Body

The next core concept is the principle that infants enter the world with a sense of body, from which they initially perceive their surroundings and that they use to express themselves. Building upon Stern's(1985) experientially based sense of a core self, sense of body relates to the infant's experience of its own body, interpersonal relationships, and the emergence of individuality. It functions from the notion that physical experience and emotional, cognitive, and perceptual experiences are linked (Piaget,1962, 1970; Piaget & Inhelder, 1970). It was developed based on the tenet that an infant's earliest experiences occur through the body. These experiences are initially registered on a somatic, kinesthetic, sensorial level (Gaensbauer, 2002, 2004). Body-oriented experiences shape how the infant begins to make sense of its surroundings and how it begins to develop as a feeling, acting, moving, communicating, cognizant being in the world.

Through body sensing, which includes sensing one's own body as well as the body of others, the infant first begins the dance of relating (Stern, 1977, 1985, 2004). The body and this interactional dance of relating are continually intertwined, informing and developing one another. Therefore, the therapist regularly thinks about how the child's way of experiencing the world from a very physical level is affecting how that child receives, reacts, and responds to experiences. I developed this view based on a thorough investigation of early childhood research and theories, which will be briefly discussed later. How I use this concept of a sense of body is exemplified in my processing notes as I review an activity Timothy and I created during a later session.

I am intrigued by the way in which Timothy intertwines his arms and pulls them toward himself, clutching his fingers and creating a tight upper body container. From this tense posture his fingers suddenly extend and flex with an intermittent jagged grasp, quickly ending again in a tight clutch. I choose a piece of music with a steady beat to capture and sustain the momentary pulsing beat he creates with his hands. This excites Timothy, evidenced by the way in which he pulls his arms in, creating an even firmer pulsing gesture that seems to dissipate into a fixed hold. *Witnessing*: How interesting. His actions match his verbal expressions—he quickly jumps from thought to thought and seems to get stuck, perseverating on an idea, losing the spontaneous turn-taking exchange of conversation. *Kinesthetic seeing*: As I try on this gesture I note how I become consumed by the sensation of my arms and hands, acting as a rigid shield from the outside world.

I place my hands over his, matching his sporadic beat for a few measures. Holding his hands, I add a more rhythmic emphasis to the pulse to suggest the beat of the music while also taking steps with my feet. He steps with me two steps before he is overcome by a surge of tension that stops us. Timothy beams his bright blue-eyed smile as he looks directly up at me. *Kinesthetic empathy*: I feel a surge of excitement well inside me. We have taken our first dancing duet steps. His enthusiasm is palpable too. *Witnessing*: The start-and-stop manner of his gesture seems to be compulsive rather than purposeful, much like his language use. So I must continue to add movements that create fluidity and continuity—this will enable him to physically and emotionally feel sustained social engagement.

This rhythmic dance grows over the next 6 months as Timothy continuously steps to the beat while holding my hands, dancing around the whole room. We begin to also dance to waltz music, further developing his kinesthetic experience of flow and fluidity. His idiosyncratic arm- and hand-tightening gesture occurs less and less, and his conversation begins to become more connected; I am able to see how each thought is linking to the next thought in creative and associative ways, and his ability to respond to a question or comment begins to emerge.

Core Principles and Strategies That Guide a Session

The therapist asks three questions as each session unfolds:

1. How does the child's way of relating and moving color that child's experience?
2. What does it feel like to experience the world through that child's particular structuring of his or her movements?
3. How can I structure an environment that enables the child to experience his or her own way of relating and functioning while simultaneously enabling the child, through that experience, to explore new ways of interacting with the environment?

The answers to these questions are found by experiencing the child's movement style during the session noting the *feeling tone, energy level* and *overall essence in the air*. The feeling tone refers to the child's emotional mood. Evaluating the actual body and movement actions the child performs in relation to the amount of concentration the presenting activity demands assesses the energy level. The child's energy level may be categorized as high, neutral or calm, low, or lethargic. The essence in the air refers to the overall feelings and emotions that are present and palpable in the room when the child—and other significant caregivers who attend sessions— enter and engage in interactive activities during the session. These elements are assessed keeping in mind that they are largely based on the therapist's subjective interpretations influenced by the therapist's own projections, misunderstandings, or an inability to perceive some aspect of the child at any particular moment. The self-observation procedure (discussed above) is specifically designed to reveal how such subjective reactions may be influencing the therapist's observations, perceptions and actions.

Creating experiential therapeutic activities to engage the social and emotional dialogue occur through a four-part procedure:

1. Match—feel the quality of the nonverbal cues through attunement or mirroring
2. Dialogue—create a dialogue through the use of these movements
3. Explore and expand—explore, expand, and develop these movements
4. Nonverbal to verbal—move the communication from nonverbal to verbal exchange—if communicative skills are available

Attunement and mirroring are the two essential methods used to try on a child's movements. During attunement, the therapist matches a particular quality of the child's movement without completely depicting the entire shape, form, or rhythmic aspect of the action in exact synchrony or simultaneity with the child. A characteristic of the action is portrayed but may not occur with the same body part, spatial attention, or intensity. In mirroring, the therapist embodies the exact shape, form, and movement qualities of the child's actions, creating a mirror image of the mover. This qualitative matching includes depicting and connecting to the emotional expressivity of the child's movements. Because exactly mirroring movements is very difficult, I have developed three categories of mirroring to more accurately represent what happens during the mirroring process: *mirroring modified, mirroring exaggerated,* and *mirroring diminished.* In mirroring modified, the overall style of the movement is still intact but some aspect may be modified slightly. During mirroring exaggerated, the therapist enlarges the child's movement qualities while the overall sense and style of movement remains intact. In mirroring diminished, the therapist reduces some aspect of the child's movement qualities, but the overall sense and style of the movement is still present.

Assessment of Movement Qualities Using Laban Movement Analysis

Five elements of the LMA system are used to analyze the nonverbal qualities of the child's movements (Bartenieff & Lewis, 1980; Laban, 1976). These five elements are effort, body, space, shape, and phrasing. Briefly described here the qualitative elements of a movement refer to the specific descriptive components of a physical action. These qualitative elements provide information about how (effort) an action is performed; what (body) body parts execute the action; and where (space) the action occurs in reference to others and the surrounding spatial environment. The shape of the movement describes the forms the mover's body makes in space. It reflects how the mover creates changing body shapes in relation to one's self and others in the surroundings. Phrasing refers to how the movements are clustered together over a period of time, creating a flow, pulse, rhythm, and melody, as the actions start, continue, pause, and stop. Phrasing marks the unfolding flow of the movement sequence. These details color the child's experiences and impact nonverbal expressions. It is these qualitative elements that construct a nonverbal language of movement.

Dynamic Processes

During sessions, a dynamic process occurs through the use of the body, movement, and dance-based activities. The term dynamic is used here from a systems theory perspective to emphasize that the nature of the session and the changes and growth in the sessions can occur simultaneously, rather than in a hierarchical manner. Four dynamic processes govern a session:

Dynamic Process I: Establishing Rapport—Each session strives to enhance the child's social/ emotional and communicative development and attachment.

Dynamic Process II: Expressing Feelings—Each session fosters the expression and exploration of feelings, emotions, traumas, and conscious and unconscious past and current events.

Dynamic Process III: Building Skills—The body, movement, and dance aspects of the session enable the enhancement and development of physical, cognitive, and coping skills in tandem with the inherently psychologically based social, emotional, and communicative focus of a dance movement therapy session.

Dynamic Process IV: Healing Dance—Through each session the child is able to explore the intrinsically healing and joyful experiences of dance, movement, and multisensory discovery.

Intervention Tools

There are a wide variety of ways the body, movement, and dance activities are used in a session. In the service of brevity, the reasoning behind the most common and basic dance movement therapy activities are simply outlined here.

- *Movement*—observe the actual actions the mover chooses to use (which may be a conscious or unconscious choice). Specifically noting how a movement is performed can reveal a great deal of information about that person.
- *Dance*—emphasizes lyricism. Looking at movement and interaction as a dance shifts the therapist's vision into seeing how movements link together.
- *Drama and Storytelling Dance-Play*—The use of movement, pantomime, and dramatic expression are very useful tools with toddlers and older children, facilitating imagination and enabling the symbolic exploration of feelings.
- *Exercise and Yoga*—these specific organized movement forms can be used to add structured movement exploration to improvisational aspects of session.
- *Relaxation and Visualizations*—These experiences, often involving breath work, enable the child to gain better body awareness, calmness, and modulation and organization of the body.
- *Space*—The placement of self, other, and objects; the types of spatial pathways; and how the whole room or parts of the room are used can greatly inform and influence the progress in the session.
- *Body*—This is the primary tool the dance therapist uses to encourage the child's self expression. The therapist and parent (if present) use their bodies to mirror and attune to the child. Using the body as a therapeutic tool provides a spontaneous interactive structure. There are endless possibilities for qualitative variation through changes in facial affect, muscle tone, physical shape, the use of touch, breath, and sound.
- *Sensorially Rich Environment*—All props—such as scarves, balls, textures, streamers, pillows, mats, blankets—are open-ended, fostering the child's own imagery and use.
- *Music and Rhythm*—There is an extensive use of a wide variety of music and rhythmic styles that can be used to affect the environment. Rhythms can be developed with and without music. These elements can change the overall mood of the room or the participating individuals. It can create a sense of calm and relaxation; stimulate expression and memory; or mobilize, energize, and regulate the mover.

Interfacing with Child Development

A strong component of this program utilized early childhood development research. I have concentrated specifically on research that focuses on infant memory, the acquisition of language, early brain development, multisensory experience, and the development of attachment through detailed nonverbal analysis of parent–infant dyads. This research has provided insight into what exactly might be happening through the nonverbal activities used during dance movement psychotherapy sessions that support children's improved relating skills and heightened ability to express their inner feelings.

Attachment theory has greatly informed much of the program. Bowlby (1969), considered the father of attachment theory, states that the mother's role is to create a safe haven, a solid base of support from which the infant is able to receive pleasure, understanding, and comfort through her accurate reading and responding to her baby's cues. From this solid base the infant is able to explore the world and feel able to return to (mother) in times of danger. Actually, the primary factor in creating a solid and secure attachment involves the parent's ability, sensitivity, accurate reading, and appropriate and consistent response to baby's cues and signals (Ainsworth, 1978; Egeland & Erickson, 1999). This greatly supports the extensive use of analyzing the individual nonverbal qualities of the child's personal movement repertoire. This is used to gain insight into the child's experience and expression of self, the parent–child relationship, and how the child interacts with others in the environment.

The role of nonverbal interaction and the use of nonverbal activities to support interaction are further supported by the work of Hofer (1981). Hofer's (Tortora, 2004b) extensive infancy attachment research with animal models has studied how the maternal figure's behaviors and actions shape and regulate the physiological, neurophysiological and psychological functioning of her babies. His work concludes that regulators of physiology are embedded in the relationship with mother. The quality of the mother–infant relationship affects the infant's physiology, neurophysiology, and psychology.

The exchange between mother and infant unfolds during each interaction and is co-constructed at the nonverbal level involving self-regulation and interaction or co-regulation (Beebe & Lachmann, 2002). Self-regulation as described by Beebe notes how each person's ability to relate to another person is affected by his or her own behaviors and state of internal regulation. Interactive or co-regulation refers to how each member of the interaction is affected by the behavior of the other member of the interaction. The work of Porges (2004) furthers these ideas. Porges, in his studies of neurological regulation within an infant, has concluded that it is a developmental process that is contingent on social–emotional interactions. He has developed the term "neuroceptive" to emphasize the sense of safety that is established through nonverbal and vocal cues, which is necessary on a neurological level, to support an infant's social engagement.

Those researchers who have studied the development of communication and its role in the development of a strong relationship also acknowledge that nonverbal experience plays a significant role between infant and caregiver in the transformation and organization of experience into language (Bucci, 1993; Appelman, 2000). Bucci has categorized two perception-action levels of representation—a continuous subsymbolic mode and a nonverbal presymbolic categorical mode. She states that nonverbal experiences are considered subsymbolic experiences that are registered in multiple nonverbal modalities—sensory, kinesthetic, somatic—and become organized into nonverbal perceptual images. The presymbolic nonverbal modes occur before symbolization, and enable the infant to categorize events, objects, and experiences into groups of discrete prototypic images. These perceptual images become nonverbal symbols that are autonomous of language (Appelman, 2000). They are the basis from which nonverbal experiences connect to linguistic expression.

A key element of nonverbal interactions that support the development of a secure bond, noted by many of these researchers, is the importance of the infant to be able to communicate with flexibility and spontaneity. Spontaneous dynamic nonverbal interactions between caregiver and infant create mental representations that organize the experience for the infant (Bowlby, 1969). Flexibility within the relationship and in the young child's ability to navigate independently in its surroundings becomes an essential component of healthy functioning. As stated by Thelen and Smith (1994), an infant who is able to respond and explore novelty and variation within the environment demonstrates a greater range of capabilities and flexibility.

These concepts are used to create a therapeutic milieu that feels secure and safe, to understand the role of the primary relationship between significant caregivers and the child, to constantly keep in mind the role each participant plays in the interactive nonverbal dancing dialogue, and the significant use of nonverbal exchange as a primary means of developing communication and relationship. Each session is created by following the child's lead. Activities are created spontaneously by staying attuned to the child's cues and nonverbal directives. Significant caregivers often take an active role in the treatment session.

The Use of the Nonverbal and Its Role in Supporting Preverbal or Traumatic Experiences

The use of nonverbal, movement, and body-based activities also enables experiences that are early, preverbal, nonsymbolic, kinesthetic, or unconscious to naturally unfold during the treatment process. This aspect of dance movement psychotherapy is especially significant, for it provides an avenue into experiences that are typically difficult to unearth because they have occurred early in life or may be traumatic in nature.

Gaensbauer (2004) has extensively studied infancy memory with a particular emphasis on traumatic events that occur during the early years. He states that during infancy the baby perceives and links emotional and somatic experiences, developing a preverbal and sensory-based memory system. Early experiences form memories that are registered and organized through somatic, sensory, kinesthetic, and nonverbal modalities. From these experiences perceptual images are created and represented through "perceptual-cognitive-affective-sensory-motor schemata" that translate these experiences into observable personal actions. This process links emotional and somatic experiences, developing a preverbal and sensory-based memory system.

This knowledge has greatly informed the Ways of Seeing method. The therapist must constantly keep in mind how previous experiences may be influencing patients' behaviors, observable in their personal nonverbal movement style, the activities they choose to do, how they relate to others, and the storylines that develop during the therapeutic dance-play. The therapist must also be mindful of how current experiences may affect the individual's continued development and will be revealed in similar ways. Nonverbal, kinesthetic, and felt-sense memories occur throughout life. These experiences greatly impact and can alter how an individual develops a personal body image and a sense of self. Focusing on early and felt-sense kinesthetic memory has been especially influential in the development of the program in a medical setting working with pediatric cancer care.

Medical Dance/Movement Therapy for Pediatric Oncology

Medical dance therapy defined by Goodill (2003, p. 17) as "the application of dance movement therapy services for people with primary medical illness, their caregivers and family members" has been developing as a specialization of the field since the 1970s. I have developed a dance movement psychotherapy program for pediatric patients at a metropolitan cancer care hospital since 2003. This program is offered through the department of Integrative Medicine Services. Treatment is provided on both the inpatient and outpatient units of the hospital. These services include individual sessions at the patient's bedside and group sessions in the playroom. The patients who have received dance movement therapy range in age from several weeks to 32 years old. Many of these sessions, especially with the very young children (birth to 5 years) also include family members who are often present with the child. The goals of these sessions include

1. Pain relief/management and comfort
2. Strengthen body awareness and body/self image in relation to the changes in the patient's body due to treatments

3. Develop relaxation techniques
4. Decrease anxiety in relation to treatment procedures and hospitalization
5. Create an environment that supports emotional self-expression about the patient's experience of his or her illness, through symbolic imagery and improvisation using movement, dance, and music
6. Enjoy the fun, pleasurable, and healing aspects of actively using one's body through creative dance expression
7. Provide emotional support, information and movement activities with family members that provide them with additional ways to engage their child

Four-Question Protocol in Medical Settings

The three-question protocol stated earlier is slightly modified in the medical setting to support the patient to consider how the illness and medical treatments may be impacting his or her pre-existing sense of self and ways of relating. The therapist has the added task of trying to detect who the patient "is" underneath this layer of illness, and how the onset of the illness may be influencing the current presenting behaviors. The ultimate goal is to help patients feel as comfortable within themselves as much as possible, portraying their familiar or natural self.

1. How does the patient's unique way of relating and moving reflect his or her experience of his or her illness?
2. How does the patient's experience of this illness color his or her unique way of relating and moving?
3. What does it feel like to experience the world through that patient's particular expressive movement repertoire?
4. How can a therapeutic environment be structured to enable the patient to experience his or her nonverbal expression as a communicative tool, while simultaneously enabling the patient to use that experience to explore new ways of coping with this illness?

These questions are easily illustrated through the following vignette. Due to the confidential nature of this work, the cases provided from the hospital represent a composite of individual dance therapy sessions.

Francesca

I enter the room of Francesca, a 3-year-old girl, who is hooked up to several tubes through a port on her chest. I have danced previously with this normally bright-eyed, spirited girl, but today she is quite still. Her father tells me she has not moved for 24 hours. Francesca entered the hospital yesterday for a quick outpatient procedure but had to be admitted due to an abnormality in her blood. They want to observe her and do more tests. She was despondent when I first suggested we dance. I note her sadness, and wonder if I sense a tinge of anger as she looks away. I put on a tango song that has a compelling, medium tempo beat and a mysterious beckoning melody, and sit across from her. Francesca cannot help but begin to bounce her leg to the rhythm. Staying aware of my own kinesthetic empathic reactions, I sense her action as an act of defiance, as I attune to her beat, clapping my hands in tempo with her leg. I create the quick flick of her leg with a short clip to my clap. She increases her motion. I increase the strength of my clap, as a way to further acknowledge her feelings. But, as often happens with such attunement, we can't help but begin to relate. The anger melts as our dancing dialogue becomes more and more playful. Suddenly Francesca jumps up and down on her bed to the rhythmic beat of a tango song, holding the tubes connected to her body up high as an arching bridge to go under and around. A nurse enters and is swept into the dance, circling around as she waves her arms in the air. Francesca's papa is thrilled and joins in too. We end our session with a calming waltz, all holding hands and swaying to the undulating beat. As I leave I overhear Francesca asking, "Papa can you play a game with me?"

Adding a Multisensory Approach to Medical Dance Movement Psychotherapy

As dance movement therapists, our primary tool for intervention is the body—which is a multisensory organism. Combining my years of experience using the body as a tool for expression and change with my training as an early childhood development specialist, a natural progression of my work has developed specifically related to caring for patients whose principal issues are medical. This approach builds upon the basic principles of dance movement therapy and incorporates the important role that multisensory experience plays in early childhood development. This treatment takes into consideration how multisensory experience impacts how individuals receive and take in information, express themselves, and store these events through memories that are registered on multiple levels, including nonverbal, felt-sense, kinesthetic modalities.

Adding a multisensory focus to medically related illness is essential for the invasive and painful treatment methods. The life-threatening nature of a cancer diagnosis is a potentially trauma-forming event in the pediatric patient's life. Despite the tenderness and kindness of the medical professionals caring for these patients, they experience a constant barrage of assaults on their bodies as treatment requires both internal and external probing, poking, and surgical investigations that can include the removal of body parts and the ingestion of unpleasant-tasting medicines. Often there are tubes attached to the children's bodies through medical ports that are inserted most commonly in their upper torso; or intravenous infusions (IV line) in which medicine is administered through a needle inserted in a vein, usually in the arm, wrist area, or hand.

These treatments frequently impede full body movement. Physically, the children go through periods of feeling weak, nauseated, or lethargic. Emotionally, their reactions cover the whole spectrum, including increased attachment to significant family members, withdrawal, fearfulness, discomfort, shyness, depression, defiance, and anger. These conditions may compromise normal developmental progressions on all levels—physical, emotional, social, communicative, and cognitive. These medical experiences are occurring during a stage in their lives when their body image and sense of self is naturally forming. It has the potential of greatly informing how they construct these aspects and perceptions of their inner self.

The multisensory approach promotes an increased awareness of self and one's body. It enables patients to gain a sense of control over their bodies and the medical experiences. This is essential because the invasive and unpredictable nature of the medical treatments and the illness can leave the patients feeling like much of what happened to them is not in their control. Using this multisensory approach during the time the patient is feeling ill or during painful medical treatments can bring great relief, by shifting the focus of awareness away from the specific painful or unpleasant body experience. The patient develops emotional and physical coping strategies. This work provides ways to express feelings that are felt but difficult to verbalize.

Multisensory Approach to Pain Management

Applying this multisensory approach to pain management has been especially successful in helping both the young patients and their families cope with particularly painful medical treatments. The specific protocol I have developed for these conditions is based on all the principles of Ways of Seeing, with the addition of techniques from the practices of hypnosis (Olness, 1996), meditation (Kabat-Zinn, 1990) and pain management (Gorfinkle, 1998). From these fields, I have incorporated the concepts that concentrated breathing techniques, guided imagery, and focused attention can be used to hold a child's focus, redirecting it away from pain. Here the young child's natural propensity for fantasy and imaginary play are also especially useful. Based on the Piagetian notion that young children first learn about and experience the world through multisensory means, this treatment uses all seven senses (taste, touch, sound, olfactory, vision, proprioceptive, and vestibular) to create an environment that stimulates, redirects and relaxes the child on a physical and visceral level. This supports even the youngest child's management of pain. The importance of the primary attachment with significant family members parents especially comes in to play during this treatment; parents and significant caregivers (often grandparents) are welcomed and significant members of the treatment protocol.

Multisensory Tools Used during Painful Medical Procedures

The specific tools used for this multisensory technique include the following:

1. Touch—massage, rhythmic rocking
2. Breath awareness
3. Creating stories (toddlers)
4. Recorded music—relaxing, rhythmic
5. Musical instruments—drum, ocean drum, rainstick, tone bar
6. Vocalizing through pain
7. Use of the therapist's voice—including vocalizations, tone, choice of words—soothing, undulating, hypnotic, empathic, matching child's distress vocalizations or monotone repetitive vocalizations
8. Physical props that are sensorial such as tactile—scarves, stuffed animals, small plastic animal figures, blankets, other objects from home; visual—light sticks, softened lighting in room, visuals on TV or computer screen
9. Medical: Oxygen, heated or cold pads, cool drinks
10. Participation/assistance of parents, including teaching them the techniques

Composite Case Examples

The following descriptions will best exemplify how these tools are used for pain management. Again, the cases provided here represent a composite of individual dance therapy sessions.

Ernest (age 24 months)

Ernest was having difficulty managing the pain induced by a particular treatment. This treatment protocol involves a 50-minute period during which medicine is typically administered through a medical port in the upper chest. The treatment is known to be painful for most children, with the degree of pain often likened to labor pains. The administration of several pain medications has been the typical method for pain relief, however, it does not fully alleviate the pain. It has been very difficult for Ernest's mother to watch her son enduring such pain, leaving her feeling helpless. During the most painful moments that can last for 20 to 30 minutes on a difficult day, Ernest will cry, scream, fling his limbs, roll up into a ball, kick, and hold his breath. The breath holding is especially problematic, for it diminishes Ernest's oxygen level, requiring further medical intervention.

I enter the session and begin to engage Ernest in playing with my colorful sheer scarves. We billow them up and down with our arms, and kick them with his feet, to support the active mobilization of his limbs. It can be helpful to keep the body moving and engaged. We play with images of the wind as we take deep breaths to blow the scarves, and our arms soar like bird wings as we spread our arms wide. We stomp through the ocean waves as Ernest vigorously kicks the deep blue scarf. I place my hands against his feet to stimulate stronger kicking from time to time. Other times we slow our actions down, breathing gently as we float on the top of the ocean waves, and then soar up into the sky as birds free in flight. As these activities stimulate his imagination and his mind, we are also creating impressions both mental and sensorial that we can call upon later on when the pain sets in. I put on ocean wave music with a lyrical orchestra accompaniment in the background. Mom participates in all aspects of the play. At some point, Ernest's actions become less vigorous and he begins to withdraw, pulling his legs into him. This happens suddenly. He becomes quiet and motions that he wants Mom to hold him on her lap in the chair. While he is on Mom's lap, I instruct Mom to rock Ernest in a small, pulsing, yet monotone manner. Ernest begins to moan. I mirror the moaning sound but modify it by extending the length of the tone, keeping it continuous, while taking deep breaths. Ernest matches his cry to my tone, and Mom follows as well. We are rocking and toning together to the music, providing auditory, vestibular, and tactile input. Ernest settles into the rhythm, but then feels a jolt of pain, indicating it is in his legs as he flings them wildly. I offer my hands to push against and he readily responds. We create a strong pulsing push, and soon he relaxes again, returning to the verbal toning as Mom begins to rock his whole body again. This time, Ernest closes his eyes and seems to settle more deeply. This is observable in his whole body, as it molds more deeply into Mom's form, hugging her close. He appears to be in a meditative state, as Ernest is absorbing and concentrating on all the sensory stimulation—almost asleep, but not. This is confirmed by the event that follows. A nurse comes in to ask Mom if she would like the second application of the pain medication that they typically do around this time in the treatment. Mom declined this second narcotic, feeling Ernest is "riding the pain" well. This momentary conversation causes Mom to stop the rocking. Ernest opens his eyes and begins to stir and whine. This immediate reaction to the momentary pausing of one of the sensory stimulations tells us he is deeply connecting to each element. It is the whole that gets created by each sensory element that enables him to stay comfortable and pain free, creating a complete sensory environment that consumes his focus and blocks the pain. He and Mom continue in this state for the rest of the session, as I rock beside them, alternating the vocal toning with verbal affirmations I whisper to Mom, to say to Ernest, "Take a breath in and out and go to sleep… breath in and out and rest …you are relaxed and safe in Mommy's arms. …" Both mother and child drift off to a place of calm and comfort. The medical treatment ends in this serene state. They feel peaceful and connected to each other. Later that day Mom reports that Ernest was able to jump back into his active self with far more ease and energy than previous treatments. They are empowered by their success in battling the pain and approach the consecutive treatment feeling they now have the tools to work through the experience. Our multisensory activities become their ritual, which they practice each night and employ each treatment session.

Zabaar (age 5)

Zabaar is from a foreign country and has few English words. He has been working hard to manage his pain with the same treatment that Ernest receives, but he is having trouble. He is a friendly boy who generally appears strong. He is very dismayed by his inability to overcome the pain that comes upon him by surprise. Deep in troubled thought, when we begin our session he is very quiet. I take out the ocean drum, a large drum that has small metal beads that are contained yet visible inside the drum. The beads roll along the drum cloth as one tips and tilts it, fast or slow or in between, creating the sound of the ocean waves, tumbling gently or powerfully, depending on how it is played.

Zabaar hits the drum and the beads shake. He seems to feel powerful from this crashing sound and begins to play it very vigorously. He experiments with different sounds. At some point we begin to blow on the surface of the ocean drum, tipping the beads inside of it as he blows. It is mesmerizing. Zabaar is able to blow with vigor and consistency. He seems to connect deeply into himself. When the pain sets in he lays his head down on his mom's lap. Mom rubs his back in a circular motion, and at times his head as well, circling cool oxygen (from a tube) above his head.

A multisensory dance continues to evolve as Mom and I work silently but together, providing auditory, vestibular, and tactile input. I add more sound layers to fill the room. I roll the ocean drum over his head, then diagonally to his side above his head, then in front of him, too. He seems to tune into the sound. Then I add quiet lullaby recorded music, and add my vocal tones to match his occasional whimpering. A resonance is heard through the room. I massage his feet, continuing to provide him resistance to push against when he moves his feet and kicks. I hold his feet at times, creating a heel-coccyx rocking full body action. As we massage his body, Mom and I keep our own breath flowing as a stimulus for him to follow.

Afterward, I contemplate the session. Witnessing my experience I write in my notes:

This layering of sensory input seems to be very key; as well as how the additional multisensory inputs all work in the same soothing fluid rhythm—we are truly creating a full sensory environment. This soothing, multisensory stimulation is countering, or distracting Zabaar from the painful sensory input of the medical treatment.

Conclusion

The Ways of Seeing dance movement psychotherapy approach has been developed through the integration of many fields of study specifically focusing on research and theories that support the primacy of movement and nonverbal communication in early childhood development. Built upon the notion that our bodies tell stories that speak of our experiences (Tortora, 2004), these experiences start to accumulate from the beginning of life, as each infant enters the world with a developing sense of body. This principle emphasizes that bodily sensations, reactions, expressions, and experiences of all children come from their keen physical receptivity to sensations—these are their earliest experiences of self—these body experiences define and continually inform them about who they are. From this understanding, intervention focuses on: (1) how a child's sense of body impacts his or her experience; (2) how the child's nonverbal style influences the "whole child," looking at the development of all aspects of self, emotionally, socially, intellectually, physically, and communicatively; (3) how to transform and elaborate on a child's existing sense of body as reflected in his or her nonverbal style, to support the development of more complex and functionally adaptive styles of behaving and relating that will incorporate all aspects of self; and (4) how an understanding of the role of multisensory experience can be used to support a young child through pain due to medical illness. Nonverbal observation, music, dance, movement, body awareness, and play are the key intervention tools of this dance therapy method that trained psychotherapists can use to best support growth and change in young children.

References

Adler, J. (1987, Winter). Who is witness? *Contact Quarterly XII*, 1, 20–29.

Adler, J. (2002). *Offering from the conscious body: The discipline of authentic movement*. Rochester, VT: Inner Traditions.

Ainsworth, M. D. S. (1978). *Patterns of attachment: A psychological study of the Strange Situation*. Hillsdale, NJ: Erlbaum.

Appelman, E. (2000). Attachment experiences transformed into language. *American Journal of Orthopsychiatry*, 70, 2, 192–202.

Bartenieff, I., & Lewis, D. (1980). *Body movement: Coping with the environment*. New York: Gordon and Breach.

Beebe, B., & Lachmann, F. (2002). *Infant research and adult treatment: Co-constructing Interactions*. Hillsdale, NJ: Analytic.

Bowlby, J. (1969). *Attachment and loss: Vol. 1. Attachment*. New York: Basic Books.

Bucci, W. (1993). The development of emotional meaning in free association. In J. Gedo & A. Wilson (Eds.), *Hierarchical conceptions in psychoanalysis* (pp. 3–47), New York: Guilford Press.

Egeland, B., & Erickson, M. F. (1999). Findings from the parent–child project and implications for early intervention. *Zero to Three: Bulletin of National Center for Clinical Infant Programs*, 20, 2, 3–16.

Gaensbauer, T. J. (2002). Representations of trauma in infancy: Clinical and theoretical implications for the understanding of early memory. *Infant Mental Health Journal*, 23, 3, 259–277.

Gaensbauer, T. J. (2004). Telling their stories: Representation and reenactment of traumatic experiences occurring in the first year of life. *Zero to Three*, 24, 5, 25–31.

Gorfinkle, K. (1998). *Soothing your child's pain: From teething and tummy aches to acute illnesses and injuries—How to understand the causes and ease the hurt*. Lincolnwood, IL: Contemporary Books.

Hofer, M. A. (1981). *The roots of human behavior: An introduction to the psychobiology of early development*. San Francisco: W.H. Freeman.

Kabat-Zinn, J. (1990). *Full catastrophe living: Using the wisdom of your body and mind to face stress, pain, and illness*. New York: Bantam Doubleday Dell.

Laban, R. (1976). *The language of movement*. Boston: Plays, Inc.

Olness, K. (1996). *Hypnosis and hypnotherapy with children*, 3rd ed. New York: Gilford.

Piaget. J. (1962). *Play, dreams and imitation in childhood*. New York: Norton.

Piaget, J. (1970). *Science of education and the psychology of the child*. New York: Penguin Books.

Piaget. J., & Inhelder, B. (1969). *The psychology of the child*. New York: Basic Books.

Porges, S. (2004, May). Neuroception: A subconscious system for detecting threats and safety. *Zero to Three*, 24 (5), 19–24.

Stern, D. (1977). *The first relationship: Infant and mother*. Cambridge: Harvard University Press.

Stern, D. (1985). *The interpersonal world of the infant*. New York: Basic Books.

Stern, D. (2004). *The present moment in psychotherapy and everyday life*. New York: Norton.

Thelen, E., & Smith, L. (1994). *A dynamic systems approach to the development of cognition and action.* Cambridge, MA: MIT Press.

Tortora, S. (2004a). Our moving bodies tell stories, which speak of our experiences. *Zero to Three,* 24 (5), 4–12.

Tortora, S. (2004b). Studying the infant's multisensory environment: A bridge between biology and psychology: An interview with Myron Hofer. *Zero to Three,* 24 (5), 13–18.

Winnicott, D. W. (1982). *Playing and reality.* New York: Tavistock.

CHAPTER 10

Dancing with Hope

Dance Therapy with People with Dementia

HEATHER HILL

Contents

Abandon all hope, ye who enter here

—**Dante**, *The Divine Comedy*

Since the latter part of the 20th century, Alzheimer's disease has come to join cancer as one of the great health threats of our time. Indeed, it may be an even greater threat than cancer has been. Whereas cancer is a pathological process attacking our physical being, Alzheimer's is seen to be a process that attacks the mind, the very essence of our humanity. Alzheimer's is not principally about potential death of the body, but about death of the Self.

The dominant model of care in the field of dementia has been, and remains, the biomedical, with the bulk of government funding going to biomedical research and practice. However, in the last 20 years, there have been challenges to this model from psychosocial approaches, in particular person-centered care. These two models differ significantly in their understanding of dementia, the person with dementia and the focus of care.

Biomedical Perspectives on Dementia and Alzheimer's Disease

Alzheimer's disease is only one of at least 60 different types of dementia, but is the most common. In the course of the last century, since Alois Alzheimer first identified it, Alzheimer's disease has gone from being viewed as an uncommon pathological process in younger (that is, middle-aged) people ("pre-senile dementia"), differentiated from senile dementia, which was seen as a normal part of aging, to being identified as one disease to which ever more older people are falling victim. It is seen as a veritable epidemic that can only worsen with the increase in the aging population. Key aspects of dementia from a biomedical perspective are listed below.

Understanding of Dementia

Dementia is viewed as the result of a series of pathological changes in the brain. It is progressive and irreversible. The person with dementia inevitably loses functions in all areas—mental, social, and physical. "Alzheimer's increasingly shuts down the vital cross talk (among brain cells) that make us who we are" (Snowdon, 2001, p. 93).

The Person with Dementia

Within this understanding of dementia, the person—the self—is notably absent. The progression of the disease means that bit by bit the person is dismantled until nothing is left. It is a "death that leaves the body behind" (Kitwood, 1997), a complete "dissolution of the self" (Symonds, in Gidley & Shears, 1987). The person is therefore a helpless victim of a pathological process and the person's behavior is nothing more than a symptom of the disease.

Focus of Dementia Care

There are now drugs which can be given in the early stages of dementia to slow the process and possibly delay entry to an institution. However, there is still no cure, and once the person is institutionalized, the best that can be offered is good physical care, keeping the person from self harm or from harming others and controlling difficult behaviors, often through medication.

While there is now more awareness of the need for life-enhancing activities such as social events, arts therapies, and so on, essentially these are "add-ons" to the real management of care, which is about physical care and control of symptoms.

A Personal Journey: Finding the Person in Dementia

My very first job as a dance therapist was at an old-style psychiatric hospital. It was drab and dreary and inhabited by masses of aging, spiritless bodies sitting around or pacing restlessly. Yet that job started a lifelong passion for working with people with dementia, for despite the grimness of the place and the diagnosis, I found in the dance therapy sessions creativity, humor, feeling, passion—I found people. Dancing with people with dementia became one of the most exciting, challenging, and creative areas of dance therapy practice for me. Yet this all happened within an overall context of hopelessness.

To find the gold in seemingly "lost" people was understandable in terms of my dance therapy training and my individual philosophy, but it seemed to make no sense within the dominant model of care in dementia. It was therefore with great excitement that I eventually came across the work of Kitwood (1997) and later Garratt and Hamilton-Smith (1995) on person-centered care.

The person-centered model, while acknowledging the impact of brain pathology, suggests that many other factors affect the experience of dementia, factors such as personal history, coping style, personality, culture, current environment and, most importantly, current relationships with caregivers. Person-centered theorists posit that the self of the individual with dementia does in fact persist, and that with support from others around them, people can achieve a state of well-being. Furthermore, the person is viewed as an active participant in trying to make sense of his or her world. While the behavior might appear meaningless to us, it might well be meaningful in terms of the fragmented and confusing reality of the individual. By entering and co-constructing this reality, we could support the person's own efforts to achieve meaning and a sense of well-being. Not only does this approach give hope to the person with dementia, but also hope to the caregivers that they in fact can make a difference to the life of the person.

Kitwood (1997) therefore suggested that the key psychological task in dementia care within a person-centered perspective was the maintenance of personhood. Of course, this includes having the best of physical care, but places emotional and social care on an equal footing, rather than as an added extra.

I seized on the person-centered philosophy with delight, for here was an approach that enabled me to make sense of what I was experiencing in my dance therapy work in dementia. Most importantly, the underlying philosophy fit with my own deeply held beliefs and values as an individual and as a dance therapist. Dance therapy and person-centered practice appeared to have much in common:

- An overall humanistic and holistic approach, which works with people rather than diagnoses, and facilitates rather than manages and controls
- Recognition and acceptance of the person with dementia as a creative individual regardless of cognitive abilities. View of the person with dementia as an active participant, rather than a patient or victim
- Acceptance of the person's reality and working with that reality
- The valuing of presence and the use of self (relationship) to promote well-being and growth in others

Thus, my involvement with person-centered care helped sharpen the focus of what I was doing as a dance therapist in dementia, which was essentially to concentrate on the sense of *Self*—something present in all therapy work no doubt, but given the extreme challenges to the self in dementia, totally central. I came to see dance therapy as contributing to the overall goal of the maintenance of personhood, this being about nurturing the individual's sense of self and fostering a state of well-being. By incorporating my dance therapy principles within a wider framework, I believed that I not only had a clearer focus, but that it enabled me to expand the work I was already doing.

Practice of Dance Therapy in Dementia within a Person-Centered Framework

The principal aim of person-centered care is the maintenance of personhood, this comprising two main parts: (1) supporting and nurturing the self of the individual with dementia and (2) fostering a sense of well-being. In reality, these two aims are not separate, but are integrally connected—a strong sense of self is vital to an individual's well-being.

In this section, I will discuss dance therapy practice as I have developed it within the field of dementia, drawing on both dance therapy theory and that of person-centered care.

Space: A Space to Be Myself

That little room gave us a whole lot of room to be ourselves.

—nursing home resident

Garratt and Hamilton-Smith (1995, p. 33) offer the following view of the construction of self and the challenges (written in brackets) it faces that arise through the process of dementia:

- *Identity* (Who am I?)
- *Relationships to Important Others* (Where are my important others?)
- *Memory* (I can't remember—fragmentation of memory)
- *Self-Esteem* (I feel useless, out of character, dependent)
- *Reality Orientation* (Where am I, why am I here?)
- *Abilities* (why can't I do it?)

This then is the "space" inhabited by the person with dementia—one where everything about oneself and the world one inhabits is thrown into doubt, is fragmented and meaningless.

As dance therapists, we need to bring the person into a different space. The creation of the "dance space" is a cornerstone of dance therapy work. It must offer a safe, holding environment that allows, indeed facilitates, the possibility of transformation. In dementia, this means an environment that has focus, and can contain and hold the person; a coherent, rather than a fragmented space. It is a setting of acceptance of the person and his or her reality, which allows freedom to be (within safe limits) and which invites the individual to emerge, to express, to communicate. In Laban terms, the quality of movement inhabiting this space would be in spell drive (weight, space, flow), a mesmerizing, drawing in, flowing through, catching up, joining together. It's about being (weight), strong focus (space), and ongoing magnetic energy that draws people to it. It must create a strong holding environment for the fragmented self.

Relationship with the Therapist

In the field of dementia—while in no way diminishing the value and necessity for skills and knowledge—the willingness of the therapist to engage in his or her total humanity is paramount. Kitwood (1997) talks of the necessity, using Buber's terms, of an I-thou relationship, rather than an I-it relationship. I-thou signifies a relationship of equals, a walking beside

(Buber, 1965). It is through this I–thou relationship that the person is enabled to "get together" the self.

Through a trusting relationship with the dance therapist and the flow of the movement, the individual may be able to reach beyond this relationship to other people. Fostering a social experience is certainly one of the goals of the dance therapy session.

Nurturing the Self

Kitwood (1997) identified actions—Positive Person Work—that enhance personhood and well-being: recognition, negotiation, collaboration, play, timalation (working with the senses), celebration, relaxation, validation, holding, facilitation. To these, he added creating and giving on the part of the person with dementia. The inclusion of the latter two reminds us that it is important that the person with dementia gives as well as receives. In a dance therapy session, the interventions proposed by Kitwood are manifested in the following key activities:

- Lengthy warm-ups that include much greeting of individuals, and a slow progressive warm-up of the whole group. Rhythmic music (2/4 or 4/4) and waltz music (3/4) often seem the best. The session finishes with lengthy goodbyes.
- Body/self awareness. Promoting feeling of one's self through movement, touching, and being touched.
- Control, mastery—through expanding sense of the self using one's personal space and oneself in space through breath work, stretching.
- Feeling oneself through the use of strength (Laban Weight factor)—pushing, pulling. Older people are delighted to discover and show their vigor and strength.
- Use of voice to free up and assert "I am here!"
- Singing. Where there's a culture of community singing, this is a way to bring people together and also promote movement.
- Use of props to focus and ground the person (feeling sense of self in the body), as well as for sensory enrichment. Bright colored scarves can attract attention and offer a physical link to others, as can hula hoops. Stretchy materials promote the exploration of different qualities of relationships such as pulling and stretching away from. I have found a large piece of blue Lycra˚ fabric to be one of my most valuable props—as a visible connection and focus for a group, as a "blue lung" to physicalize a group breathing experience and as an environmental representation of the sea in its changing moods.

- Flow activities that foster communication, a sense of presence, and that bring people together to engage with each other, to enable release and relaxation, to hold the person in the moment. These include clapping, shaking, swinging individually and with partners and dancing with scarves and saris.
- Using aspects of dance/movement that encourage focus and coherence—direct use of space, rhythm, physical contact.
- Being seen, being acknowledged by others. An important part of my sessions is to have participants show the group a movement they have created.
- Affirming and validating the person as above and in every way possible, e.g., using his or her movement idea in the group, tapping into personal memories, and encouraging the participants to share in movement as well as words.
- Accepting the feelings as they appear. There is sadness, nostalgia, longing alongside happier emotions and humor. People need to be able to express and feel the former as well as the latter.
- Very importantly, the person with dementia is regarded as a dance partner rather than a patient (though obviously someone who may require extra support to be able to fulfill that role).
- A session with those with more advanced dementia often means working one to one within a group setting. In such situations, it is still important for the therapist to hold the idea of a group/social experience, even if much or most of the work is with individuals. Although sessions may be shorter or longer depending on how established the group is, I allow an hour for each session. This may include only 45 minutes of active movement, for with older people more extended hellos and goodbyes are necessary. Within the session, pacing the activities is very important, in terms of allowing periods of recuperation between more active phases. However, do not underestimate the energy and passion that is possible in older people.

Promoting Well-Being

Kitwood (1997) identified basic human needs that are particularly under threat in dementia:

Attachment
Identity
Comfort
Meaningful occupation
All in a context of Love

Clearly, dance therapy meets these needs through an empathic, holding relationship that offers a sense of safety and belonging through affirmation of the person, and offering an activity that taps into what is personally meaningful. To give a clearer picture of what is written above, I will present a case study that was the subject of a master's dissertation on the experience of dance therapy for a person with dementia. In the study, I purposely focused on the woman's experience rather than clinical benefits of dance therapy, because even now, the voice of the person with dementia is mainly missing from research studies.

Case Study: Out of the Cupboard ... to the Brightness

This was a phenomenological study of four individual sessions of dance therapy with Elsie, an 85-year-old woman with dementia, who was at that time a patient in a geriatric-psychiatry hospital. I chose not to plan the sessions, but to work improvisationally from what emerged. A music therapist provided mainly improvised music in response to what he observed in our movement interactions. A few hours after each session, Elsie and I sat down together to watch the video of the session—and this in turn was videotaped, thus allowing me to gain access to verbal and nonverbal responses of Elsie to what she saw. Watching the session video thus enabled Elsie to reflect on what she'd done in the dance—a reflection that would have been difficult to talk to her about by simply questioning. Out of all this data, I selected significant moments of session one for study, plus the transcripts from all the video viewing meetings, and on these were based my conclusions about Elsie's experience. The choice to study the first session in depth was a good one, in that it clearly demonstrated much about the development of the relationship through dance and the journey Elsie had embarked upon. Elsie had come to the session rather tired that day, and while she had opted to come, I felt some ambivalence—and guilt—that I had allowed her to do so. At the same time, I struggled with anxiety about whether I'd get any useful data for my research (which in turn made me feel even guiltier). In the meantime, Elsie battled with tiredness and her desire to be helpful to me. It was only at the moment of letting go (very physically, through deep sighing and stroking down touch), and accepting the tiredness and that nothing might happen, that things started to happen. The dominant movement quality that then emerged was that of strength, with Elsie pushing and pulling against me, as if testing herself and me. This finally resolved itself when strength dissolved into flow. The music took the role of a holding environment, with us only sometimes moving, but by and large just being together and strongly connected.

Overview of the Significant Moments from Session 1

The first two significant moments introduced elements—relationship, tiredness, bursts of energy, testing strength, humor—that were explored more fully in the last significant moment. In the early stages, tiredness interfered with E's natural impulse to respond to humor, contact and strength. It was indeed the very acceptance of this tiredness by both H and E that seemed to liberate E in some way from its power and that established the relationship on a more equal basis. Without this self-acceptance and trust in the relationship with H, it is doubtful E could have undertaken the more risky testing out that occurred in the final significant moment.

In significant moment 3, she fully tested herself and H, and was very much in control of the action. E revealed herself to be a person of high energy, strength, and humor, who enjoyed being in control but also felt confident enough to share power. The final resolution of the session comes in the scene of being friends, the emphasis resting on the word "being." No longer, is there a need to do, to act, to test out, to prove. There is simply acceptance and self-acceptance.

E has made a significant journey in this session. No longer is she the tired, uncertain, unsure E of the early part of the session. Tiredness itself is no longer the enemy. It has been accepted and transformed into relaxation, ease of being. E is no longer a patient, a follower, but an equal partner in a friendship (Hill, 1995, p. 60). ("Friendship" in this context signifies a relationship of equality and reciprocity between partners)

What emerged clearly from the experience was that through the dance relationship Elsie was able to have moments when she was more "together," more sure and stronger. These, I believe, were moments of dance, when she was totally involved, totally at one with herself and with me. The transcripts from the video-viewing sessions greatly expanded my understanding of her experience, because it took me into a process that went beyond the quality of brief moments. Through Elsie's words, I came to see that through the entire progression, she had renewed contact with herself and that her sense of self was strengthened and self-esteem increased. This was very evident in the way she spoke about the images she saw on the video. The woman dancing in session one was someone else—*"I'd like to have done that work but it's just not me on there"* (Hill, 1995, p. 181)—Elsie spoke of her in the third person and heartily rebuffed any suggestion to the contrary. By session two, Elsie had begun to sometimes use the first person. By session three, she had completely owned the person on the screen and identified this person with her "old" self. This occasioned much reminiscence. Interestingly, when talking to her daughter about our sessions, she referred to "fights in the water," which harked back to a significant childhood memory, one she often spoke about to others. It would seem that through the dance therapy process and the opportunity to reflect on it by watching the video, Elsie grew in self-esteem and confidence over the period of the study. She connected with her strength and humor (*"I'm glad I'm strong,"* Hill, 1995, p.188) which had always been part of her, and also connected with her past and brought those positive feelings into her present. She realized the role the dance experience and our relationship had played in this process: *"It's brought the dullness out from me ... to the brightness* "(p. 204); *"So that's brought me out of my cupboard"* (p. 202). *I'm glad I met you* (p. 205) (Elsie's words at the last session). The strong bond we had forged in dancing together remained long after the sessions ended. Some months later, when I visited Elsie at her new nursing home, while Elsie may have forgotten exactly who I was, she did remember I was someone significant—an old friend who had shared something special in the past.

The Essence of Dance/Therapy Work in Dementia

Dance therapy in dementia is essentially "self" work. It is not about working with pathology, but about drawing out and nurturing the person. It is about offering a space where the scattered, fragmented self can find acceptance, holding and coherence, and an opportunity to achieve a more ease-ful state of being.

Other Contributions of Dance Therapy

Nolan et al. (2002) have suggested that we should move beyond person-centered care to a more inclusive model that captures "the interdependencies and reciprocities that underpin caring relationships" (p. 203). This approach, it is suggested, reflects a highly individualistic view that does not take into account the mutual impact of families, professional caregivers, and the person with dementia. For this reason, they suggest the term "relationship-centered" care. In this wider arena, dance therapists may also play a useful role.

Work with Families and the Person with Dementia

There is, of course, immense need for family caregivers to have opportunities for self-nurture and sharing with others in the same role. This is an area where dance therapy skills could make a valuable contribution in working on relaxation and release of tension, fun, social interaction, as well as dealing with issues of frustration, grief, anger, sadness, letting go, and so on. However, I see that another very important role for dance therapy is in helping families and the relative with dementia find satisfying ways to spend time together. For married couples, for instance, a diagnosis of dementia means an almost immediate change in relationship—from husband and wife to caregiver and cared for. The changes brought with this illness bring great emotional and psychological challenges to the individual, but also create huge feelings of loss for their partner, not to mention the emotional and often physical burdens associated with the role of caregiver. The greatest desire of the family is for the partner or relative to go back to the way he or she used to be—an impossibility—and they are at a loss as to how to relate to this "new" person. Contact becomes uncomfortable and at times unbearably sad. Dance therapy can offer families a space where they can be together as people. It does this by its inclusiveness—people with and without dementia are all equal participants; its structure supports their interactions—and its "aesthetic"—people are engaged in a creative endeavor that is enriching, meaningful, and touches some of their deepest feelings.

Being Husband and Wife Again

As part of a community program, four husband-and-wife couples (one partner in each couple having dementia) came together for a "movement and relaxation" session. At one point in the session I, as facilitator, got husbands to sit across the circle from wives and then we explored reaching out across the circle to our partner. Suddenly Arthur (who was the ill partner) got out of his chair, knelt down and walked upright on his knees across the circle to his wife. He took her hand and gave her a kiss. Words fail to express the emotions we all felt witnessing this. The feedback from participants and my own observations underscored the value that this sort of experience had as it enabled people to have the opportunity to be husbands and wives again. The dance therapy space gave them a language in which to communicate with their spouses, a language that did not necessarily involve words. Even when we got to the more verbal context, when we had afternoon tea together, the relationships remained more equal and it seemed like just any social event involving couples interacting with other couples. After the session, the organizer, who had also attended it, wrote to me: "J., who was the last caregiver waiting for a taxi, commented that she's on antidepressants but after today she commented she'll sleep without problems and had such a fun afternoon and she did a little step dance as she said it."

Training of Staff: Toward an I–Thou Caring Relationship

Bridges (2006) has drawn attention to the fact that we as dance therapists have a lot of skills that can be relevant beyond our specific work. She suggests it is important to identify those unique skills that we can therefore apply to the issues and needs within the wider contexts in which we work. I believe this is very true in dementia care. Training in this area has tended to focus on facts—nature of dementia (in terms of the biomedical model)—and skills. However, this has not been enough to significantly impact on work practices to render them more person-centered. Sheard (2002) suggests that we need to move beyond facts to real feelings and real life. Staff needs to connect in a real way with people with dementia so that they see the latter as just the same as themselves, except of course that they are struggling with an illness. Professionals need to be able to walk in the shoes of such a person to understand more about their experience and why they might do what they do. I have suggested in a doctoral thesis (Hill, 2005) that learning should go beyond the verbal/cognitive and work through embodied learning, not only in the sense of working on the development of empathy, but as an effective learning medium for all aspects of dementia care. Embodied learning touches the human being at a deeper level than if restricted to the cognitive, because it grounds it in the experience of the body. Todres (2007) notes that "the lived body thus grounds understanding by intimately participating in a world that can show new horizons and meanings …(it) gives to understanding the textures and aliveness of a 'fleshly' world that is relevant to persons" (p. 2). In other words, it brings understanding closer to the person than mere abstract facts.

Dance therapy philosophy and knowledge suggest the following underlying values in learning:

- Acknowledging in the first place that learning and knowing come through many modalities including the body
- Recognizing what a person already knows and accepting where that person is
- Facilitating movement in order to offer options and new possibilities
- Encouraging questioning, reflection on the part of the person

In person-centered care, the emphasis is on the self, in particular the self in relationship. Dance therapists are well placed to work with caregivers on awareness of themselves in relationship and on development of such skills, especially bearing in mind the importance of the nonverbal in this illness. Gibson (1998) suggests that people with dementia are if anything more sensitive to the affective, the nonverbal atmosphere. They need caregivers who can relate to them at this level. It is important that training therefore takes into account both the embodied nature of learning and of relationship. This is something dance therapists are well acquainted with.

Conclusion

I believe that dance therapists may play an absolutely important role in dementia care because of their skills in working with the embodied person, their empathy and sensitivity to nonverbal aspects of relationship and environment. I also believe that these professionals can make a huge contribution in applying their skills and awareness to wider issues in the field of dementia, such as the work with families and with professional caregivers. By emphasizing the humanity in all of us, dance therapy can be a powerful voice for all who live and work with this ailment, acknowledging everyone's pain and difficulty but also offering a vision of hope. I think the following from two American dance/movement therapists, Liat Shustik and Tria Thompson (2001), sums it up:

> Dancing and moving with others can open hearts not only to the fears and frustrations of life, but also to the magnificent strength and beauty manifested in bodily expression and communal bonding. Those persons with dementia have a gift of hope to share with us. Through their simplicity, vulnerability and deep wisdom, they lead us in an everlasting dance where as partners we may share the universal choreography of life. (p. 76)

References

Bridges, L. (2006). Applying dance movement therapy: Principles in treatment settings. *Moving On, 4*, 4, 21–23.

Buber, M. (1965). *The knowledge of man: A philosophy of the interhuman.* New York: Harper & Row.

Garratt, S., & Hamilton-Smith, E. (Eds.). (1995). *Rethinking dementia: An Australian approach.* Melbourne: Ausmed Publications.

Gibson, F. (1998, October–November). Unmasking dementia. *Community Connections, 6–7.*

Gidley, I., & Shears, R. (1987). *Alzheimer's.* Sydney: Allen & Unwin.

Hill, H. (1995). An attempt to describe and understand moments of experiential meaning within the dance therapy process for a patient with dementia. Master's dissertation, Latrobe University, Bundoora, Australia. Available online: http://www.lib.latrobe.edu.au/thesis/public/adt-LTU20041215.100826/index.html.

Hill, H. (2004). Talking the talk but not walking the walk: Barriers to person centered care in dementia. Doctoral dissertation, Latrobe University, Melbourne. Available online http://www.lib.latrobe.edu.au/thesis/public/adt-LTU20041215.100826/index.html.

Kitwood, T. (1997). *Dementia reconsidered: The person comes first.* Buckingham, UK: Open University Press.

Nolan, M., Ryan, T., Enderby, P. & Reid, D. (2002). Towards a more inclusive vision of dementia care practice and research. *Dementia, 1* (2), 193–211.

Sheard, D. (2002). Beyond mechanistic dementia care training are real feelings and real life. *Signpost to Older People and Mental Health Matters, 7* (2), 10–12.

Shustik, L., & Thompson, T. (2002). Dance/movement therapy: Partners in person-hood. In A. Innes & K. Hatfield. (Eds.), *Healing arts therapies and person-centered dementia care* (pp. 49–78). London: Jessica Kingsley.

Snowdon, D. (2001). *Aging with grace: What the nun study teaches us about leading longer, healthier and more meaningful lives.* New York: Bantam Books.

Todres, L. (2007). *Embodied enquiry: Phenomenological touchstones for research, psychotherapy and spirituality.* Basingstoke, Hampshire: Palgrave Macmillan.

CHAPTER **11**

Dance/Movement Therapy and Acquired Brain Trauma Rehabilitation

CYNTHIA BERROL

Contents

Introduction

Imagine, if you will, a young adult male (Ted) speeding along the highway one evening at 65 or 70 miles an hour when he suddenly loses control of his vehicle, careens off the road, and smashes head-on into a tree. As the car is stilled, the youth's head bangs forcefully against the windshield. Like a jelled pudding, his brain, enclosed in a rigid container, sloshes back and forth, hitting the anterior and posterior portions of his skull in a coup (direct) and contre coup (rebound) assault. In addition, the temporal lobes are jabbed by the contiguous bony projections along the lateral aspect of his skull.

Discovered unconscious, Ted is rushed to a hospital for treatment. Miraculously surviving the accident, upon awakening from coma 2 weeks later he has no recollection of what has happened, wonders what he's doing in a strange place, in hospital garb, surrounded by strangers. Ted has acquired a severe, diffuse, closed head injury affecting, in varying degrees, all domains of his behavior and performance.

In contrast, a more discrete injury, such as a penetrating wound from a shotgun causing an opening in the skull (open head injury), would be expected to produce more focalized lesions. Stroke, another form of acquired brain injury (ABI) differs in terms of etiology in that it is an internally induced event affecting one of the cerebral hemispheres. The functional ramifications would differ somewhat from Ted's, whose more diffuse damage presents the potential for serious secondary complications associated with closed head injury. Patients with Ted's type of traumatic brain injury (TBI) typically awake from coma with no memory of the event; their last recollection of themselves is that of an intact, functional individual (Berrol, 1984).

By definition, the diagnosis of severe closed head injury is determined by length of coma, that is, 6 hours or longer. Prognosis is commonly based on two factors, length of coma and length of posttraumatic amnesia (PTA) (Rosen & Gerring, 1986; Cook et al., 1987). Thus, for an individual in a coma of 10 hours' duration, the probability of a good recovery would be much better than for Ted, comatose for 2 weeks. The second variable of outcome, PTA, refers to the inability to remember events or to store information subsequent to the injury. The shorter the time span between this form of amnesia and the ability to consistently recall post injury events in addition to being oriented to time and place, the better the outcome. Memory of the accident is, however, irretrievable—i.e., permanently lost.

This chapter explores the nature of ABI, traumatic injury (closed and open), and stroke, that is, etiology, cerebral mechanisms of injury and recovery, and the manifested sequelae that impact the mind/body. In all three types of brain insult, although various domains of function are compromised, they differ in terms of their respective neuropathology, functional sequelae, and outcome. Three case exemplars are incorporated to illuminate how dance/movement therapy (DMT) has been conducted in both group and individual interventions. The first concentrates on individuals with severe TBI, the second on brain injury (BI) due to stroke and the last, on an individual with neurotrauma caused by a penetration wound.

Overview: Brain Anatomy and Function

Weighing approximately 3 pounds, the surface of the brain resembles a "soft wrinkled walnut." A rather vulnerable structure containing between 20 and 100 billion neurons, it lies protected, encased in a bony skull (Restak, 1984). Topographically, the brain can be mapped into three global zones, the cerebral cortex (the outermost and newest layer), the brain stem (comprising the midbrain, medulla and pons), and the cerebellum.

Moreover, the brain is divided into two seemingly symmetrical hemispheres joined together by the corpus callosum, a large collection of nerve fibers that maintain neuronal communication between them. Subdivided further, each hemisphere contains four lobes differing in location and function—frontal, parietal, temporal, and occipital. The association areas—nerve cells lying contiguous to the lobes and nonspecific in function—are assumed to be intimately involved with the integration of complex behaviors rather than with specific sensory or motor operations (Thompson, 1975).

Stuss (1988) points out that the frontal lobes have hookups to all areas of the brain and thus play a role in all aspects of cognitive, physical, and emotional behavior. The connections of the frontal lobes to the limbic system, the "seat of emotions," control the balance between intellect and the primary emotions. In frontal lobe injury, this balance can be destroyed, resulting in alterations of affect and emotional stability. In addition, Luria (1970) contends that lesions in the association areas of the frontal lobes (cerebral cortex), responsible for integrating inputs from different neuronal sources, could cause severe cognitive disturbance such as the inability to conceptualize, to plan, to make reasonable decisions, or to carry out a simple sequence of actions. Unfortunately, in most cases of severe diffuse neurotrauma, the frontal lobes are significantly involved.

Mechanisms of TBI

The brain, considered the driving force underlying all human behavior and function, manifests as an intertwining mass of soft wrinkly convolutions of grey and white matter. In an automobile accident such as Ted's, injury occurs when the head strikes a rigid surface (i.e., a windshield), and the series of shock waves set into motion within the brain causes diffuse neuronal damage. In the instance of a bullet's penetrating the skull and brain, a focal force is created in which the extent of damage is dependent upon the areas of the brain impacted. In either case, if the individuals survive the trauma, a number of factors will determine whether the damage is classified as mild, moderate, or severe.

In contrast, a stroke or cerebral vascular accident (CVA) arises from an internal source. Triggered by various vascular conditions, the essential feature is an interruption of blood flow to the brain, by either a blocked or ruptured artery. In both instances, nerve cells in the surrounding areas are destroyed. If only one of the cerebral hemispheres sustains damage due to the blockage of blood flow, physical symptoms (paralysis, partial paralysis, or weakness in muscle tone) will be manifested on the opposite side of the body. Survival and prognosis are dependent upon the location and extent of the cerebral damage (National Stroke Association).

Incidence and Demographics in Brief

According to the Centers for Disease Control (2005) and the Brain Injury Association of America (2006), of the 1,400,000 individuals who sustain traumatic head injuries each year, 50,000 die and 235,000 are hospitalized. The causes range from motor vehicle crashes (39%, 19% pedestrian related), to falls (28%) and assaults, including use of firearms (18%). Gunshot wounds—many self inflicted—are the leading cause of death in TBI. Bicycle accidents, the predominant form of recreational injury for children ages 5 to 14 years, send 350,000 to emergency rooms annually. Regarding gender, males are one and a half times more likely to sustain an acquired TBI than females. The two age groups at highest risk are 0–4 years, and 15–29 years. Falls and stroke are the most common causes of BI in older individuals past 75 years of age.

Although considered the leading injury due to the wars in Iraq and Afghanistan, the incidence of TBI reported for military combatants are not factored into civilian data. The Defense and Veterans Brain Injury Center estimates that "from 10 to 20% of troops serving in Iraq and Afghanistan have suffered some type of brain injury" (U.S. Department of Veterans

Affairs, 2008, p. 1). Regarding U.S. combatants, nearly 5,000 have been medically identified as having sustained brain injuries over the past 5 war years. However, according to self-reports (anecdotal), the number of TBIs due to "blast exposure" is thought to be as high as 300,000 for the same 5-year period (Sayer et al., 2008; Tanelian & Jaycox, 2008).

Sequelae of ABI

In the aftermath of moderate and severe neurotrauma, all domains of human function—physical, cognitive, and psychosocial—are disrupted in varying degrees. As noted earlier, one of the benchmarks for determining severity of damage as well as for predicting outcome is length of coma. For individuals emerging from coma, regardless of duration, memory of the event is forever lost. Unable to fathom what has occurred, he or she awakens to a strange new world—disoriented, confused, agitated, and often frightened; it is a time of behavioral fragmentation.

Then, the slow process of recovery begins, spanning weeks, months, years, sometimes a lifetime. Yet, no matter how significant the progress, severe brain trauma precludes complete restoration to one's former state of being. Personality, behavior, cognition, emotions, physical attributes are all affected in some measure. Family and friends, unprepared for the sequelae, cannot easily recognize this altered person nor readily accept the metamorphosis. Although individual pathophysiology varies in severity and degree, the debilitating long- and short-term symptoms require the services of an interdisciplinary team of health professionals to assist in the process of habilitation and rehabilitation for the injured as well as the significant others in his or her life. (Di Joseph, 1981; Generelli, 1984; Berrol, 1984). Following the acute medical phase, rehabilitation specialists may include traditional therapies such as psychological, physical, occupational, and speech, as well as complementary approaches such as DMT.

The physical, psychosocial, and cognitive hallmarks of ABI outlined below are important for dance/movement therapists (dmts) to be aware of as well as to understand how they can impact every aspect of a survivor's life.

Physical

Motoric problems are common in ABI. The extent and severity of impairment is dependent upon the location and scope of brain damage. Dysfunction may include paresis (e.g., partial paralysis), severe musculoskeletal weakness or abnormal muscle tone in one or more body parts, or even paralysis (total loss of motor function) in one or more areas of the body. The more diffuse the brain damage, the greater the arenas of dysfunction.

Perceptual Motor

Potential problems with visual-motor perception span spatial orientation and judgment, eye–hand coordination, right–left discrimination, depth perception, visual field cuts (blind spots in segments of the visual field), body scheme (e.g., awareness of body parts and location in reference to the self), et cetera.

Sensory

Sensory impairments may include a loss or diminution of sense of touch, pain, pressure, or temperature. The opposite problem may present as well, that is, heightened sensitivity to touch, pain, pressure, or temperature.

Cognitive

Although loss of memory of events pre- and post-trauma are typical sequelae of ABI, a major degree of return is expected. In instances where areas of the brain related to short-term, long-term or retrieval memory are damaged, corresponding functional limitations may perpetuate. Memory and problem solving issues (the latter due to prefrontal lobe damage, the region that controls abstract thinking) combine to form psychosocial difficulties. In addition, associated problems such as short attention span and learning disabilities are common manifestations, particularly with school-age children (Rosen et al., 1986; Berrol & Katz, 1985).

Psychosocial

While families more easily accept the physical impairments of TBI, the changes in personality are particularly disruptive to their personal relationships. The person they knew and loved is now transformed into a stranger, someone no longer familiar. Most frequently reported of the psychosocial difficulties 1-year post-injury are aggressive behavior, stress management, depression, emotional lability, and impulsivity (Baguley et al., 2006; Centers for Disease Control, 2005).

In a recent study examining aggressive behavior in 228 patients with moderate to severe injuries, Baguley et al. (2006) employed a research design that combined cross-sectional and longitudinal (5 years) methodology. Measurement indices included the Glascow Coma and Outcome Scale, Duration of Coma, The Overt Aggressions Scale (OAS), The Beck Depression Scale, and the Low Satisfaction with Life Scale (LSL). The OAS and Beck Scale were administered three times post injury: at 6 months, 35 months and 60 months. Most were victims of vehicular accidents (66%), followed by falls (17%), assaults (12%) and other (5%). Of particular interest, levels of aggression did not alter over time and neither injury-related impairments nor severity nor premorbid (preinjury) factors were significant predictors of aggressive behavior. Moreover, the findings revealed that the younger the age at injury, the higher the incidence of aggression and lower the satisfaction with life. Of particular importance, a significant and consistent correlation was recorded between aggressive behavior and depression. Thus, the authors concluded that management of depression is an important factor to address in treatment.

Brain Plasticity: A Neurophysiologic Mechanism of Injury and Recovery

Current theories of human physiological development and function emphasize a dynamic system of innate properties of self regulation, self-organization, and homeostasis (Campbell, 2000; Schore, 1994; Stern, 1985/2000). In other words, internal mechanisms are constantly at work to maintain a balance of the neurophysiologic systems. Similarly, after brain trauma, mechanisms are operating in attempts at self restoration. Within the cerebrum, neural-plasticity is the overarching means facilitating dynamic reorganization, an ongoing process that facilitates recovery. Although brain plasticity slows with age, various types of enrichment and stimulation trigger new neuronal connections and may strengthen weakened ones as well. The three forms reviewed below are diaschisis, collateral sprouting, and denervation supersensitivity (Bach-y-Rita, 1981; Di Joseph, 1981).

Diaschisis

Defined as "swelling and altered cerebral blood flow" (Di Joseph, 1981), diaschisis is one of the basic mechanisms related to recovery. Precipitated by the initial shock of injury, it leads to a disruption and depression of brain operation. As this type of interference within the neural system gradually resolves, sometimes over a period of years, a gradual restoration of associated functions occurs.

Collateral Sprouting

Another type of neuroplasticity, this is a process by which axons of intact regions of the brain send dendritic shoots to damaged areas to form new synaptic connections—i.e., reactive synaptogenesis. Although considered a factor advancing healing, it may also act as a maladaptive deterrent, namely, when the new connection is incompatible with receptors of the damaged site.

Denervation Supersensitivity

This neuronal response refers to a phenomenon in which intact fibers at the damaged location subsequently become hypersensitive to neurochemicals at synapses that transmit sensory information. Under normal circumstances, the reduced number of nerve fibers would not react to the stimuli; under these altered conditions, a hyperexcitablity develops, meaning that the remaining neurons are empowered to respond to stimuli formerly the responsibility of an entire region.

Other Considerations

Age, environment, and drug treatment are other factors affecting the dynamic reorganization of the brain. There's general agreement that the younger the individual, the better the prognosis and the more rapid the rehabilitation (Rosen & Gerring, 1986). Bach-y-Rita (1981) notes that an enriched dose of social stimulation—i.e., increased opportunities for positive interactions—maximizes the potential for recovery. In addition, specific drugs can be administered to help stabilize central nervous system (CNS) function.

Important to consider, as well, is that varying degrees of spontaneous recovery occur, especially in the first year post injury, as the CNS seeks self regulation via the innate mechanisms of neuralplasticity. In stroke, the parameters of prognosis are generally more circumscribed and predictable than in TBI. For instance, progress in speech (often a consequence of left hemisphere damage) begins to slow 4 months post stroke and for the most part plateaus after the first year (Wikipedia, 2008). On the other hand, although improvement slows considerably in TBI 1 year post injury, increases in function, albeit unpredictable, may be ongoing for years—especially in closed TBI where confounding sequelae may gradually begin to subside over time. A full complement of rehabilitation services may be necessary to maximize the restoration of function once the acute stages of the trauma have been stabilized medically.

Principles of Treatment

The diffuse dysfunction caused by moderate to severe brain insult, particularly in closed head injuries, requires a multimodal team approach to treatment to tap into the psychosocial, physical, and cognitive domains of behavior and performance. The approach focuses on simultaneous stimulation of different sensory systems to access the individual's areas of strength (e.g., tactile, visual, auditory, motoric) in an attempt to activate a weaker channel. Cross-modal learning by simultaneous stimulation of different sensory channels is a common educational technique, particularly with individuals with special needs.

Other standard principles of treatment in DMT and most other therapeutic and educational disciplines include

1. Begin at the individual's current level of function.
2. Build on the familiar and what has been overlearned (tantamount to a conditioned response) and consistent with premorbid styles.
3. Motivate by presenting stimuli that are meaningful to the individual. The CNS is believed to respond to emotionally charged situations—i.e., what is perceived as either threatening or personally arousing. What is perceived as neutral tends to be filtered out (Di Joseph, 1981).
4. Encourage active and proactive participation (a common feature of DMT). Treatment effects tend to be increased and of longer duration with proactive rather than passive or reactive participation.
5. Develop a structured, consistent format that incorporates ritual and repetition plus some variation to avoid habituation (i.e., tuning out).

Initially, with this population, a directive, therapist-motivated approach is recommended. As familiarity and trust are engendered in the therapeutic relationship, greater patient–client initiative is encouraged.

Areas of Intervention

It is within the framework of the principles of treatment that the targeted areas of intervention are addressed. Therapeutic goals are derived from the sequelae common to ABI and classified below as psychosocial, physical, and cognitive (see Table 11.1). These areas of function will be amplified in the sections that follow.

Depending on whether one is the patient with TBI or his or her loved ones, rehabilitation goals may differ. For the latter, the debilitating consequences of personality changes and cognitive impairments are often priorities. In contrast, patients tend to focus on their physical limitations—paralyses, pareses, ataxia (balance) etc.—rather than the psychosocial issues that interfere with their personal interactions and adaptation to lifestyle changes.

Table 11.1 Primary Areas of Function for DMT Intervention for Individuals with ABI

Psychosocial	Physical	Cognitive
Body Image	Movement Dynamics	Memory
Self Concept	Range of Motion	Short and/or Long Term
Social Skills	Balance	Attention/Concentration
Affect/Self Regulation	Motor Planning	Communication Skills
	Motor Sequencing	
	Spatial Awareness	
	Spatial Judgment	
	Rhythmic Discrimination	

Clinical Illustrations

The interventions below illustrate how DMT was conducted in three different types of treatment settings with three different ABI populations. The first is with a group of individuals who had sustained severe TBI, and the second with a group of older adults with stroke. The third chronicles an adult male, a survivor of a near-fatal gunshot wound. Several factors influenced DMT treatment, among them the nature and mission of the health care facility, the group and or individual's level of recovery and function, and in some instances, the goals and objectives prescribed by the rehabilitation team based on various neuropsychological and functional assessments

Group Example: TBI (Berrol & Katz, 1985)

The DMT intervention recounted here took place in a transitional living center (i.e., residential) whose purpose was to provide a concentrated program of rehabilitation services to individuals who had sustained severe TBIs. Clients resided in and received most of their services in a large, former single-family residence converted into a rehabilitation facility. The overarching goals were to enhance psychosocial and daily living skills so as to maximize the clients' capacity for community living and to improve their overall quality of life.

This sampler provides an overview of the format and content of the DMT sessions conducted one day a week over the course of a year. The group comprised eight participants ages 20 to 60-plus years (seven males and one female) who were between 6 to 10 months post injury. In the group portrayed here, two of the residents were nonambulatory, and most had speech and expressive language problems. All possessed varying degrees of memory deficits, difficulties with planning and judgment, and organizational and conceptualization problems. Likewise, they displayed a general lack of initiative and self motivation. In varying degrees, these participants exhibited classic impairments associated with severe brain damage. The format for each session included a warm-up, theme development, and closure.

Warm-Up The warm-up served a number of purposes: to organize the group and the body, to stimulate cognitive processing, to facilitate group awareness and interaction, and to enable the therapist to assess the immediate tenor and needs of the participants. Bach-y-Rita (1981) stresses the importance of social and cognitive stimulation via group interaction. In my role as therapist, I would typically begin in a circle formation to demarcate a visible boundary and create a central focus of attention. With the external rhythmic support of music, I would initiate, picking up observed movement

(Chacian style; see Chaiklin & Schmais, 1993) and then encourage the participants to alternate leadership in follow-the-leader fashion. In this way, we would employ nonlocomotor movement using body parts, first in isolation and then progressing to a more coordinated use of the entire body—bending, stretching, swinging, swaying, et cetera. Incorporating standard movement dynamics, we would explore various ranges and qualities—e.g., quick–sustained, strong–light, big–small, open–closed and so forth.

To kindle cognitive function, basic imagery offered a vehicle to jog symbolic processes. Some basic questions such as: "What does this movement feel like or remind you of" might draw responses like "swatting flies," or "I'm swimming," "waving good-by," "throwing a ball," etc. Similarly, imagery served as a stimulus to heighten particular qualities and ranges of movement.

Theme Emergent themes enabled the group to explore common issues of concern through movement. A recurring problem for these residents as well as for most survivors of severe brain trauma is loss of control over one's life, a phenomenon tantamount to a loss of sense of self. While the thrust of rehabilitation is to prepare individuals for greater independence, paradoxically, the rehabilitation process can unwittingly perpetuate dependency. The reality is that a direct approach in a highly structured environment is frequently warranted as a result of the individual's impaired judgment and ability to plan, or, sometimes, make even the simplest decisions. Factors such as the magnitude and extent of neuropathology, the stage of recovery plus environmental conditions will, for the most part, determine the degree of cognitive, psycho-affective and social disorganization.

During one of the sessions, working in dyads, each of a pair alternated roles, either as the active or passive mover. The active person applied tactile manipulation to resculpt the partner's posture. During the second part of the activity, the task of the previously passive person was to resist being moved. Interestingly, those individuals who were characteristically compliant found difficulty sustaining motoric resoluteness and gave in with only minimal effort. We followed with a collaborative venture. Dividing into two groups and taking turns, one half worked together to mold the other half into a group frieze.

Verbal processing followed. The participants were asked several questions related to their experiences: whether the active or passive role felt more comfortable, whether they could recall a situation in which they had felt passive or manipulated, what it felt like to resist, what it felt like to join together in a group effort. Diverse responses ranged from the comfort of passivity and lack of ideas about what to do next to finding satisfaction with both roles to discomfort with resisting. As the discussion progressed, one resident commented. "People just push you around." Another remarked, "You have to be for yourself." A third said, "I like being with everybody; it makes me feel good." All expressed enjoyment of the cooperative experience engendered by the group frieze.

Closure   The concluding portion of this and other sessions typically comprised quiet time, a time to refocus on the body, and a time to reflect on and recapitulate the session. Reviewing the shared experiences through recalling and sequencing the components of the session (either verbally or via movement) are important cognitive tools for bolstering memory. Likewise, relaxation and breathing techniques were often incorporated to facilitate sensory-motor awareness, augment body image, enhance concentration, and stimulate inner reflection.

Group Example: Stroke

Extrapolated and adapted from a federally funded research project (Berrol et al., 1997), the following intervention represents DMT with older adults whose neurotrauma was caused by a stroke. Although sessions were conducted for 5 months across five different geographic regions of the United States, the clinical sampler recounted here took place in a senior day care center in San Francisco, California. A group of eight African American seniors, all at least 60 years of age, gathered twice a week for 45 minutes of DMT. Although they exhibited varying levels of limitations with mobility (several used wheelchairs or walkers), all had functional speech. The therapeutic domains targeted for therapy for this research study included physical function, cognition, mood, social interaction, and daily living skills. Congruent with the previous group example, and intrinsic to this intervention as well, each session contained a warm-up, development and closure. Described here is a summation of one session I observed during the final month of the project.

Warm-Up   Adapting to the physical limitations of the group, the warm-up concentrated mostly on non-locomotor movement, progressing from simple body part isolations to motoric actions requiring more generalized coordination. Ritual, an important element, was incorporated throughout. Seated in a circle for check-in, the session opened with what constituted a how are you feeling today ritual (and then repeated as the closing "check-out" ritual). Feeling states were communicated individually via gesture—from palms of hands touching to arms spread 180 degrees apart, along with corresponding spoken numbers. For example, number one—palms touching—symbolized the lowest mood level; number 10—arms spread 180 degrees—represented the highest mood level. Each person's check-in was amply supplemented with verbal commentary.

Theme From a leisurely, therapist-led warm-up with individual body parts, the activity progressed to more global movement. A theme emerged as leadership spontaneously transferred to group members. When one person opted to change from sitting to a standing position, all rose and actively engaged in the rhythmic movements, whether supported by a chair, a walker, or a neighbor's arm. As an observer of the session, I noted that, as the group took more active leadership, the therapist slipped into a participatory role, assisting and guiding unobtrusively, becoming more directive only when the collective energy waned. The prevalence of music throughout—swing, jazz, and blues—seemed a unifying catalyst for synchronous movement that energized the group and sparked their imaginations. At one point, all pretended they were members of a band playing different instruments—piano, guitar, horn, drum, and finally, impersonating the conductor.

Closure Affording a time for refocusing and reflection, the group members communicated their experiences and shared feelings and memories. They gave and received mutual positive feedback and group support. Instances of integrating touch were exhibited through self massage—rubbing/patting body extremities, holding hands or shoulders, pushing hands, et cetera. A spontaneous sequence evolved when one person initiated a hugging movement; the others immediately mirrored, joining in a chorus of, "I love myself." This sequence evolved into a synchronous rocking movement in which all simulated rocking a baby. While continuing to rock, a dialogue ensued concerning their own children and how many each one had.

The closing check-out ritual now revealed arms perceptibly more open and corresponding numbers substantially elevated. At this point, increased verbal expression and lively interactive dialogue were evident. Group members responded to each other's augmented check-out levels, clapping, laughing, uttering supportive and empathic remarks such as: "Atta girl;" "You're going to make it!" "You're doing better and better;" "You looked much stronger today;" "Come on, you can do it. I couldn't walk after my stroke and look at me now. You can do it too."

Individual Example: Gunshot Injury

The intervention documented here took place in an intensive day treatment program for adults with ABI within a university setting in Copenhagen, Denmark, where I was initiating and conducting a DMT treatment program for both groups and individuals. The rehabilitation team included several neuropsychologists, two special educators, one physical therapist, and one speech therapist. Only eight "students" (as they were called) were accepted for each treatment period, a duration of 4 months—the equivalent of a school semester. For acceptance, individuals were carefully screened on the basis of the following criteria: potential for employment, academic or vocational training, partially preserved ability to communicate, some insight into his or her condition, motivation for treatment, and the ability to ambulate.

Profile of L.G.   A 35-year-old male, L.G., had sustained a severe head injury inflicted by his spouse via a bullet to his right temporal lobe that ultimately became encapsulated between his brain stem and cerebellum. Subsequent to a 1-month period of coma and a 3-month hospitalization, he received 1 year of inpatient rehabilitation. Four years post injury and with minimal intervening treatment, he entered the day program. Although living with his sister, who assisted him with shopping, housekeeping and meal preparation, L.G. was independent in terms of self care and activities of daily living. He used public transportation to and from the treatment center.

Particular presenting problems included a general lack of initiative and difficulty with auditory and cognitive processing. For example, when listening to a brief radio newscast, he would become overwhelmed, not able to filter out more than one piece of information at a time or attend to more than one task at a time, such as listening and taking notes. Delayed reaction times were also reflected in L.G.'s verbal and physical responses. Interestingly, short-term memory appeared intact; once a piece of information was learned, although with much repetition, it was retained and easily retrieved.

L.G. exhibited a low tolerance for frustration, giving up easily on tasks. Typically, his reaction was to abruptly cease an activity, stating, "I can't do that." In terms of affect, he displayed no emotion when presented with potentially emotionally charged issues such as his former wife and the shooting incident. Although he would talk about the event, when asked how he felt about it, his usual reply was, "nothing." L.G. expressed doubts about himself in relation to his life, relating that he felt as if he were standing still, suspended in time. Hopelessness about himself and his future seemed a predominant concern.

On the physical level, L.G. displayed significant balance and postural problems. His gait was uneven due to weakness of the left side, his steps small and halting. His movement was very tentative and controlled, lacking in any dynamic variation. He was unable to coordinate or replicate even a simple motoric sequence. With head and upper trunk habitually rounded forward, his focus was perpetually down, whether seated or standing, whether still or mobile. However, when engaged in one-on-one verbal interactions, he consistently established eye contact.

The psychosocial, cognitive, and physical goals of treatment established by the rehabilitation team along with input from L.G. shaped the priorities of the DMT sessions. When questioning him about his habitual downward gaze, L.G. averred that he kept his head down to see where he was going—that is, where his feet were (obvious symptoms of proprioceptive and balance issues due to his injury). As an adaptive pattern of nearly 4 years, L.G. believed this was the only way he could successfully ambulate; that without this visual cue as an aid, he would fall. L.G. stated that he wanted to work on his balance and physical weaknesses. Thus, the physical domain became the motivating stepping stone and prime conduit for addressing his psychosocial and cognitive issues

Format of Sessions To stimulate cognitive processing—an important component of his treatment plan—we would generally begin with verbal interchange, reviewing what we had worked on during the previous session as well as discussing a possible agenda for the current one. As a cognitive reinforcement strategy, these items were listed on a chalkboard, prominently displayed. To ensure a stable and secure environment, familiar movement activities were incorporated each week, amplified with variations and modifications.

Generally, we started with some sort of proprioceptive activity to allow L.G. to sense his body weight more fully—to feel "more grounded." Assuming a variety of postures, we pushed against each other physically. The challenge of trying to throw the therapist off balance proved an effective motivator. On occasion, the addition of a weight secured to his left (weak) ankle was used to augment sensory input. Included regularly into the sessions were explorations utilizing eye focus and shifting tempos. In the early weeks, music was an important external rhythmic organizer to establish a steady underlying beat to which he could connect. While L.G. walked, keeping time, he had the challenge of focusing straight ahead (eye level) and later, on specified objects in the room. Oral counting soon replaced the music. After setting an initial beat, L.G. would continue, counting aloud and moving. Later, he shifted to mental counting, finally internalizing more fluid and varied walking patterns and postures. He varied tempos, added changes of direction and focus. Increasingly, L.G. was taking responsibility for making the spatial and temporal decisions regarding his movement—an example of proactive participation.

Appreciating this newly discovered control over his body, L.G. would be seen rushing down the hallways of the facility with a singular, purposeful focus, as if late for an appointment—in Laban terms, quick and direct movement. The staff was quick to note and comment on his dramatically changed gait and demeanor. In processing how he felt about his progress, L.G. remarked that he was now able to look at the outside world, to see the things around him when he walked down the street. "I feel freer now."

Addressing his difficulties with body scheme, his limited kinesphere and movement repertoire, we often explored movement variations involving mirroring. Alternating roles, we sometimes moved in synchrony like a mirror image, or echoed—a delayed response—or altered movement qualities—e.g., reproducing the movement faster or slower, lighter or more forcefully, bigger or smaller, et cetera. Consistently, when initiating, L.G. reverted to slow, symmetrical patterns. A breakthrough occurred during one of our final meetings, when I repeatedly modeled asymmetrical and quick movements. In contrast, as leader, L.G. would slow the pace and return to his habitual symmetrical postures. At some point, a shift occurred when he spontaneously picked up his pace, offering a variety of odd shapes for me to mirror. L.G. was at last beginning to reflect an expanding range in both the qualitative and quantitative components of his movement.

During our concluding session, when asked what had been most meaningful about DMT, he replied, "I discovered I had a body."

Staff Observations   The staff attributed L.G.'s physical and behavioral progress, in large measure, to the DMT intervention, noting how it had generalized to other facets of the program. In group sessions, L.G. now sat upright in his chair, was a more active participant in discussions in contrast to his limited communication early in the program. He was consistently attentive and affable, even displaying a good sense of humor. The special educator remarked that he seemed more confident, willing to persevere with cognitive tasks previously rejected, that he was not as easily frustrated. The psychologist with whom he regularly worked conceded that in L.G.'s case, the movement experiences had been a catalyst for his psychological and cognitive improvement, that for L.G., his physical being appeared keyed to his psychic state.

With L.G.'s awareness of his improved motoric state and the realization that he could control his physical function, a more positive self image and sense of self surfaced.

Follow-Up   Two years post treatment, records revealed that L.G. was living independently, shopping, and cooking for himself. Although not gainfully employed, he was successfully undertaking personal projects such as painting and fixing up his apartment. Attending the equivalent of a community college, he was earning better than passing grades. In short, L.G.'s life appeared to be gaining purpose and meaning.

Summary and Conclusions

A review of the overarching constituents of ABI reveal that its global effects can dramatically impact both the individuals who sustain neurotrauma and their loved ones. Rehabilitation thus requires a multidimensional process, that is, a well coordinated team of health care providers. DMT has, in some settings, been a part of that collaboration.

This chapter was intended to address key facets related to working with survivors of ABI in the rehabilitation setting. Spanning a broad spectrum of issues relevant to DMT, the subject matter included the nature and neuropathological mechanisms of ABI (specifically, TBI and stroke), etiology, and demographic data, the ubiquitous functional consequences of injury, neurophysiological factors that impact healing, and the principles as well as target areas of treatment. The final section presented three case exemplars of DMT interventions: the first addressed a group housed in a transitional living center for individuals with severe neurotrauma; the second focused on a group attending a day-care center for older individuals with impairments due to stroke; and the final case chronicled an adult male whose neuropathology was inflicted by a gunshot wound. Somewhat unique, this last intervention took place in a brain injury center located in a university, that is, an educational setting rather than a medical milieu.

While all three used props at times, the two group interventions shared more commonalities by virtue of the inherent nature of a group process. These were characterized by: (1) use of the circle and music to organize the participants, and to promote interactive communication and personal expression through rhythmic movement; and (2) a consistent format of a warm-up evolving into the theme and culminating with some form of closure.

The one-on-one DMT intervention was circumscribed by the goals of the rehabilitation center with an emphasis on cognitive and psychosocial issues, yet configured by the "student's" overriding concerns with his movement limitations and strong motivation to work on related problems. As L.G. gained control of his physical being, corollary improvements were manifested in the psychosocial and cognitive domains. This case offers an observable demonstration of the potential power of movement as a mind–body enhancer and facilitator of human behavior and function.

In rehabilitation programs in which DMT plays a role, it is essential that the therapist possess a basic understanding of the various types of brain injuries and the corollary functional implications. Likewise, from a psychotherapeutic perspective, it is important to be aware of the confounding dimensions of neurogenic pathology. Specifically, in some instances, problems of neurogenic origin can obscure psychogenic issues; on the other hand, organic issues may be mistakenly identified as psychogenic. These variables not only help determine the potential for habilitation and rehabilitation, but guide the formulation of treatment goals as well as impact the therapeutic process. As a healing modality predicated on the mind–body process, DMT affords a valuable contribution to the rehabilitation of individuals and groups who have sustained neurotrauma.

References

Bach-y-Rita, P. (1981). Central nervous system lesions: Sprouting and unmasking in rehabilitation. *APMR, 62*, 413–17.

Baguley, I., Cooper, J., & Felmingham, K. (2006). Aggressive behavior following traumatic brain injury. How common is common? *The Journal of Head Trauma Rehabilitation, 21*(1): 45–56.

Berrol, S. (1984). Coma management in perspective. Paper presented at Braintree Hospital's Fifth Traumatic Head Injury Conference, October 1984. Braintree, MA.

Berrol, C. F. (1990). Dance/movement therapy in head injury rehabilitation: *Brain Injury, 4*(3), 257–65.

Berrol, C. F., Ooi, W. L., & Katz, S. S. (1997). Dance/movement therapy with older adults who have sustained neurological insult: A demonstration project. *American Journal of Dance Therapy, 19*(2): 135–160.

Berrol, C. F., & Katz, S. S. (1985). Dance/movement therapy in the rehabilitation of individuals surviving severe head injuries. *American Journal of Dance Therapy, 8*, 46–66.

Brain Injury Association of America. Causes of brain injury. Accessed 1/30/06 from: http:www.biausa.org/pages/causes_of_injury.html.

Campbell, S. (2000). The child's development of functional movement. In S. Campbell, D. V. Linden & R. Palisano (Eds.), *Physical therapy for children* (2nd ed., pp. 3–44). Philadelphia: S.B. Saunders.

Centers for Disease Control (2005). Traumatic brain injury in the United States: A report to Congress. Accessed 2/7/2006 from http://www.cdc.gov/doc.do/id090001f3ec800101e6.

Chaiklin, S., & Schmais, C. (1993). The Chace approach to dance therapy. In S. Sandel, S. Chaiklin, & A. Lohn (Eds.), *Foundations of dance/movement therapy: The life and work of Marian Chace* (75–97). Columbia, MD: Marian Chace Memorial Fund of the American Dance Therapy Association.

Cook, J., Berrol, S., Harrington, D. E., et al. (Eds.). (1987). *The ABI handbook: Serving students with acquired brain injury in higher education*. Sacramento, CA: California Community Colleges.

Di Joseph, L. (1981). *Traumatic head injury: Mechanisms of recovery*. Paper presented at the Coma to Community, Workshop presented at Santa Clara Valley Medical Center, San Jose, CA.

Generelli, T. (1984, October). *Recent developments in acute pathophysiology of head injury*. Paper presented at Braintree Hospital's Fifth Traumatic Head Injury Conference, Braintree, MA.

Kay, T., & Lezak, M. (1990). Debunking Ten Myths of "Recovery." D. W. Corthell, (Ed.) *Traumatic Brain Injury and Vocational Rehabilitation*. University of Wisconsin-Stout: The Research and Training Center.

Luria, A. R. (1970). The functional organization of the brain. *Scientific American, 222*(3): 66–78.

National Stroke Association: What is stroke? http://info stroke.orf/siteInfo. (Retrieved 2/7/06).

Restak, R. (1984). *The brain*. New York: Bantam Books.

Rosen, C. D., & Gerring, J. (1986). *Head trauma: Educational reintegration.* San Diego: College Hill Press.

Sayer, N. A., Chiros, C. E., Sigford, B., Scott, S., Clothier, B., Pickett, T., & Lew, H. L. (2008). Characteristics and rehabilitation outcomes among patients with blast and other injuries sustained during the Global War on Terror. *Archives of Physical Medicine and Rehabilitation, 89*(1): 163–70.

Schore, A., N. (1994). *Affect regulation and the origin of the self: The neurobiology of emotional development.* Hillsdale, NJ: Lawrence Erlbaum.

Stern, D., N. (1985; 2000). *The interpersonal world of the infant: A view from psycho-analysis and developmental psychology.* New York: Basic Books.

Stuss, D. (1988, April). *What the frontal lobes do.* Paper presented at Rehabilitation: Coma to Community, San Jose, CA.

Tanelian, T., & Jaycox, L. H. (Eds.), *Invisible wounds of war: Psychological and cognitive injuries, their consequences and services to assist recovery.* Santa Monica, CA: RAND Corporation, MG-720-CCF, 2008, 492 pp., available at http://veterans.rand.org/.

Thompson, R. F. (1975). *Introduction to physiological psychology.* New York: Harper & Row.

U.S. Department of Veterans Affairs (2008). Understanding the effects of blasts on the brain. *VA Research Currents*, May-June, 1.

Wikipedia. *Stroke Recovery,* http://en.wikipedia.org/wiki/Stroke_rehabilitation. (Accessed June 11, 2008).

Aspects Integral to the Practice of Dance/Movement Therapy

CHAPTER 12

Laban's Movement Theories

A Dance/Movement Therapist's Perspective

ELISSA QUEYQUEP WHITE

Contents

Introduction

In the early 1960s, Marian Chace began teaching her famous 3-week course in dance therapy in New York City at Turtle Bay Music School. Upon completion of the course, Chace met with individual students and evaluated their progress in the class. After that, students were left to their own devices. Some were fortunate enough to further their studies by apprenticing with Chace at St. Elizabeth's Hospital in Washington, D.C. Others found institutions where they could volunteer, practice their newly found craft, and arrange to meet with fellow students to discuss what took place in their dance therapy sessions.

This scenario lent itself to questions such as: What am I doing? How will I know if I'm doing anything helpful? How can I explain what I am doing? Am I doing more harm than good? For former dancers, it became an imperative to go back to resume dance classes in order to understand their moving bodies, i.e., to see what they were expressing and communicating as they danced. As dancers, the concern was with form and technical correctness. Now, the questions were different: What are patients seeing and experiencing as I move? Am I expressing with my body what I think I am saying? Can I communicate with patients through my movements? Is my body expressing feelings clearly? Am I able to "pick up" others' movements clearly enough for people to follow? The questions were endless.

Development of Early Training

While these questions were floating around in the minds of novice dance therapists, Irmgard Bartenieff began teaching courses in Effort-Shape (Bartenieff & Davis, 1965), at the Dance Notation Bureau (DNB) in New York City, about the same time Chace was giving her courses in New York City. Bartenieff trained Martha Davis and Forrestine Paulay and together they began a certification program in Effort-Shape at the DNB. Effort-Shape movement analysis is a system to observe, notate, and analyze movement. It is based on the movement theories of Rudolf Laban, in particular the motion factors or efforts (Laban, 1960; Laban & Lawrence, 1974). Their shape correlates were conceptualized by Warren Lamb (Dell, 1970). Prior to the introduction of Effort-Shape in the United States, Laban's system for notating dance, Labanotation (Laban, 1956), was fairly well-known in dance circles and was taught at the DNB. In 1978, the Laban/Bartenieff Institute of Movement Studies (LIMS), became an entity in and of itself and currently houses the certification program known as Laban Movement Analysis (LMA) which incorporates Effort-Shape. I was in the first certification class, completed in 1971, when it was housed at the DNB.

Use in Dance/Movement Therapy

The notion that one could learn to observe, notate, and analyze the substance of movement using a system other than that of Labanotation appealed to novice dance movement therapists. Through Effort-Shape we would be able to inform ourselves about patients and inform and educate other mental health staff about what occurs with patients in dance therapy sessions. Effort-Shape could be a tool with which these "nonverbal" sessions could be discussed with one another using this common language, presuming everyone studied it.

In early 1968, I was asked to conduct a workshop with dance movement therapists (dmts) and to teach them what I was learning in Effort-Shape. I had been employed as a dance therapist for over a year. After assessing this workshop experience, I realized that Effort-Shape was not just a useful tool for us to be able to learn and assess what we saw when we were dancing/moving with our patients but that it could enable us to know our own preferred movement proclivities (movement repertoire). Would not a movement analysis for dance therapists be akin to psychoanalysis for budding psychoanalysts (Schmais & White, 1968)? It was believed that the system of Effort-Shape could help dance therapists know their strengths and their limited and persistent movements' patterns, and learn how to develop and make use of a more varied movement repertoire. This increased range of movement would enable a dance therapist to relate in dance movement to a greater segment of people, as well as to empathize, pick up, and develop the more subtle aspects of a patient's movement expression.

In DMT, therapists are concerned with the dance/movement dialogue that occurs between them and the patients. I will mostly be referring to group dance therapy; although I believe that similar phenomena occur while working with individual patients. During sessions, dance movement therapists need to be concerned with what they see while dancing. As this dance progresses they "pick up" or develop "empathic reflection" (Sandel, 1993) while sharing a patient's dance movements. Feelings expressed through patients' movements then become available to dmts as the dialogue continues. How they choose to choreograph these dance movements to reflect feelings back to a patient, depends on their sensitivity through tuning in to what the patient seems to be expressing and what in the therapist's movement repertoire will support and involve the patients in a more defined picture of what they are communicating in the dance. Many times, verbalization of symbolic images accompanies these definitive movement statements and helps the patients become aware of what they are expressing or feeling (Stark & Lohn, 1993) and moves the patients toward healthier functioning. Verbalizations are constantly being used in a dance therapy session to encourage and support the patient's movement and emotional process.

Further Use of Laban's Work

Rudolf Laban's philosophy that life is movement and movement is life formed the basis for his interest in creating and systematizing Labanotation, also known as Kinetography (Laban, 1956), Space Harmony (Laban, 1966) and Effort or the motion factors (Laban, 1960). He was a dancer, creator of dances, and movement choirs; an artist, architect, mathematician, and teacher.

Laban traveled freely through artistic and scientific circles, giving him the freedom and knowledge to conceptualize theories and notation systems about movement. As a teacher, he encouraged all of his students to use and develop their potential and this resulted in his followers' further developing the material in ways that interested them. Thus, we have Warren Lamb, who was instrumental in developing the "shape" and "shaping" aspects of Effort-Shape (Dell, 1970). He developed Laban's material for use in assessing and training of personnel in business (Lamb, 1965). Marion North's *Personality assessment through movement* (1972) informs us of the many gradations and meanings of each motion factor (efforts) and their combinations. Judith Kestenberg, a psychoanalyst who studied and worked with Warren Lamb and Forrestine Paulay, devised the Kestenberg Movement Profile together with her Sands Point Child Development Group (Lewis & Loman, 1990). Further, Laban's work with dancers such as Mary Wigman, Hanya Holm, Kurt Jooss, and their disciples, have had a profound influence on modern dance.

Categories of Observation

The aspects of LMA, which I have found useful for both the teaching and practice of dance therapy, are delineated below. The three categories of observation—body, space (space harmony), and efforts (motion factors)—are descriptive for what could occur during a dance therapy session. Laban devised symbols for body parts, spatial designations, and the motion factors and these can be found in publications by and about the Laban material (Bartenieff & Lewis, 1980; Bartenieff & Davis, 1965; Dell, 1970; Laban, 1960; Laban & Lawrence, 1974; Lepczak, 1989; North, 1972; Preston, 1963). Once familiar with the symbols, a kind of shorthand, it is more efficient and quicker to observe and notate movement as it happens rather than to translate movement into words. Although the teaching of Effort-Shape when I studied it began with our learning about the efforts, the order here is reversed. When we initially began teaching Effort-Shape to dance therapy graduate students, we noted a tendency for students to use effort terminology—e.g., "float," "punch," "light" "direct," etc. This proved to be counterproductive, because the students would use the effort terms as a defense against allowing feelings, images, and metaphors to evolve from the movement. They relied on the cognitive use of the effort terminology to describe the movement/actions rather than delve into their feelings to illuminate what they saw. Thus, teaching about space or aspects of space harmony first enabled students to "rely" on the verbalization of images and symbolism that arose in subsequent semesters of teaching students.

As indicated above, the three categories of observation presented herein are "body," "space" and "effort." Laban (1960), referring to the body, states: "The flow of movement is strongly influenced by the order in which the parts of the body are set in motion" (p. 21). Given this premise, Marion North, at a workshop in the early 1970s, indicated how the observations of body, space, and effort overlap. However, even though these three aspects can be looked at separately during an observation, she indicated that the "body" category is often observed first. These three areas will be discussed separately, although they are eventually integrated into a whole assessment.

Body

Body Part Usage and Origination

Generally speaking, people begin movement phrases with the same body parts time after time. This is also true of phrases in a dance therapy session, e.g., a dance therapist may usually begin a session with the feet doing only weight shifts in a rhythmic pattern. When the same dance therapist begins with another part of the body, say arms, this may have been observed and picked up from a group member. When a patient initiates a movement with a different part of the body this could be indicative of many things. For the dance therapist to become aware of this new usage could turn out to be significant—perhaps an indication that change may be on the way. Knowing Laban's observational and analytic system for the body parts is important as one learns to see which body parts initiate movement and this can be significant.

Body Shape

There are four distinct body shapes—narrow, wide, curve, and twist (North, 1972). These shapes can either change or be static (fixed) and can be seen in the torso. One would think that a narrow body shape would be found in thin or slim people, just as a wide body shape might be seen in a heavy person, but close scrutiny of these types of body shapes show that a wide shape can be found in a thin person and the reverse. Curve and twist shapes are more obvious, as observations of these types are quite literal. A common curve shape can be seen in people whose appearance is that of being "burdened." Photographs of fashion models generally display a twist shape. Shape changes in the body can also be significant. A common example of a body shape change usually occurs when one is physically ill and the shape becomes more of a curve, even if one's normal shape is curve. The observations of body shape are of particular concern with regard to psychiatric patients. Their body shapes are static and fixed and when movement is observed going through the torso (where body shape is seen), it is possible that this is an indication of change soon to occur.

Gesture–Posture

The names in this category are quite explicit. Gestural movement refers to a movement that appears in one part of the body and does not affect movement in the rest of the body. Gestural movements can also be done with several parts of the body simultaneously and not affect the rest. A postural movement is one in which movement may begin in one part of the body and then travel through the entire body. When working toward full body action in dance therapy, this would necessarily incorporate postural movement, indicating a fuller expression of emotions. "There is a close relationship between the integration of postural changes and the shift of psychic attitudes" (Chaiklin & Schmais, 1993, p. 77).

Simultaneous–Successive Movements.

Simultaneous movements refer to two (or more) parts of the body that move at the same time, such as having both arms reaching forward for an object. Successive movements generally are those that start in one part of the body and sequentially move to another part. For patients, experiencing these successive movement patterns allows for a greater range of feelings and emotions.

Space

All of Laban's work occurs within the "sphere of movement" or kinesphere (Laban, 1950, 1966). There are many ways in which the body can move harmoniously and flowingly through space going from one designated point to another (26 in all, with the 27th point being "in place"). The ways in which the body can move from one point to another signify the many abilities of the body to bend, straighten, change shape, be flexible, etc. (Laban, 1950,

1966; Preston, 1963). These 26 points are found in several scales. Only three of the scales that are part of Space Harmony will be presented here and shown in their very elementary connections. Further study can be found in *Choreutics* (Laban, 1966), his second book on space harmony.

The scales are most useful for dmt students, for they help them incorporate different pathways of moving through space aside from their habitual ways. These points on the scale open many possibilities of helping patients make explicit what their dance movements are expressing. For example, a movement phrase with significant emotional content may be quite expressive, and to repeat this phrase in the same pathway could initially be a very intense experience. The dance therapist needs to understand when this moment has reached the apex of feeling and cognition, yet be aware that the patient may need to have a fuller experience and understanding of the expression. A different spatial pathway could provide this "apex" for the patient.

Kinesphere

This is the space that is used all around the body by the limbs standing still or in motion. It is commonly said that your kinesphere goes with you wherever you go. Another image would be for a person to imagine the body in a "bubble," with limbs moving around the body in "near" space, "middle" space or "far reach" space. A mover who uses near space would not reach for an object (using far reach space) but might move the body to get the object. It is sometimes very difficult for patients to use far space, such as when fully stretching above the head or extending themselves toward someone across a circle. A patient in one of my dance therapy sessions, when asked to reach out across the circle to another person, walked to that person instead of using far reach space. Some examples of the use of kinesphere in daily life can be seen: using the computer would be near space, sweeping a floor probably entails use of middle and near space, and stretching for an object on a high shelf is an instance of using far reach space.

Spatial Designations

Experience has shown that using symbols instead of language for points in space helps to identify these areas. The designated points are quite specific and once identified, the dmt can move easily to areas in space between points that are not customarily used. In DMT sessions, it helps the therapist to identify more clearly which areas are frequently or less frequently used. For example, in many cultures "forward" (F) space usage is the norm and use of "back" (B) space is neglected.

Basic Areas of Space

The three basic areas of space around the body are

High (H)-up and above the body
Medium/Middle (M)-around the body
Deep (D)-below the body's waist

Other space designations are

To the left (L)
To the right (R)
Forward (F)
Backward (B)
Center (C)

Space is divided into three planes (picture the body in the middle of each plane), and coincides with the three-dimensionality of the body—Vertical, Horizontal, and Sagittal. Each plane has two dimensions, primary and secondary (Figure 12.1).

Primary dimensions are
Vertical (H to D)
Horizontal (L to R)
Sagittal (B to F)

Secondary dimensions are

Horizontal (L to R) for the Vertical plane
Sagittal (B-F) for the Horizontal plane
Vertical (H-D) for the Sagittal plane

Where primary and secondary dimensions of each plane meet in space they form four "corners" of a plane and are referred to as the Door, Table, and Wheel (Preston, 1963).

Vertical: Door—high right (HR), deep right (DR), deep left (DL), high left (HL)
Horizontal: Table—right forward (RF), left forward (LF), left backward LB), right backward (RB)
Sagittal: Wheel—forward high (FH), forward deep (FD), backward deep (BD), backward high (BH)

Although we use all planes in everyday life, some of us have a tendency to consistently move in and be comfortable in one or more of the planes. A person who is comfortable in the use of the door plane can be said to be in a presentation mode. One who uses the table plane is more into

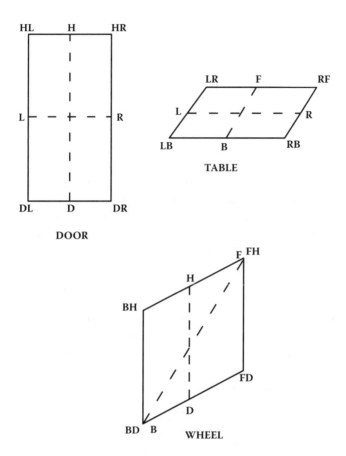

Figure 12.1 The three planes, their corners, and primary and secondary dimension.

communication, whereas the person who uses the wheel is more likely to be into action.

Dimensional Scale

The spatial areas in the Dimensional Scale (Preston, 1963) sometimes called the three-dimensional cross (Laban, 1950), or Defense Scale (Bartenieff, 1980), are connected in a sequence that starts with the right side leading: H (high), D (deep), L (to the left), R (to the right), B (backward), F (forward).

This sequence allows the body to feel the single dimensions of space and comes from the center of the body. It is done in a continuous motion (using the right arm) rising (H), sinking or falling (D), crossing the body (L), opening away from the body (R), retreating (B), advancing (F). The transitions from one point to another can create different feelings of moving in space depending on whether you go through the center of the body or connect the designations peripherally. This basic scale helps one to feel the full dimensionality of the self as much as is possible in the up–down or vertical dimension of the body, the side–side dimensions and the forward–backward dimension. Moving into these dimensions again can show where one is comfortable in the area of space, or whether one tends to avoid or bypass a dimension.

A Scale

The A Scale consists of each of the four corners of the planes following the sequence of Door, Wheel, Table. The transitions from one place to another in space are peripheral, and if one were to draw a line connecting all the points, one would see the shape of a figure with 20 faces called an icosahedron (Figure 12.2). Following is the sequence of the A Scale leading with the right arm and side of the body. Although this is the customary beginning, it can be started at any "door" point:

(LB starting point) HR, BD, LF, DR, BH, RF, DL, FH, RB, HL, FD, LB

Depending on the path from one point to the next, the inclinations felt by the body are designated as "flat," "steeple," or "transverse." With each of these inclinations the torso and limbs, because of the peripheral transitions from point to point, will experience ways of twisting, expanding, full reaching, and traveling (Preston, 1963; Bartenieff & Lewis, 1980) not

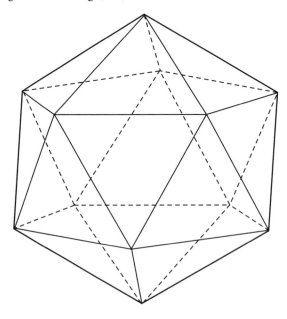

Figure 12.2 Icosahedron.

common in everyday movement. This scale gives more options for the dmt to introduce to patients different and unusual ways of moving through space. The dance becomes more interesting and pleasing when these options are available. This is a very elementary presentation of the scale and it will be helpful to study this scale more in depth in Preston (1963) and Bartenieff and Lewis (1980).

Diagonal Scale

This scale comprises one of each of the primary dimensions of the planes and where these dimensions meet in space. Because of the way humans are built, one cannot do this scale precisely, as our bodies get in the way of some of the diagonals, so one attempts an approximation. This scale lends itself to the most mobility in space. If you picture the body within the center of a cube, the points go from one top corner of the cube to the opposite bottom corner, giving us eight destinations or four complete diagonals. The pathways in this scale go through the center of the body and thus are defined as central transitions. The importance of this scale for DMT is that it helps to move a person into full body action as espoused by Marian Chace (Chaiklin & Schmais, 1993). When accompanied with full effort actions (to be discussed later) everyday movements such as chopping, rocking, sports movements, or household tasks are easily attainable and supported during a session.

The scale is

HFR (high, forward, right) to DBL (deep, backward, left)
HFL (high, forward left) to DBR (deep, backward, right)
HBL (high, backward, left) to DFR (deep, forward, right)
HBR (high, backward, right) to DFL (deep, forward, left)

Let me reiterate that for the dance movement therapist, learning the scales through practice can prove to be invaluable. This body knowledge can provide harmonious, varied, interesting, and spontaneous ways to move in space. One of the hazards of being a practitioner is that we all get stuck in our movement patterns and certainly the majority of the people we work with are non-educated in movement and sometimes their limitations reflect their illnesses. This type of dialogue sets up limited patterns and, at best, repetitious movement in space. I am not an advocate of the notion that people change if and when one alters their movement patterns. My experience is that people change when they are ready to do so. Subtle indications of change are when the dmt can see and feel a "difference" in someone's movement. It is at this point that the dmt can use what has evolved to explore the possibility of introducing new ways of moving. For example, the dmt working with a patient whose movements display only a variation of up–down in the vertical plane can, when the patient becomes involved in the rhythm of the movement, begin to encourage movement in one of the diagonals. By doing this, the patient can begin to have access to a different area of space, providing for a greater range of movement and expression.

Effort–Motion Factors

The expressive and communicative aspects of bodily movement are discernible and can be notated and codified using the many variables of Laban's spatial locations and motion factors, referred to as "Effort." "A person's efforts are visibly expressed in the rhythms of his bodily motion" (Laban & Lawrence, 1974, p. 2). Laban, together with Lawrence, who was a management consultant, worked to help those working in factories in England during World War II make the most effective use of their movements. Although effort training was utilized in a particular way for their industrial studies, Laban believed that the principles of Effort were also relevant applied to the arts of dance and mime (Laban, 1960; Laban & Lawrence, 1974).

When people begin to move, their bodies go through space in ways that offer significant qualitative differences that yield expressions of distinctive styles or personalities. These qualitative or dynamic aspects of movement are described in effort terms. As an analogy, in music the written notes can be seen as the structure (spatial locations) and the qualities called for (i.e., pianissimo, forte, andante, allegro, etc.), can be equated to efforts. For the dmt, knowing and understanding one's predominant efforts can be invaluable when tuning in and "picking up" the unique movements of a patient. This ability to carefully tune into and respond to a patient in this nonverbal manner establishes a trusting relationship necessary for the therapy process. This demonstrates the principle that Marian Chace so profoundly expounded: meeting the person where they are.

In Effort theory, there are four motion factors: space, weight, time, and flow, with each factor having two polarities. To Laban, these motion factors are the ways in which inner impulses and energies are manifested in movement, whether conscious or unconscious (Laban, 1950). They are done with intention and substance, and are not passive movements (Laban, 1950, 1960; Laban & Lawrence, 1974; North, 1972; Preston, 1963).

The *space* motion factor consists of the elements of "direct" or "flexible" (sometimes referred to as indirect). A direct movement has the appearance of having a straight path whereas flexible movement is a path that can be roundabout, wavy, or undulating. Threading a needle is an example of being direct. The maneuvering or meandering through a crowd is indicative of a flexible or indirect approach.

The *weight* factor consists of "strong" and "light." Strong is sometimes referred to as "firm" and can be seen as forceful or energetic movement. In daily life, strength can be seen in movements that are punching, stomping on the ground, or lifting heavy objects. Light or fine-touch movement can give the appearance of being delicate, sensitive, or gentle. Examples of lightness can be seen in the caress of a newborn infant, or gentle tapping on a shoulder to get a person's attention.

The *time* factor, "sudden," sometimes referred to as "quick," exhibits a sense of instantaneousness or urgency, whereas "sustained," sometimes referred to as "slow," gives a sense of lingering, endlessness, or leisureliness. An example of sudden or quick movement is that of touching a hot stove or jumping out of the way of danger. Sustained or slow movement is often seen in an unhurried walk or a lingering stretch.

The *flow* factor of movement can either be bound or free. Movement that is controlled, restrained, or that can be stopped during midstream is referred to as bound flow. This type of flow is useful in the careful stepping on uneven rocks or in the careful approach to picking up tiny objects. Movement that seems to be difficult to stop or is fluent or ongoing with ease is called free flow. Swaying and rocking are movements that exemplify free flow, as does the gushing of enthusiasm when two friends unexpectedly meet. With many psychiatric patients, either because of medications or their illnesses, the flow of their movement is mainly bound. Many times, this can be seen in the torso as if there is an attempt to be held together.

According to Laban (1960), "The person who has learnt to relate himself to Space and has physical mastery of this, has Attention. The person who has mastery of his relation to the Weight factor of effort has Intention, and he has Decision when he is adjusted to Time" (p. 85). The ease or restraint or the preciseness of actions is controlled by Flow.

The material in this effort section is abstract and cannot be learned from merely reading about it—one has to "move" it and kinesthetically experience the sensations that each of the effort elements produce as you move. Extended research and study of Space–Attention, Weight–Intention, Time–Decision, Flow–Precision is presented by North (1972) and it provides us with refined meanings of the degrees of the motion factors that are seen in movement.

A person's daily movement phrases fluctuate between combinations of two or three motion factors. The combinations of two motion factors "reveal inner states of mind" (North, 1972, p. 246) reflecting a mover's inner attitude. They are briefly presented here with their inner states: space and time (awake), flow and weight (dreamlike), space and flow (remote), weight and time (near), space and weight (stable), time and flow (mobile) (Laban, 1960, Preston, 1963) The combinations of three motion factors are called drives. There are four of these: "passion" (with no use of space), "vision" (no weight), "spell" (no time), and "action" (no flow). Free or bound flow often accompanies the action drive and it is then called a full effort action

Table 12.1 Basic Effort Action Drives

Effort Action	Name	Spatial Affinity
Light, Flexible, Sustained	Float	HRF (high, right, forward)
Strong, Direct, Quick	Punch or Thrust	DLB (deep, left, backward)
Light, Direct, Sustained	Glide	HLF (high, left, forward)
Strong, Flexible, Quick	Slash	DRB (deep, right, backward)
Light, Direct, Quick	Dab	HLB (high, left, backward)
Strong, Flexible, Sustained	Wring	DRF (deep, right, forward)
Light, Flexible, Quick	Flick	HRB (high, right, backward)
Strong, Direct, Sustained	Press	DLF (deep, left, forward)

(Bartenieff & Lewis, 1980). Explanation of these are beyond the scope of this chapter, but we all move in these inner states and drives as part of our everyday movement life and they are seen often in DMT sessions.

An interesting aspect of Laban's theories that has been orally passed down is the concept that motion factors are more natural or easier to do in certain spatial areas and are referred to as space and effort affinities. Laban (1950) does state that the

"three-dimensional cross can ... be seen to relate to the motion factors of weight in the up–down dimension (light–strong), of space in the spreading of the side–side dimension (direct–flexible), and of time in ... activities producing the forward-backward dimension (slow–quick)." (p. 125)

The motion factors are more easily done and learned with their spatial affinities, although the efforts can be done in any area of space.

For the purposes of DMT, the eight basic efforts sometimes called the Basic Effort Action Drive (Laban & Lawrence, 1974; Bartenieff & Lewis, 1980) have proved very worthwhile because of the DMT principle of supporting and encouraging full body action (Table 12.1). These actions more easily bring into awareness feelings being expressed and communicated in a patient's movements. This action drive (Space, Weight and Time) when done with their spatial affinities, gives the mover the most dynamic movement and mobility in space. This is learned and practiced as if one were inside a cube linking the eight diagonal directions in space with the eight effort actions (See Figure 12.3).

It is common during a DMT session for the dmt to support "quick" movements that could be expressive of aggressive or angry feelings by encouraging repeated and rhythmic "punches" or "stamping." But, it is also true that slashing, wringing, or pressing movements are expressive of different aspects of anger. With wringing or pressing movements the sustainment involved can bring about feelings of anguish or of power. It is

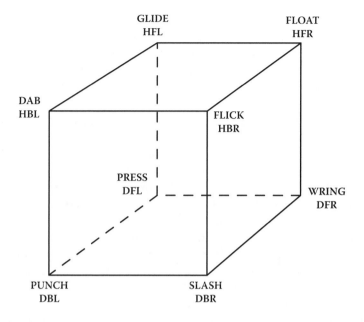

Figure 12.3 Diagonal scale with effort actions.

sometimes necessary for people to feel the freedom of slashing out. Because of the fundamental use in rhythm and form in a DMT session this slashing out can be very safe and controlled.

Transitions

An important ingredient for maintaining the DMT process is the use of transitions between motion and emotion events. If one were to experience a DMT session, there would be several high points (interventions accompanied by symbolism, body action, and verbalizations) with transitional movements in between these high points. There are many possibilities for transitions. Transitions can consist of gradual, less gradual, or abrupt transitions (Preston, 1963). An example of a gradual transition would be going from "float" to "glide" where only one motion factor, space, changes from flexible to direct. Less gradual would be changing two motion factors, such as in float to dab, where space (flexible to direct) and time (sustained to quick) are changed. Finally, abrupt transitions are where three motion factors would change—float to punch (light, sustained, flexible to strong, quick, direct). Each of these types of transitions, depending on what the dmt is reflecting back, produces different motions or emotions. An important feature of being aware of transitions is to be able to use a person's comfortable movement proclivities to help him or her experience movements that may not be easily accessible. For example, observing that a patient always moves in an action drive pattern such as "punch" (strong, direct, quick) the dmt can maintain the efforts of direct and quick and change one element. Changing the element of strong to light will give the experience and expression of gentleness or sensitivity and becomes a "dab." As with all of the Laban material presented here, it is necessary to "move" through these effort actions to experience and understand the power of this "drive." It cannot be learned by the written word.

Transitions are important to understand and master for they allow moving from one dance movement event (or dance action) to another. These are valuable in keeping the process of the DMT session continuous so that the e/motion(s) revealed are based on an organic and understandable development. For example, an abrupt transition between "float" (sensitive/light, lingering/sustained, and indulging/flexible in space)—a feeling of being above it all, and "punch" (firm/strong, to the point/direct and quick)—a feeling of making yourself known and hitting your mark—brings about different emotions compared with a gradual transition of "float" to "glide," where the sensitivity and lingering feelings are maintained, but the flexible attitude becomes direct, bringing about an exact awareness of where you are in space.

A patient with whom I worked danced/moved with the constant use of the motion factor time. The element that was so predominant in her movements was the use of "quick." She also had bound flow and the space element of "direct." This is a difficult pattern to be in because "quick" has to be constantly renewed—this was not a question of keeping a beat but her constant state was one of urgency and franticness. While moving with her it was clear that she was aware of this state and when I asked her what would happen if she were to slow down, she said that slowing down would allow her to become aware of her feelings. Inasmuch as she was in this vision drive (no weight), it was very difficult to encourage her to change or lessen the elements of quick, bound flow, and direct. The strong element of the motion factor weight was introduced periodically during our dance together. This was not a conscious choice on my part, but, because of my training in dance and because Laban's work is so ingrained in my body, introducing the strong element was the "easiest," least disruptive and body-coherent path to take rather than changing what was so predominant in her movements. It was only afterward, while recording my notes, that I understood what occurred. During the dance I knew it was important and would be easier for her to feel a sense of intention or self prior to giving up or lessening the sense of urgency and franticness. I believe that when one is tuned in and picking up movements, allowing oneself to be totally empathic in the dance, one's body memory, or unconscious will lead to where one needs to go.

Conclusion

The continuous dance within a DMT session does not allow time for notating or even minutely analyzing movements. What is extremely important is that dance therapists be able to incorporate kinesthetically into their bodies (muscle memory and feeling states) the dance movements of the patients in order to recreate or recall these after a session has ended. A dmt is then able to keep records of dance movements for future reference and assistance in the recording of a patient's progress. The expertise that one acquires through the training in Laban's theories enhances this body-and-movement understanding because the observation of movement while dancing and the process of empathic reflection (Sandel, 1993) become one.

The inspiration for becoming a dmt is the awareness of what dance has meant to the person. In countless applications of potential students entering graduate programs, the most common theme has been "dance has transformed my life." It is hoped and sometimes assumed that this kind of transformation through the dance can be made available to others. What practicing dmts face in due course is how to keep this dance alive both in themselves and for the people with whom they work. With the knowledge of Laban's theories, this is possible, because one can learn so many dynamic and spatial choreographic options during the dance.

Marian Chace (1993) referred to the dance in DMT as "basic dance." "The term ... has been coined to differentiate it from the artificial and elaborate forms of dance which depend upon physical *tours de force* as a means of entertainment, rather than communication" (p. 410). While teaching, Chace would refer to the art and aesthetics of the dance for both therapist and patient and she felt that gracefulness was an indication of health. She cautioned us to work with the healthy part of the patient. Dance/movement therapists need to have a strong dance background because that is the basis for the language that enables us to communicate in this nonverbal manner with our patients even though we use verbalizations. It is ironic that during DMT training students must learn to "let go" of the techniques of the specific dance training yet maintain the principles that make up the dance—phrasing, rhythm, sentence structure (how to put steps together), etc. Laban's work helps to further this understanding by giving us infinite possibilities using spatial patterns and dynamics. With this movement knowledge one is able to automatically focus on the expression and communication of the patients' movements and thus instantaneously give life, understanding, and meaning to their dances.

> What one experiences through movement can never be expressed in words; in a simple step there may be a reverence of which we are scarcely aware. Yet through it something higher than just tenderness and devotion may flow into us and from us. (Laban, 1975, p. 35)

References

Bartenieff, I., & Davis, M. (1965). *Effort-shape analysis of movement: The unity of function and expression.* New York: Albert Einstein School of Medicine.

Bartenieff, I., & Lewis, D. (1980). *Body movement: Coping with the environment.* New York: Gordon and Breach Science.

Chace, M. (1968). Talk for Louisiana State Community Ballet Group Conference. In S. Sandel, S. Chaiklin, & A. Lohn, (Eds.) (1993). *Foundations of dance/movement therapy: The life and work of Marian Chace.* Columbia, MD. The Marian Chace Memorial Fund of the American Dance Therapy Association. 408–414.

Chaiklin, S., & Schmais, C. (1993). The Chace approach to dance therapy. In S. Sandel, S. Chaiklin, & A. Lohn, (Eds.) (1993). *Foundations of dance/movement therapy: The life and work of Marian Chace.* Columbia, MD: The Marian Chace Memorial Fund of the American Dance Therapy Association.

Dell, C. (1970). *A primer for movement description using effort-shape and supplementary concepts.* New York: Dance Notation Bureau, Inc.

Laban, R. (1950). (Revised by Ullman, L. 1988). *Modern educational dance.* London: Northcote House.

Laban, R. (1956). *Principles of dance and movement notation.* London: Macdonald and Evans.

Laban, R. (2nd ed. by Ullman L., 1960). *The mastery of movement.* London: Macdonald and Evans.

Laban, R. (1966). *Choreutics.* London: Macdonald and Evans.

Laban, R. (1975). *A life for dance.* London: Macdonald and Evans.

Laban, R., & Lawrence, F. C. (1974). *Effort: Economy in body movement.* London: Macdonald and Evans.

Lamb, W. (1965). *Posture and gesture.* London: Duckworth.

Lepczak, B. (1989). Martha Graham's movement invention viewed through Laban analysis. Overby, L. Y., & Humphrey, J. H. (Eds.) *Dance: Current selected research,* (Vol. 1). New York: AMS. 45–62.

Lewis, P., & Loman, S. (1990). *The Kestenberg movement profile: Its past, present applications and future directions.* Keene, NH: Antioch New England Graduate School.

Lovell, S. M. (1993). An interview with Warren Lamb. *American Journal of Dance Therapy, 15* (1): 19–34.

Newlove, J. (1993). *Laban for actors and* dancers. New York: Theatre Arts Books.

North, M. (1972). *Personality assessment through movement.* London: Macdonald and Evans.

North, M. (1990). *Movement and dance education.* London: Northcote House.

Preston, V. (1963). *A handbook for modern educational dance.* London: Macdonald and Evans.

Preston-Dunlop, V. (1970). *Readers in Kinetography Laban: Motif writing for dance.* London: Macdonald and Evans. Series B, Books 1–4.

Sandel, S. (1993). The process of empathic reflection in dance therapy. In S. Sandel, S. Chaiklin, and A. Lohn, (Eds.) (1993). *Foundations of dance/movement therapy: The life and work of Marian Chace.* Columbia, MD: The Marian Chace Memorial Fund of the American Dance Therapy Association.

Schmais, C., & White, E. Q. (1968). Introduction to dance therapy. Proceedings, Postgraduate Center for Mental Health Conference on Research in Dance Therapy. Reprinted (1986), *American Journal of Dance Therapy*, 1, 23–30.

Schmais, C., & White, E. Q. (1968). Movement analysis: A must for dance therapists. Proceedings, Fourth annual conference of the American Dance Therapy Association. Reprinted (1989) *A collection of early writings: Toward a body of knowledge.* (Vol. 1). Columbia, MD: American Dance Therapy Association. Columbia, MD: The Marian Chace Memorial Fund of the American Dance Therapy Association, 120–135.

Siegel, M.B. (1968). Effort-Shape and the therapeutic community. *Dance Magazine,* June.

Stark, A., & Lohn, A. F. (1993). The use of verbalization in dance/movement therapy. In S. Sandel, S. Chaiklin, & A.F. Lohn (Eds.), *Foundations of dance/movement therapy: The life and work of Marian Chace.* Columbia, MD: The Marian Chace Memorial Fund of the American Dance Therapy Association.

Thornton, S. (1971). *Laban's theory of movement: A new perspective.* Boston: Plays, Inc.

White, E. Q. (1974). Effort-shape: Its importance to dance therapy and movement research, *Focus on Dance, VI,* I: 33–38.

CHAPTER 13

Applying the Kestenberg Movement Profile in Dance/Movement Therapy

An Introduction[*]

SUSAN LOMAN and K. MARK SOSSIN

Contents

---

[*] This chapter is an updated version of Sossin, K. M. & Loman, S. (1992), Clinical applications of the Kestenberg Movement Profile. In S. Loman & R. Brandt (Eds.), *The body mind connection in human movement analysis*. Keene, NH: Antioch New England Graduate School.

The Kestenberg Movement Profile (KMP) is a complex instrument for describing, assessing, and interpreting nonverbal behavior. Over many years, Kestenberg pursued an enduring inquiry into the nature and significance of nonverbal behavior, beginning with her training with Paul Schilder (1950). In the early 1950s, she devoted extensive study to Effort/Shape Analysis, which is based on the work of Rudolph Laban's motion factors (Laban & Lawrence, 1947; Laban, 1960) and Warren Lamb's (1965) interpretation of their use and structure (Ramsden, 1973). By 1953, Kestenberg had begun longitudinal studies of the movement patterns of three children, who were each followed for 20 years. Later, Kestenberg's investigations into the role of nonverbal behavior in treatment and assessment were pursued further within the collaborative context of the Sands Point Movement Study Group. Kestenberg made important clinical and theoretical contributions through her observation of infants, children, and adults.*

The original interpretive framework associated with the KMP is Anna Freud's developmental psychoanalytic metapsychology (Freud, 1965); this has evolved over many years alongside contributions to developmental, clinical, and psychoanalytic research and theory. The original group realized that little was known about movement from a psychoanalytic perspective, and even less was standardized. Moreover, they were concerned not just with adults but also with preverbal infants and children, and sought a methodology that would apply comparable measures to the infant, child, and adult. Those applying the newly evolving method notated infants on neonatal units, as well as children in nursery schools and well-baby clinics. As the KMP emerged, children were also observed and followed on Israeli kibbutzim. From 1972 through 1990, the Center for Parents and Children of Child Development Research on Long Island applied, and developed new methods of primary prevention for children prebirth through 4 years of age, with special attention paid to nonverbal and movement processes, the parent–infant/toddler dyad and family relations. Families would begin their participation during pregnancy. At the Center, the largest number of KMP assessments was made from live observation, film, and video recordings, because periodic movement observations were a regular part of the ongoing assessment. The KMP assessments provided opportunities to apply and clarify the diagnostic utility of the KMP in relation to clinically known adults and children.

The KMP evolved during more than 30 years of research by Kestenberg and her colleagues (Kestenberg, 1975; Kestenberg et al., 1971; Kestenberg & Sossin, 1979, Kestenberg Amighi, Loman, Lewis, & Sossin, 1999). Their findings linked the dominance of specific movement patterns with particular developmental phases and psychological functions. Movement observation complements Kestenberg's (1975, 1976, 1980a, 1980b) investigations of multiple facets of development, including gender, pregnancy and maternal feelings, trauma, and obsessive-compulsive disorder. The dominant focus of much research has been the development of techniques for the primary prevention of emotional disorders, in addition to bearing upon psychotherapeutic technique and developmental psychoanalytic theory. The KMP's specialized movement language, and its body of theory and research, can only be summarized in this chapter, which draws primarily on the work of Kestenberg et al. (1999), a text attempting an accessible elucidation of the KMP method and associated theory. The KMP's information about intrapersonal psychological functioning is applicable to all age groups; some patterns may even be studied in the womb (Loman & Brandt, 1992; Loman, 2007). Any two or more profiles (e.g., mother and child) can be compared with each other to yield information about areas of interpersonal conflict and harmony. At the Center for Parents and Children, the profile was used to assess the interpersonal dynamics (e.g. harmonies and conflicts) among family members, as well as to evaluate congenital movement preferences, levels of developmental achievement, as well as developmental arrest or regression, and factors indicative of cognitive and social abilities.

Summary of the KMP

The KMP contains nine categories of movement patterns representing two lines of development. System I, or diagrams on the left side of the KMP, documents a line of development beginning with movement patterns available to the fetus and newborn and continuing throughout life. Tension-flow rhythms pertain to inner needs and bear a special correspondence to developmental phase organization, and tension-flow attributes describe those affects most readily associated with temperament (and pleasure/displeasure feelings). System I evolves to pre-effort and effort diagrams reflecting more advanced patterns in response to learning modes and environmental challenges. Pre-effort movements bear correspondence to what have traditionally been deemed defenses, and effort patterns are linked to adaptations and masteries. System II, reflected by the diagrams on the right side of the KMP, documents a line of development dealing with relationships to people and things. The top diagrams, bipolar and unipolar shape-flow, represent movement patterns available to the fetus and newborn that continue throughout life. They describe, respectively, symmetrical and asymmetrical dimensional body expansion and contraction. Bipolar shape-flow patterns are linked to experiences of comfort and discomfort, while unipolar patterns bear more upon approach and withdrawal. Next, shape-flow design represents movement pathways toward and away from the body, followed by shaping in directions representing patterns that form linear vectors, and finally, shaping in planes represents elliptical designs within one or more spatial planes. The KMP graphically depicts 120 distinct movement factors (across 29 polar dimensions) and includes a body attitude description and qualifying numerical data. With regard to pre-effort, effort, shaping in directions, and shaping in planes, distinctions are made between patterns that are gestural and those that are postural (following Lamb, 1965). Each of the nine KMP diagrams refers to a specific kind of movement pattern (Figure 13.1 is an example of a blank KMP profile). The observational, developmental and interpretive characteristics of the KMP's movement patterns are summarized below.

Tension-Flow Rhythms

The KMP's view of development proceeds through a sequence of developmental phases, corresponding to the tension-flow rhythms (see Kestenberg & Amighi et al., 1999). As development proceeds through each phase, preferences for different movement patterns surface and change and are reflected in the qualities of movement that are most likely to be used. Variations between free and bound flow are rhythmic, although irregular, in their intervals. Ten rhythmic patterns have been identified, corresponding in pairs to the five major developmental phases: oral, anal, urethral, inner-genital, and outer genital (Kestenberg, 1975). The ten basic rhythms are sucking, snapping/biting, twisting, strain/release, running/drifting, starting/stopping, swaying, surging/birthing, jumping, and spurting/ramming (Table 13.1). At the height of each phase, we expect to see the largest proportion of rhythms typical for that phase, but all of the rhythms are still available to the individual. For example, the oral/sucking

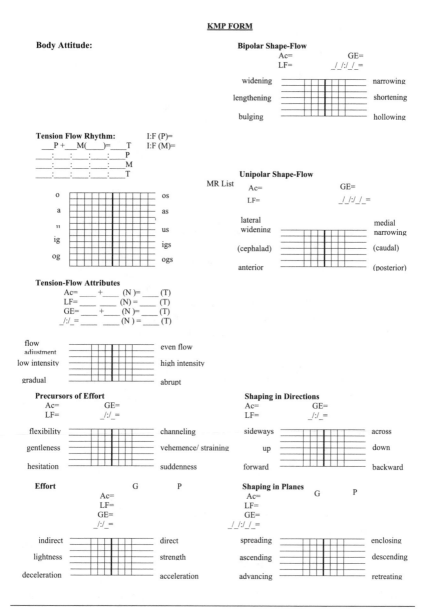

Figure 13.1 Blank KMP form.

rhythm would be most prominent rhythm in the oral indulging phase. All body parts can show all rhythms, and all rhythmic patterns are evident (to greater or lesser extents) at all phases. Frequency distributions appear to reflect consistent individual differences. Other body parts, such as the fingers or toes, may also show these rhythms, and the different areas of

Table 13.1 Understanding KMP Diagrams

Tension-Flow Rhythms	Pure Rhythms
o	oral sucking
os	oral snapping/biting
a	anal twisting
as	anal strain/release
u	urethral running/drifting
us	urethral starting/stopping
ig	inner genital swaying
igs	inner genital surging/birthing
og	outer genital jumping
ogs	outer genital spurting/ramming

Note: *Pure rhythms* are motor expressions of specific needs. They are directed to satisfying needs in a fashion that is clearly organized and adapted for functioning in their zone of origin. *Mixed rhythms* tend to reflect individual predilections and adaptations to specific contexts. Such mixtures may reduce optimal functioning or may help adjust the way a need is met.

the body may express consistent or inconsistent rhythmic patterns. In addition to the 10 basic rhythms, there is great variety of mixed rhythms, combinations of two or more rhythms. Individual preferences for specific tension-flow rhythms indicate their preferred methods of drive discharge. Comparison of tension-flow rhythm patterns in interpersonal relationships, such as between mother and child, reveals the areas of potential complementarity or conflict in the relationship in terms of needs.

Tension-Flow Attributes

Tension-flow is a manifestation of animate muscle elasticity. Bound flow is a restraining movement pattern that occurs when agonist and antagonist muscles contract simultaneously. Free flow is a releasing movement that occurs when a contraction of the agonist muscles is not counteracted by the antagonists. Neutral flow refers to a limited range of flow observed in limpness, de-animation, or numbing; neutral flow increases as a function of constricted affective state or compromised health. Tension-flow can also be classified in terms of its attributes (or intensity factors), which describe tension changes along three dimensions: even or adjusting, high or low intensity, abrupt or gradual. Tension-flow attributes (TFA) pertain to fighting or indulging patterns of arousal and quiescence. Preferences in TFAs are present from birth (and even before); they show increasing stability as the individual matures, influenced by both developmental factors and individual temperament. Although tension-flow patterns are meaningfully evident throughout life, they tend to become subordinated over time, especially in purposeful actions, to more advanced movement factors.

Interpretively, tension-flow is linked to affect regulation: bound flow and fighting attributes are associated with cautious feelings, while free flow and indulging attributes are associated with carefree feelings. More subtle or complex affects are related to combinations of tension-flow attributes.

Precursors of Effort

Laban used the term *effort* (1960; Laban & Lawrence, 1947) to describe movement changes (including tension-flow) in relationship to space, weight, and time. Efforts are developmentally preceded by precursors of effort (used interchangeably with the term *pre-effort*), affectively charged ways of manipulating the external environment, which become motor counterparts of defense mechanisms and styles of learning. The KMP denotes six pairs of precursors of effort: channeling vs. flexible, straining and vehemence vs. gentle, and sudden vs. hesitating. The first element of each pair is fighting, while the second element is indulgent. For example, channeling keeps tension levels even to follow precise pathways in space; this has a fighting character. Its opposite, the flexible precursor of effort, changes tension levels to meander around in space, and is thus more indulgent. In terms of defense mechanisms, isolation (a protective separating of thought/action from associated feelings) can take the form of channeling, employing an even flow of tension. Avoidance may be put to defensive use in the form of flexibility. Like defenses themselves, precursors of effort can subserve problematic or constructive ends; isolation can be indicative of affective disassociation (possibly amplified by neutral flow) or of objective thinking. The precursors of effort are both body-oriented, in terms of bound and free tension-flow alternations, and reality-oriented, in terms of space, weight, and time; hence, they mediate between tension-flow and effort.

Effort

Efforts are the motor components of coping with external reality in terms of space, weight, and time. In space, direct and indirect are distinguished; in weight, strength and lightness; and in time, acceleration and deceleration. Direct, strength, and acceleration are fighting effort elements, while indirect, light, and deceleration are more accommodating ways of dealing with space, weight, and time. The line of development of an effort element may be traced back to a specific precursor of effort and, even further, to a specific tension-flow attribute pattern. The individual's mature constellation of effort elements shows their preferences in terms of attention, intention, and decision-making.

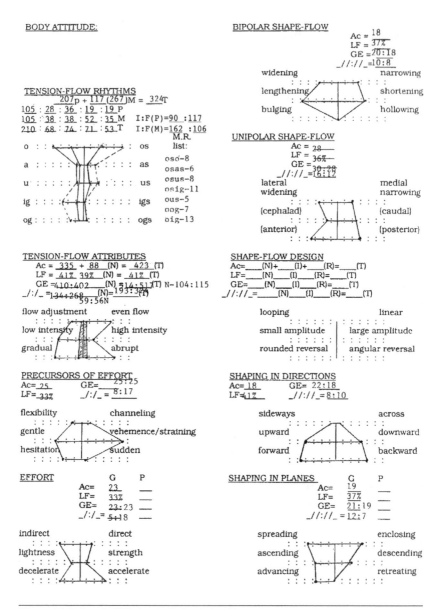

Figure 13.2 Sample KMP of typically developing 16-month-old boy.

Bipolar Shape-Flow

Changes in shape-flow express shifts in affective relations with objects in the environment. Bipolar shape-flow is the symmetrical growing and shrinking of the body in response to environmental stimuli. In terms of breathing,

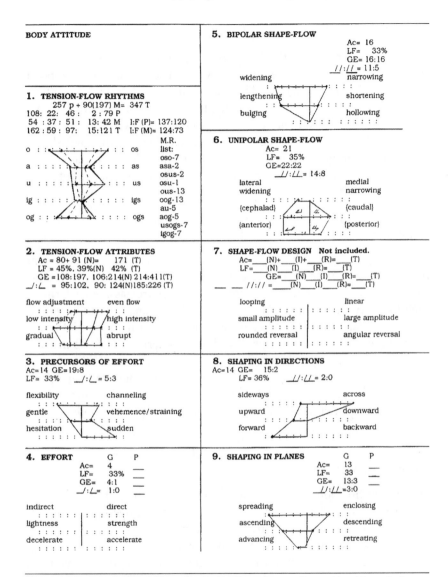

Figure 13.3 Sample KMP of 17-month-old girl with cardiomyopathy, post heart transplant.

for example, we grow with inhalation and shrink with exhalation. Growing and shrinking occur in three dimensions: horizontal (width), vertical (length), and sagittal (depth). Bipolar shape-flow expresses the individual's emotional response to the environment, and structures their discharge of fighting and indulging drives or motives. As mentioned, bipolar shape-flow is especially expressive of affects of comfort and discomfort (e.g., with our real or imagined surroundings). Hence, self-in-the-world feelings are conveyed through bipolar shape flow.

Unipolar Shape-Flow

In unipolar shape-flow, the body grows and shrinks asymmetrically, expressing attraction or repulsion toward discrete stimuli. Unipolar shape-flow also occurs in three dimensions: horizontal (lateral vs. medial), vertical (cephalad vs. caudal), and sagittal (anterior vs. posterior). In a vertical unipolar movement, the body grows only upward or downward (vs. a vertical bipolar movement, which lengthens both upward and downward). Unipolar shape-flow evolves from reflexive behavior and contributes to a system of extending the body in space (shaping of space in directions).

Shape-Flow Design

Along with changes in body shape, body movement also creates designs in personal space. These movements can be either away from the body (centrifugal) or toward the body (centripetal). They are classified in terms of their linearity, their degree of amplitude, and their angularity. Shape-flow design is notated somewhat like tension-flow, but utilizing spatial rather than tension parameters. Shape-flow design patterns reflect the individual's style of relating and feelings of relatedness. They are influenced by cultural conditioning, congenital preferences, developmental stages, and situational factors. A methodological challenge of shape-flow design pertains to the two defining poles (toward and away from the body) within three-dimensional reality.

Shaping of Space in Directions

Shaping in directions is formed by the linear projection of the body into dimensional space. These directional movements bridge distant objects with the self. Directions in space include moving across the body and moving sideways (horizontal), moving downward and moving upward (vertical), and moving backward and moving forward (sagittal). Directional patterns are associated with precursors of effort, defenses against external stimuli, and environmental learning responses. Closed-shape directions (moving sideways, upward, and forward) form the outer limits of bodily access, creating new boundaries. For example, moving across the body creates a shield against frontal and side attack, while moving sideways eludes attacks from the back and side. Learned responses are linked to these interpersonal defenses; for example, moving backward, a defense against frontal attack, is associated with suddenness, allowing the mover to quickly avoid an aggressor.

Shaping in Space in Planes

Shaping in planes configures space by creating concave or convex shapes. Horizontal shaping encloses or spreads, vertical shaping descends or ascends, sagittal shaping retreats or advances. However, each spatial plane includes a principal and an accessory dimension. In the horizontal plane, the accessory dimension is sagittal; spreading and enclosing are used in exploration. In the vertical plane, the accessory dimension is horizontal; ascending and descending are used in confrontation. In the sagittal plane, the accessory dimension is vertical; advancing and retreating are used in anticipatory actions. Interpretively, shaping of space in planes expresses multi-dimensional relationships with people as well as some inanimate objects linked to representational experience and their internalized images.

The Two Systems

The tension-flow/effort system (System 1), shown by the diagrams on the left side of the KMP (Figure 13.1), depicts developmentally evolving patterns of dealing with internal and external reality. The shape-flow/shaping system (System II), shown by the diagrams on the right side, depicts developmentally evolving patterns of spatial movement expressing growing complexity of object relations. The two systems resonate interpretively: fighting tension-flow/effort patterns are affined (fit well) with shrinking shape-flow and closed shaping; pleasant and indulging tension-flow/effort patterns are affined with growing shape-flow and open shaping.

Other Integral Features of the KMP

The KMP is statistically constructed, and organized to optimize its use as a descriptive tool; however, it can only summarize the complex processes involved in human movement. The raw notational data supplements the profile, especially with the individual's characteristic patterns of phrasing. Certain patterns may appear more in the introduction, main theme, ending, or transition of a phrase.

Movement can occur in gestures, using just one part of the body, or in postures, involving the entire body (Lamb, 1965, 1987; Ramsden 1973). Movement phrases sometimes show the same patterns, first in a gesture and then in a posture, or vice versa. These sequences are called gesture-posture or posture-gesture merging, and are generally not integrated until adolescence. Interpretively, postures indicate a more whole-hearted involvement than gestures, because they require greater bodily participation. Actions influenced by conscience and aspirations are likely to be evidenced in postural movements.

The load factor is a statistic that shows the complexity of movements in each subsystem by indicating how many elements are included in an action. The range of the load factor is between one (33% load factor) and three (100% load factor). It compares the relative complexity of each subsystem.

Another important statistic is the gain–expense ratio, which compares the number of movement elements (gain) per subsystem to the number of movement flow factors (expense). The gain–expense ratio is interpreted in relation to other subsystems, and indicates the relative degree of affective control (nonflow movement patterns) vs. affective spontaneity (flow patterns) in each domain. This affective component is further broken down into a ratio of free flow (ease) to bound flow (restraint) or a ratio of growing (comfort) and shrinking (discomfort) in Systems I or II, respectively.

Flow Factors

Both tension-flow and shape-flow are fundamental in the experience and expression of affect. Bound flow corresponds to inhibition, discontinuity, and to affects related to danger (anxiety), whereas free-flow corresponds to facilitation of impulses, continuity, and to affects related to release and safety.

Tension-Flow Attunement

Affect attunement (sharing of feelings) can be measured using the KMP. The relative similarity or difference in tension-flow is a basic measure of attunement. Attunement in tension-flow appears to be a key manifestation of empathy between individuals, such as caregiver and child (Kestenberg, 1985). Higher attunement is deduced from higher concordance of the tension-flow attribute diagrams between two individuals (Sossin & Birklein, 2006; Birklein & Sossin, 2006) regarding statistical approaches to such measurement, and this can be seen more directly in temporal coding bearing directly on interpersonal contingencies.

Clashing represents a form of non-attunement. For example, a client may move and speak using the tension-flow attributes of high intensity and abruptness. The clinician who responds to this client in low intensity and graduality will present a clashing, non-attuned pattern. Though each therapist brings his or her own temperament to bear, it is intrinsic to the therapeutic process to interact with the client with a reasonable degree of attunement; too great a breach of attunement will interfere with the client's understanding of the therapist's communication. An upset child who becomes highly intense may not respond to the clinician who is speaking and moving in low intensity. Once the therapist attunes to him in high intensity, the child may follow the therapist into a less intense, calmer state (Loman, 1998). Challenges to down-regulation often bear on specificities and nuances of movement. The KMP offers a schematic and graphic rendering of those patterns employed in parent–child and therapist–child co-regulation (Sossin & Charone-Sossin, 2007).

Shape-Flow Adjustment

Through the expansion of growing and the contraction of shrinking in bipolar shape flow is found the physical basis of primary narcissism (Kestenberg & Borowitz, 1990). From these bipolar patterns, one can assess feelings of well-being. Ideally, the parent grows into the child as the child grows into the caregiver, creating shape-flow adjustment. In the absence of parental responsiveness and mutuality of interaction, the child may show an excessive growing out into the world, i.e., an excessive degree of neediness.

Empathy and Trust

While empathy is attunement to another's needs and feelings, as expressed in tension-flow, trust is the adjustment of one's responses to create coordination and predictability, as expressed in shape-flow (Kestenberg & Buelte 1977a, b). The inherent parting and reuniting promoted by coregulated shape-flow between parent and infant creates a reciprocal expectedness that is at the heart of trust, and that anchors later progress along the developmental line of separation-individuation. Perfect harmony in shape-flow is not the goal because it is through titrated misalliances that differentiation evolves. A safe holding environment is necessary, however, before either empathy or trust can be created and maintained, whether in the therapeutic alliance or in a caregiver–child relationship. The dyadic therapist, encountering a relational misalliance, tries to facilitate the development of empathy and trust. This requires being translator, mediator, and protector for both members of the parent–child dyad, and creating a holding environment (sometimes literally) for the parents, so that they, in turn, can provide it for the child. As Kestenberg and Buelte (1977a) have observed, holding another without being held oneself is not conducive to healthy development. Trust develops, alongside mirroring and identification, from patterns of mutual relatedness identifiable in shape-flow rhythms. Similarly, the therapy process proceeds differently via "readjustments of relatedness" or interpretation depending on whether the patient is benefiting from identificatory/mirroring experiences or those that serve differentiation. Trust involves predictability in the domains of comfort–discomfort and approach–withdrawal regulation.

The child's spatial configurations are modeled on the caregiver's shaping in planes in the embrace and support of the child. Trustful and mistrustful feelings develop in shape-flow. For example, a bipolar shape-flow skewed toward narrowing, shortening, and hollowing, with little growing, is suggestive of problematic narcissistic development, and small, uneasy, or empty feelings about self. Continued healthy development will involve conflict (seen in dyadic movement discordances, especially in flow) as well as attunement (seen in dyadic movement concordances, especially in flow) between caregiver and child, depending on the child's stage of maturity (Kestenberg, 1965a, 1965b, 1975). Complete attunement and tension-flow synchronicity becomes maladaptive in development.

Since Kestenberg's original contributions, significant research on infant–caregiver interaction has highlighted the importance of rhythmic coupling/coordination in organizing early communication (Trevarthen, 1998), and has underscored the link between a midrange interactive coupling and optimal social communication (Beebe et al., 2000); while these approaches have usefully discovered the temporal/contingency factors at play, the KMP still offers a special window into other qualities of movement patterns that meaningfully pertain to their personal and interpersonal meanings. It is important to remember that clashing and individuated patterns are necessary for the construction of healthy ego boundaries. Some patients with significant relational disturbances may actually show an uncanny empathy in their ability to identify the needs and feelings of others (including the therapist). Their capacity for affective merger is over-developed and inappropriately directed; their tension-flow attunement is extreme, one-sided, and generally unsustainable.

To see how such skews may occur, take the example of a mother holding her baby in bound flow and high anxiety. Her anxiety flows only one way, toward her child, and limits her ability to receive emotional feedback. Her baby's ability to attune with her is therefore restricted; she can feel the child's emotion only when it is the same as hers. Lacking true empathy, the baby experiences a one-sided attunement, encouraging the development of a false sense of self (Winnicott, 1965). This interactive perspective can be applied to patients across the diagnostic spectrum. In severe disturbances, the patient's one-sided empathy also lacks feelings of trust and comfort. A sense of sameness develops without a sense of relatedness, because the other person is not experienced as reciprocally adjusting. This, in turn, requires defenses against these frightening feelings.

The therapist wishes to communicate not only empathy and understanding, but also support, structure, and confidence. An enraged client in high-intensity even flow who hears a response in low-intensity flow adjustment such as "don't worry, it's all right," is unlikely to feel understood. On the other hand, a therapist who becomes equally enraged and anxious destroys the therapeutic holding environment. The KMP provides a framework for understanding the complexity of this situation, and for outlining steps toward therapeutic complementarity and concordance, by taking into account developmental lines of movement as well as general affinities and matching between Systems 1 and 2.

The KMP in Dance/Movement Therapy

The dance/movement therapist who is trained in the KMP and movement development uses it as a framework to understand the sequence of typical movement patterns in evaluation and treatment planning. The therapeutic procedure begins with the establishment of trust and rapport with the patient through tension-flow attunement and predictability. The aim of this section is to present some aspects of the KMP that are useful in diagnosis and treatment planning, with special emphasis on applications in dance/movement therapy. The authors will draw vignettes from their work with both children and adults in preventive and therapeutic settings.

Dance/movement therapists have increasingly drawn upon psychodynamic and developmental models in framing their clinical interventions (Dosamantes, 1990; Goodill, 2005; Kornblum, 2002; Lewis, 1984, 1986, 1990, 2002; LeMessurier & Loman, 2008; Loman, 1998, 2005, Loman & Foley, 1996; Loman & Merman, 1996; Sandel, 1982; Siegel, 1974, 1984; Tortora, 2006). The KMP offers a developmental framework that can be used to encourage and measure growth, and to integrate progressive interventions with the developmental process (La Barre, 2001). It describes the typical developmental process in movement terms that aid in identifying deviations from the norm as well as strengths and latent potentials. Though the KMP can be used as a descriptive tool separate from any wedded interpretive approach, the evolved and multifaceted psychodynamic framework that has grown alongside use of the KMP provides information about drive development, affects, defenses against drives, defenses against objects, ego and superego functioning, object relations, narcissism, and areas of conflict or harmony in dynamics and object relationships.

The diagnostic/interpretive application of the KMP can lead to the detection of specific early developmental deficits and areas of psychic conflict, and suggests which movement patterns will be likely to foster resolution and growth (LeMessurier & Loman, 2008). For example, the profile can indicate delayed, missed, distorted, or prematurely induced developmental milestones by showing scant or overabundant amounts of phase-appropriate movement patterns. Specific problems caused by trauma, such as abuse, separation, or illness during a specific phase of childhood, may affect the shape of diagrams in the KMP. When children experience these difficulties, they feel a sense of inadequacy that affects their self-image and often endures into later life. Body-image distortions, restrictions of movement, and accident-proneness may all be remnants of childhood trauma. The KMP identifies the specific movement patterns that are most relevant to the early conflicts between a specific caregiver and the child (such as inadequate holding and support or constitutional temperamental differences) that had, or are having, a formative impact upon the child's movement repertoire and psychosocial experience.

Once a deficit or challenge area in movement patterning is recognized in the KMP, various channels of intervention can be explored. By offering a systematic way to discern an individual's movement repertoire, and to correlate it with psychological experience, the KMP offers a strategy for approaching treatment. Dance/movement therapists often use tension-flow attunement to develop affective empathy and shape-flow responsiveness to develop trust (Kestenberg & Buelte, 1977a). These processes can evolve into more mature movement interactions when the patient is ready.

Dance/movement therapists operate in many different professional settings, and the KMP provides them with a powerful tool to assess patients in developmental and psychodynamic terms. To optimally use the KMP, the therapist would evaluate the patient's progress with complete pre- and posttreatment profiles. In treatment planning, the KMP would be used to identify strengths as well as deficits, guide the therapists' movement approaches, and help the therapist determine whether to use attunement, mirroring, or affined movement patterns with the patient (Loman, 1994), or even when to choose specific clashes or discordances in movement experience in the context of rupture/repair sequences.

A child or adult with a developmental delay linked to the twisting phase, for example, may lack flexibility, have difficulty adjusting to external changes, and feel insecure in unfamiliar situations. The goal of the dance/movement therapist would be to help transform this over-stability into the capacity for change and discovery. At first, the patient may be rigid, immobile, and unapproachable; time and measured exposure are needed to gain trust and establish a safe, stable environment.

Clients most often respond well to attunement, a form of movement empathy that involves kinesthetic identification with muscle tension. For example, the therapist could use palm-to-palm contact to match a patient's even tension flow. Lower and higher tension changes could be gradually introduced, and then slight twists or flow adjustments may be modeled.

The therapist might suggest movements or images involving twisting, flexibility, indirectness, exploration or scattering. Infants can be engaged in games that require flow adjustment, such as peek-a-boo, following a favorite toy with their eyes or hand, or imitating funny twisting faces. Children often respond to the idea of moving like animals, such as snakes or fish. Flexible props, such as scarves or ribbon sticks, can also be used.

There is much room for creativity on the part of the therapist in eliciting flow adjustment, flexibility, and indirectness.

Therapeutic Significance of Developmental Transitions

Developmental transitions are especially vulnerable times for children. An influx of aggression is in evidence to enable the child to garner the energy needed to master the new developmental task. This aggression is normal, but may produce behaviors that are antisocial such as biting people in the teething phase, throwing objects in the anal phase, or ramming into people and things in the outer genital phase. An over-reactive response to this fighting behavior may encourage a child to continue employing it in a maladaptive attempt to cope. Dance/movement therapists can provide acceptable outlets to express aggression. For example, safe objects for the biting tension-flow rhythm, such as a biting-toy given to a teething child, may successfully redirect a child who has bitten another. Key to the KMP approach is redirecting the aggressive behavior into creative outlets that use similar movement patterns so as not to restrict the child's use of important developmental milestones.

When a trauma occurs in childhood, typical development is disrupted; an adult patient may retain issues, defenses, and movement patterns characteristic of that stage into adulthood. If the trauma occurred during the teething phase, biting may be retained as a defense and biting rhythms may dominate or be scantily represented. Such atypicalities would be indicated in the KMP by a skewed ratio of teething-phase movement patterns.

Therapists can identify the developmental phase associated with clients' aggression, and help them express it in an appropriate, safe environment. In one group dance/movement therapy session for acute psychiatric patients, a woman with schizophrenia paced continually, as she did on the unit. The dance/movement therapist incorporated her pacing into a group movement interaction, using her abrupt rhythm of starting and stopping suddenly, which typically appears in 2-and-a-half-year-old toddlers in the urethral fighting phase of development. The patient was asked to lead a portion of the group session that involved moving to music and stopping when the music was turned off. The patient was invited to be the one to control when the music was playing and when it was stopped. She became extremely animated during this segment of the session, which was in keeping with her preferred movement quality of starting/stopping rhythms. In this way, the patient was able to channel her pacing into an appropriate movement sequence. She responded very favorably to this suggestion because it used the urethral fighting rhythm in keeping with her proclivity for this developmental level. Specific contexts, chosen tasks, and therapeutic mirroring can lead to resonant experiences in which the patient's recognition of familiarity in kinesthetic reverberations leads to affective connectedness, and to an availability for reflective linkages that would not otherwise be accessible.

KMP observations reveal the strengths and limitations in the patient's movement repertoire. The dance/movement therapist may then facilitate the patient's strengths and help develop the patient's poorly represented movement patterns in order to provide more optimal choices and balance in the patient's "nonverbal lexicon."

Therapeutic Intervention in the Caregiver–Child Relationship

In parent–child therapy and in the therapeutic nursery, clinical interventions are often directed at improving the mutual adaptation of caregiver and child by fostering mutuality, reciprocity, and attunement. According to Winnicott (1965), the therapist's place is in the "potential space" between the baby and the mother. The therapeutic nursery is a playground of this potential space, an intermediate area in which the therapeutic staff can facilitate responsivity, reciprocity and mutuality in parent–child relationships. Frame-by-frame microanalysis of early parent–child interaction (Beebe & Lachmann, 2002; Beebe & Stern, 1977; Stern, 1971, 1995; Brazelton, Koslowski, & Main, 1974) has discovered a great deal about early affective and social experience. Disruptions in mutual regulatory processes, for example, when problems in affect regulation stem from maternal depression (Tronick & Weinberg, 1997), underscore the importance of movement communication and implicit gestural communication in the sharing of affects and the transmission of stress states (Sossin & Birklein, 2006). Brazelton et al. (1975), refer to the chaotic non-synchrony in a disturbed mother–child interaction, which can manifest as severe pathology, such as failure to thrive.

The rhythm and movement attunement between parent and child is examined to determine if the mutually regulated feedback system has been distorted, possibly indicating an emotional disorder in an individual or a relational disorder in a dyad or family. Intervention begins at the point where the connection has been distorted. Children with atypical patterns or sensory dysregulation can be perceived as "rejecting" (Thoman, 1975), which can lead to problematic projective identifications. The therapist will try to use (and maximize) the potential inherent in the parent–child dyad to create corrective experiences. Movement experiences and awarenesses can be enhanced via therapeutic video feedback. The KMP provides an observational language for schematizing parent–child movement patterns, and is an invaluable tool in diagnosis and treatment planning (Sossin, 2002).

Autism and the KMP

The KMP has great potential for use in early at-risk assessment, treatment planning, and research with children with pervasive developmental disorders. Future research with the KMP can produce more definitive descriptions of children on the autism spectrum (and other diagnostic groups). Especially needed are correlational studies using other measures of descriptive appraisal (e.g., the Behavior Rating Instrument for Autistic and Atypical Children [BRIAAC]—Ruttenberg, Kalish et al., 1974; the Functional Emotional Assessment Scale [FEAS], Greenspan, Degangi & Wieder, 2001; and the Autism [Diagnostic Observation Schedule [ADOS], Lord et al., 2000). Some studies of this nature are under way. It is possible that research with populations characterized by repetitive, stereotypic movement patterns may require amended profiling procedures to account for their skewed frequency distributions (perhaps scoring stereotypic and non-stereotypic behavior separately as two distinct profiles).

Behavioral Description

Children with pervasive developmental disorders, such as early onset autism, generally show atypical, repetitive movement patterns along with gross impairment in interpersonal responsiveness and communication skills. Common autistic movements include grimacing, rocking, arm-flapping, and jumping up and down. They are exacerbated by any stimulation, such as a spinning toy (Wing, 1975). Other movements found in children with autism include rocking from back foot to front foot while bending at the waist, walking on tiptoe, body spinning, odd postures, etc. In one case, dating back to the earliest recognition of autism as a diagnosis, Kestenberg (1954) noted a boy's very " peculiar body schema ... [His legs showed fluidity and] were very much his own [while the upper part of his body was in] fixed control [and was] rejected as nonexistent and later as not belonging to him" (pp. 37–38).

Other Features of Autism

The characteristic grimaces and flapping patterns of children with autism have several other distinctive features, as defined by the KMP. Consider shape-flow. One child with autism frequently used an oblique facial gesture with unipolar shortening, hollowing, and widening of the mouth, accentuated by medial narrowing, in high intensity of tension. The discomfort of shrinking clashing with widening in fighting-high intensity signaled to others an aversion to interpersonal contact, and served to impede communication. This characteristic repulsion of interpersonal stimuli in children with autism is accompanied by a preference for shrinking patterns of shape-flow. Closed, shrinking bipolar patterns also provide the structure for inwardly directed aggression, such as bruxism (teeth grinding), self-biting and self-hitting. Exhalation is more pronounced than inhalation in the child with autism's breathing rhythm (Blau & Siegel, 1978) reflecting greater shrinking than growing patterns. Not surprisingly, children with autism show diminished shaping in planes, reflecting their lack of multidimensional object relations. Only after the development of object constancy will the child with autism begin to show shaping in planes.

Therapeutic Implications

In autism, the child's bond with the primary caregiver does not evolve typically. Treatment approaches can be based on developmental movement patterns (Adler, 1968; Kalish, 1968, Loman, 1995), such as the KMP. A treatment strategy incorporating the KMP was used for a 3-year-old boy with autism at a therapeutic nursery. It aimed to facilitate interaction between mother and child in the nursery and at home. This involved both shape-flow patterns affined with the child's tension-flow, and deliberate clashing of shape-flow and tension-flow, to direct aggression outward. Empathy was facilitated through tension-flow attunement (pushing–pulling and giving–taking games), signing, and parental psychotherapy. The boy had less neutral flow and clearer body boundaries than his mother, with spurts of initiation. The mother felt discomfort in neutral flow; this was discussed in therapy, enhancing her empathetic ability. Her growing responsiveness to flow changes led to more attunement in touching and holding her child. The boy then showed more imitation, less localization, and less isolation of flow. Improved attunement also led to increased and prolonged eye contact. Mutual breathing between mother and child was also used: rhythmic growing into and separating from each other in all body planes (shape-flow). At first the boy's responses were unpredictable and unreliable, improving as their attunement increased. The typical process of shape-flow adjustment leading to mirroring and identification (Kestenberg & Buelte, 1977a) was seen in the improved relational patterns resulting from shape-flow harmony.

Intervention methods, such as a developmental individual differences, relationship-based (DIR) model (Greenspan & Wieder, 2006), have shown astute attention to movements, gestures, and other nonverbal behaviors, but generally lack a language of movement to do so. Trevarthen (2000; Trevarthen & Daniel, 2005) highlighted the importance of "synrhythmia" in early development in the attainment of intersubjectivity, and has further pointed to the efficacy of music therapy for children with autism in facilitating experiences in which the child's behaviors move toward rhythmic emotional interaction. While such approaches appreciate factors such as intensity and timing, it is our impression that further therapeutic windows are open when identifiable types of tension- and shape-flow patterns, as well as more advanced movement patterns, involved in self-regulation and dyadic co-regulation can be specified and themselves become attended to in the treatment.

Neutral Flow in the Therapeutic Process

The typically limp body attitude of children with autism is due to their excessive neutrality of tension-flow and shape-flow, a lack of both elasticity and plasticity. This manifests as floppiness, sometimes alternating with tense inflexibility, detachment, a lack of kinesthetic animation, and inertia. Although they may episodically shift out of neutral flow, their penchant is to return to it. In adults, excessive neutral flow can be found in severe depression, in extreme catatonia, in fatigue, and in altered states of consciousness. Neutral shape-flow involves a loss of body boundaries; the child with autism's body appears to dissolve. On the other hand, children with autism often create and maintain intense bound tension on the periphery (i.e., finger twisting). Perhaps this creates body boundaries where otherwise there are none. It is normal to use some level of neutral tension-flow, particularly in relating to inanimate objects. However, children with autism appear to use neutral tension-flow to become inanimate themselves, like wheels or other spinning objects. This poses a problem for the therapist who wishes to enter this discomforting, nonfeeling world and attune with the child. According to Kestenberg, it is necessary to enter into a neutral zone to establish contact (Kestenberg & Buelte, 1977a, b). The child regulates the contact in the neutral zone, and then is able to expand contact into give-and-take games. Because children with autism show little imitation, the therapist may imitate them (kinesthetic contact is preferable to visual contact). In this attunement, both child and therapist will use the most basic tension-flow attributes before moving up the developmental line.

Other Examples of Neutral Flow in the Therapeutic Process

In the following vignette we will see how neutral flow is observed in a feeding scenario with a mother and child. Clashing patterns during early feeding experiences are particularly important, as this is when children learn to regulate their intake; the clashes may lead to eating disorders later (Charone, 1982). Consider this scenario: a 13-month-old boy is sitting face-to-face with his mother, who is feeding him with a spoon. His tension-flow expresses graduality, low intensity and flow-adjustment while his attention wanders around the room. His mother becomes frustrated by her perceived failure at feeding. She narrows her brow and shoulders, raising her level of intensity and abruptness. In bound flow, containing her impulses, she blocks out everything except channeling the spoon toward his mouth. This clashing pattern is continually repeated, especially during feeding. Sometimes it precipitates a temper tantrum, but just as often they appear to meet in the neutral zone without making true contact, and the task is completed with a striking lack of relatedness. The solution of meeting in the neutral zone is not uncommon; it is often seen when the mother is severely depressed. The child seems to find that this neutrality is the only place to connect, even minimally, with the mother.

Another example of neutral flow interaction occurred with an elderly patient with a profound loss of cognitive and memory functioning. From a movement perspective, she exhibited a lot of neutral flow exhibited through wooden or limp movement, shapelessness, and lack of body boundaries. A dance/movement therapy intervention using hand-to-hand tension-flow attunement was begun as a prelude to experimental treatment with cognitive stimulation. As a result of the intervention, her ability to establish a relationship re-emerged, she became more verbal, and her memory functioning improved significantly.

Conclusions

For the dance/movement therapist, the KMP provides a sophisticated framework for the notation, classification, and interpretation of movement patterns. Its systematic observational schema and broad scope of application in assessment, diagnosis, and treatment make it an ideal research tool. Knowledge of the KMP and its growing body of research gives the clinician a deeper appreciation and understanding of preverbal and nonverbal behavior. Many areas of potentially fruitful research and clinical application have yet to be pursued. Unlike rating scales, the KMP is a complex instrument, requiring skilled and experienced notators who have demonstrated proficiency and reliability. Further research will enable the KMP to evolve as a clinical tool; so far, its developmental model has been primarily based on hundreds of case studies, including longitudinal studies of children, adolescents, and adults (Kestenberg, 1965a, b, 1967; Kestenberg & Sossin, 1979). The KMP's interpretive framework and clinical utility will develop as it is applied to a broad spectrum of research topics. Recent studies have focused on the application of KMP regarding stress transmission in parent–infant dyads (Sossin & Birklein, 2006; Birklein, 2005), depression (Brauninger, 2005), gender and leadership, (Koch, 2006), learning styles, (Beier-Marchesi, 2007; Kestenberg Amighi, 2007), postpartum psychosis (Lier-Schehl, 2008), and mother–infant interaction in psychiatry (Koch & Brauninger, 2005). Future studies can produce norms for healthy and pathological populations across culture, age, and gender, from which a statistical outline of diagnostic indicators can be drawn (Sossin, 2003). Longitudinal research with the KMP can advance psychodynamic theory by tracing specific developmental issues (such as aggression, narcissism, superego development, or personality) from early infancy. Detailed studies of specific diagnostic populations are needed to establish the range of individual variation within groups. Other subjects for study could include premature infants, individuals with physical illnesses, role-dependent or context-dependent behavior. Research can also increase our understanding of risk factors, prevention, and early intervention approaches with vulnerable infants and children (Kestenberg & Buelte, 1983; Sossin, 2007).

Methodological research can examine the reliability of the current notation (Sossin, 1987; Cruz & Koch, 2004; Koch, Cruz & Goodill, 2002), and develop amended profiling procedures as needed for specific applications. Computer programs can facilitate scoring and correlation of profiles (Lotan & Tziperman, 1995, 2005). The validity of the current interpretive schema can be examined, and specific distributions can be related to clinically relevant variables such as IQ, depression, neurological impairment, defense mechanisms, and systemic conflicts.

The KMP-trained therapist has available the tools of a comprehensive movement lexicon to aid in communication, a system with which to validate intuitive knowledge, and with which to plan, implement, and monitor change. The KMP provides dance/movement therapists with an in-depth system for observing, assessing, and working with the nonverbal language of clients. The KMP approach can further an understanding of the sequence of movement phases typical in development and enable the therapist to provide a suitable environment in which the developmental process can beneficially evolve. Based on the information obtained from notation and profiles, specialized interventions can be designed and implemented with the uniqueness of the individual in mind.

References

Adler, J. (1968). The study of an autistic child (film and presentation). *Proceedings of the American Dance Therapy Association, Third Annual Conference* (pp. 43–48). Madison, WI: American Dance Therapy Association.

Beebe, B., Jaffe, J. Lachmann, F., Feldstein, S. Crown, C., & Jasnow, M. (2000). System models in development and psychoanalysis: The case of vocal rhythm coordination and attachment, *Infant Mental Health Journal, 21* (1–2), Special Issue in honor of Louis Sander, 99–122.

Beebe, B., & Lachmann, F. (2002). *Infant research and adult treatment, Co-constructing interactions*. Hillsdale, NJ.: Analytic.

Beebe, B., & Stern, D. (1977). Engagement–disengagement and early object experiences. In N. Freedmand & S. Grand (Eds.), *Communicative structures and psychic structures*. New York: Plenum.

Beier-Marchesi, K. (2007). Emotions and second language learning: The role of body experience and empathy in the classroom. In S. Koch & S. Bender (Eds.). *Movement analysis: The legacy of Laban, Bartenieff, Lamb and Kestenberg* (pp. 161–173). Berlin: Logos.

Birklein, S. B. (2005). Nonverbal indices of stress in parent–child interaction. *Dissertation Abstracts International, 66* (01):542B. (UMI No. AAT 3161860).

Birklein, S. B., & Sossin, K.M. (2006). Nonverbal indices of stress in parent–child dyads: Implications for individual and interpersonal affect regulation and intergenerational transmission. In S. Koch and I. Bauninger (Eds.) *Advances in dance/movement therapy: Theoretical perspectives and empirical findings.* (pp. 128–141). Berlin: Logos.

Blau, B., & Siegel, E. V. (1978). Breathing together: A preliminary investigation of an involuntary reflex as adaptation. *American Journal of Dance Therapy, 2,* 35–42.

Brauninger, I. (2005). *Tanztherapie. Verbesserung der Lebensqualitat und Stressbewaltigung. [Dance Therapy. Improvement of Quality of Life and Coping].* Weinheim, Germany: Belz Verlag.

Brazelton, T. B., Koslowski, B., & Main, M. (1974). The origins of reciprocity. In M. Lewis and L. A. Roseblum (Eds.), *The effect of the infant on its caregiver.* New York: Wiley Interscience.

Brazelton, T. B., Tronick, E., Adamson, L., Als, H., & Wise, S. (1975). Early mother–infant reciprocity. In *Ciba Foundation Symposium 33: Parent–infant interaction.* New York: American Elsevier.

Charone, J. K. (1982). Eating disorders: Their genesis in the mother–infant relationship. *International Journal of Eating Disorders, 1,* 15–42.

Cruz, R. F. & Koch, S. (2004). Issues of validity and reliability in the use of movement observations and scales. In R. F. Cruz & C. Berrol (Eds.), *Dance/movement therapists in action: A working guide to research options.* Springfield: Charles C Thomas.

Dosamantes, E. (1990). Movement and psychodynamic pattern changes in long-term dance/movement therapy groups. *American Journal of Dance Therapy, 12,* 27–44.

Freud, A. (1965). Normality and pathology in childhood: Assessments of development. In *The writings of Anna Freud (Vol. 6).* New York: International Universities Press.

Goodill, S. (2005). *An introduction to medical dance/movement therapy: Health care in motion.* Philadelphia: Jessica Kingsley.

Greenspan, S. I., DeGangi, G., & Wieder, S. (2001). *The Functional Emotional Assessment Scale (FEAS): For infancy and early childhood.* Bethesda, MD: Interdisciplinary Council on Development & Learning Disorders.

Greenspan, S. I., & Wieder, S. (2006). *Engaging autism: Using the floortime approach to help children relate, communicate, and think.* Cambridge, MA: Da Capo.

Kalish, B. (1968). Body movement therapy for children with autism. *Proceedings of the American Dance Therapy Association, Third Annual Conference* (pp. 49–59). Madison, WI: American Dance Therapy Association.

Kestenberg, J. S. (1954). The history of an "autistic child": Clinical data and interpretation. *Journal of Child Psychiatry, 2,* 5–52.

Kestenberg, J. S. (1965a). The role of movement patterns in development: 1. Rhythms of movement. *Psychoanalytic Quarterly, 34,* 1–36.

Kestenberg, J. S. (1965b). The role of movement patterns in development: 2. Flow of tension and effort. *Psychoanalytic Quarterly, 34,* 517–563.

Kestenberg, J. S. (1967). The role of movement patterns in development: 3. The control of shape. *Psychoanalytic Quarterly, 36,* 356–409.

Kestenberg, J. S. (1975). *Children and parents.* New York: Jason Aronson.

Kestenberg, J. S. (1976). Regression and reintegration in pregnancy. *Journal of the American Psychoanalytic Association, 24,* 213–250.

Kestenberg, J. S. (1980a). Ego-organization in obsessive-compulsive development: A study of the Rat-Man, based on interpretation of movement patterns. In M. Kanzer & J. Glenn (Eds.), *Freud and his patients.* New York: Jason Aronson

Kestenberg, J. S. (1980b). The inner-genital phase: Prephallic and preoedipal. In D. Mendel (Ed.), *Early feminine development: Contemporary psychoanalytic views.* New York: Spectrum.

Kestenberg, J. S. (1985). The flow of empathy and trust between mother and child. In E. J. Anthony and G. H. Pollack (Eds.), *Parental influences: In health and disease.* (pp. 137–163). Boston: Little Brown.

Kestenberg, J. S., & Borowitz, E. (1990). On narcissism and masochism in the fetus and the neonate. *Pre- and Perinatal Psychology Journal, 5,* 87–94.

Kestenberg, J. S., & Buelte, A. (1977a). Prevention, infant therapy and the treatment of adults: 1. Toward understanding mutuality. *International Journal of Psychoanalytic Psychotherapy, 6,* 339–366.

Kestenberg, J. S., & Buelte, A. (1977b). Prevention, infant therapy and the treatment of adults: 2. Mutual holding and holding-oneself-up. *International Journal of Psychoanalytic Psychotherapy, 6,* 369–396.

Kestenberg, J. S., & Buelte, A. (1983). Prevention, infant therapy and the treatment of adults: 3. Periods of vulnerability in transitions from stability to mobility and vice versa. In J. Call, E. Galenson, and R. Tyson (Eds.), *Frontiers of infant psychiatry.* New York: Basic Books.

Kestenberg, J. S., Marcus, H., Robbins, E., Berlowe, J., & Buelte, A. (1971). Development of the young child as expressed through bodily movement. *Journal of the American Psychoanalytic Association, 19,* 746–764.

Kestenberg, J. S., & Sossin, K. M. (1979). *The role of movement patterns in development (Vol. 2).* New York: Dance Notation Bureau.

Kestenberg Amighi, J. S. (2007). Kestenberg Movement Profile perspectives on posited Native American learning style preferences. In S. Koch & S. Bender (Eds.). *Movement analysis: The legacy of Laban, Bartenieff, Lamb and Kestenberg* (pp. 175–185). Berlin: Logos.

Kestenberg Amighi, J. S., Loman, S., Lewis, P., and Sossin, K.M. (1999). *The meaning of, developmental and clinical perspectives of the Kestenberg Movement Profile.* New York: Routledge.

Koch, S. C. (2006). Gender and leadership at work: Use of rhythms and movement qualities in team communication at the workplace. In S. C. Koch and I. Bauninger (Eds.). *Advances in dance/movement therapy: Theoretical perspectives and empirical findings.* pp. 116–127.

Koch, S. C., & Brauninger, I. (2005). International dance/movement therapy research: Theory, methods, and empirical findings, *American Journal of Dance Therapy 27* (1), 37–46.

Koch, S. C., Cruz, R. F., & Goodill, S. (2002). The Kestenberg Movement Profile: Performance of novice raters. *American Journal of Dance Therapy, 23,* 71–87.

Kornblum, R. (2002). *Disarming the Playground: Violence prevention through movement and pro-social skills.* Oklahoma City: Wood and Barnes.

Laban, R., & Lawrence, F. C. (1947). *Effort.* London: MacDonald & Evans.

Laban, R. (1960) *The mastery of movement* (2nd ed.). London: MacDonald & Evans.

La Barre, F. (2001). *On moving and being moved: Nonverbal behavior in clinical practice.* Hillsdale, NJ: Analytic.

Lamb, W. (1965). *Posture and gesture.* London: Gerald Duckworth.

Lamb, W., & Watson, E. (1987). *Body code: The meaning in movement* (2nd ed.). Princeton, NJ: Princeton Book Company.

LeMessurier, C., & Loman, S. (2008). Speaking with the body: Using dance/movement therapy to enhance communication and healing with young chilren. In D. McCarthy (Ed.). *Speaking about the unspeakable: Non-verbal methods and experiences in therapy with children* (pp. 45–49). London: Jessica Kingsley.

Lewis, P., (Ed.), (1984). *Theoretical approaches in dance-movement therapy, Vol. II.* (2nd ed.). Dubuque, IA: W.C. Brown-Kendall/Hunt.

Lewis, P., (Ed.), (1986). *Theoretical approaches in dance-movement therapy, Vol. I.* Dubuque, IA: W.C. Brown-Kendall/Hunt.

Lewis, P. (1990) The Kestenberg Movement Profile in the psychotherapeutic process with borderline disorders. In P. Lewis & S. Loman (Eds.), *The Kestenberg Movement Profile, its past, present applications, and future directions.* Keene, NH: Antioch New England Graduate School.

Lewis, P. (2002). *Integrative holistic health, healing, and transformation: A guide for practitioners, consultants, and administrators.* Springfield: Charles C Thomas.

Lier-Schehl, H. (2008). *Bewegungsdialoge bei Mutter und Kind.* Hamburg: Dr. Kovac.

Loman, S. (1994). Attuning to the fetus and the young child: Approaches from dance/movement therapy. *Zero To Three, Bulletin of National Center for Clinical Infant Programs. 15,* 1 August/September.

Loman, S. (1995). The case of Warren: A KMP approach to autism. In F. J. Levy (Ed.) *Dance and other expressive art therapies.* New York: Routledge.

Loman, S. (1998). Employing a developmental model of movement patterns in dance/movement therapy with young children and their families, *American Journal of Dance Therapy. 20,* (2) 101–115.

Loman, S. (2005). Dance/movement therapy. In. C. Malchiodi (Ed.). *Expressive therapies.* (pp. 68–89). New York: Guilford.

Loman, S. (2007). The KMP and pregnancy: Developing early empathy through notating fetal movement. In. S. Koch & S. Bender (Eds.). *Movement analysis: The legacy of Laban, Bartenieff, Lamb and Kestenberg.* (pp. 187–194). Berlin: Logos.

Loman, S., & Brandt, R. (1992). *The body mind connection in human movement analysis.* Keene, NH: Antioch New England Graduate School.

Loman, S., & Merman, H. (1996). The KMP: A tool for Dance/Movement Therapy. *American Journal of Dance Therapy (18),* (1). pp. 29–52.

Loman, S. with Foley, F. (1996) Models for understanding the nonverbal process in relationships. *The Arts in Psychotherapy. (23)*, (4), 341–350.

Lord, C. Risi, S., Lambrecht, L., Cook, E. H., Leventhal, B. L., DiLavore, P. C., Pickles, A., & Rutter, M. (2000). The Autism Diagnostic Observation Schedule-generic: A standard measure of social and communication deficits associated with the spectrum of autism. *Journal of Autism and Developmental Disorders, 30*, 205–223.

Lotan, N., & Tziperman, E. (1995, 2005). *The Kestenberg Movement Profile Analysis* www.deas.harvard.edu/climate/eli/KMP (revision).

Ramsden, P. (1973). *Top team planning.* New York: Halsted/Wiley.

Ruttenberg, B., Kalish, B., Wenar, C., & Wolf, E. (1974). A description of the Behavior Rating Instrument for Autistic and other Atypical Children (BRIAAC). Therapeutic process: Movement as integration: *Proceedings of the Ninth Annual Conference* (pp. 139–142). New York: American Dance Therapy Association.

Sandel, S. L. (1982). The process of individuation in dance-movement therapy with schizophrenic patients. *The Arts in Psychotherapy, 9*, 11–18.

Schilder, P. (1935, 1978) *The image and appearance of the human body.* London: Routledge.

Siegel, E. V. (1974). Psychoanalytic thought and methodology in dance movement therapy. *Focus on Dance, 7*, 27–37.

Siegel, E. V. (1984). *Dance movement therapy: Mirror of our selves and the psychoanalytic approach.* New York: Human Sciences.

Sossin, K. M. (1987). Reliability of the Kestenberg Movement Profile. *Movement Studies: Observer Agreement, Vol 2* (pp. 23–28). New York: Laban/Bartenieff Institute of Movement Studies.

Sossin, K. M. (2002). Interactive movement patterns as ports of entry in infant–parent psychotherapy: Ways of seeing nonverbal behavior. *The Journal of Infant, Child and Adolescent Psychoanalysis, 2* (2), 97–131.

Sossin, K. M. (2003, October). Recent statistical and normative findings regarding the KMP: Implications for theory and application. *Proceedings of the American Dance Therapy Association 37th Annual Conference*, Burlington, VT.

Sossin, K. M. (2007). History and future of the Kestenberg Movement Profile. In S. C. Koch & S. Bender (Eds.), *Movement analysis: Bewegungsanalyse.* (pp.103–118). Berlin: Logos Verlag.

Sossin, K. M., & Birklein, S. (2006). Nonverbal transmission of stress between parent and young child: Considerations, and psychotherapeutic implications, of a study of affective-movement patterns. *Journal of Infant, Child, and Adolescent Psychotherapy, 5*, 46–69.

Sossin, K. M., & Charone-Sossin, J. (2007). Embedding co-regulation within therapeutic process: Lessons from development. *Journal of Infant, Child, and Adolescent Psychotherapy, 6*, 259–279.

Stern, D. N. (1971). A micro-analysis of mother-infant interaction: Behavior regulating social contact between a mother and her three-and-a-half-month-old twins. *Journal of the American Academy of Child Psychiatry, 10*, 501–517.

Stern, D. N. (1995). *The motherhood constellation: A unified view of parent–infant psychotherapy.* New York: Basic Books.

Thoman, E. (1975). How a rejecting baby affects mother–infant synchrony. In *Ciba Foundation Symposium 33: Parent–infant interaction.* New York: American Elsevier.

Tortora, S. (2006). *The dancing dialogue: Using the communicative power of movement with young children.* Baltimore: Brookes.

Trevarthen, C. (1998). The concept and foundations of infant intersubjectivity. In S. Braten (Ed.), *Intersubjective communication and demotion in early ontogeny.* (pp. 15–46). New York: Cambridge University Press.

Trevarthen, C. (2000). Autism as a neurodevelopmental disorder affecting communication and learning in early childhood: Prenatal origins, post-natal course and effective educational support. *Prostaglandins, Leukotrienes and Essential Fatty Acids, 63,* 41–46.

Trevarthen, C., & Daniel, S. (2005). Disorganized rhythm and synchrony: Early signs of autism and Rett syndrome. *Brain & Development,* 27(1), S25–S34.

Tronick, E. Z., & Weinberg, M. K. (1997). Depressed mothers and infants: Failures to form dyadic states of consciousness. In L. Murray & P. Cooper (Eds.), *Postpartum depression and child development.* New York: Guilford, pp. 54–81.

Wing, L. (1975). Diagnosis, clinical description and prognosis. In L. Wing (Ed.), *Early childhood autism (2nd ed.).* Oxford, England: Pergamon.

Winnicott, D. W. (1965). *The maturational processes and the facilitating environment.* New York: International Universities Press.

CHAPTER 14

Emotorics

A Psychomotor Model for the Analysis and Interpretation of Emotive Motor Behavior[1]

YONA SHAHAR-LEVY

… For in my flesh shall I see God

—Book of Job

The body is the best picture of the mind.

—Wittgenstein

Contents

Central Concepts of Emotorics

- Emotive movement
- Paradigmatic typology of emotive movement
- Archetypal relational settings
  - Self within a parental envelope
  - Self in forceful, vertical postures in a relatively open inter-personal space
- Universal prototypes of emotive motility
  - The attachment psychomotor prototype
  - The forceful face-to-face psychomotor prototype
- Paradigmatic potentials of emotive movement vs. Personal move-ment Patterns
- Physical gravity vs. interpersonal gravitation
- Psychomotor choices
- A binary matrix of potential emotive motor elements
  - 22 Binary potentials
  - 3 Dynamic modifiers
  - Binary transitions and interweaving
- Primary motor behavior vs. secondary motor behavior
- Retrieved memory clusters

Introduction

The motor system is the overt aspect of brain functioning and psychological processes. It speaks in the language of visible body shapes, postural attitudes, tension contours, and rhythmic patterns. The basic grammar of this language consists of muscle contraction vs. muscle relaxation, of movement flow vs. movement inhibition, of body parts and joint orchestration, and of the body's varying relations to space, time, and objects.[1]

One of the paradoxes of contemporary neuroscience is that, although it has developed sophisticated methods and equipment in order to make the invisible brain processes accessible to sight, it refrains from devoting similar systematic attempts to emotive movement. The visible processes of a moving body are not treated with articulated analytic concepts and tools. Instead, only generalized terms like "behavior" "experience" "activity" are used.

A number of neuroscientists emphasize the significant role of motor processes (Evarts, 1976; Damasio, 1994; Panksepp, 2003). Panksepp contends that the core-self consists of primal interweaving between motor circuits and emotional ones:

> I assume that the most fundamental forms of affective consciousness within the mammalian brain arise from a neurodynamic scaffolding that provides a stable self-referential set of internal motor coordinates upon which various sensory and higher perceptual learning mechanisms could operate. (p. 115)

However, this understanding has not yet served as a basis for a systematic effort to define a comprehensive typology of motor behavior as well as of its core building blocks.

My own encounter with a systematic method of movement analysis was in the classes of Noah Eshkol (1956–1960) and in the Eshkol-Wachman book *Movement Notation* (1958). The Eshkol-Wachman model examines the movement of discrete body parts in relation to space (measured by axes and angles) and time. Because it offers a sophisticated tool for precise movement notation, it is used by choreographers, movement teachers, and researchers. Yet, in spite of my admiration for the Eshkol-Wachman model, I had to take another direction because it purposely left out the connections between movement and emotions.

By contrast, in the course of a 35-year dance/movement therapy (DMT) practice with children, adolescents, adults, and families, I reached the conclusion that, in final analysis, human motor behavior contains manifest or subliminal *emotive elements. In other words, human movement is always emotive movement.* "Emotive Movement" is the interwoven expression of drives, emotions, perception, and interpersonal relations through motor channels.

To expand my understanding of emotive movement I turned to developmental, relational, psychoanalytic, and neuroscientific paradigms in search of theoretical connections and correlations to the concept of Emotive Movement.

Emotorics is a psychodiagnostic model that puts emotive movement at its center. The construction of Emotorics has been guided by the premise that a systematic diagnostic tool must combine a theoretical framework regarding the general nature of emotive movement and a systematic articulation of emotive movement's building blocks.

The process of constructing Emotorics involved a dual strategy:

1. To formulate a matrix of paradigmatic premises regarding body-movement–mind connections to be used as a frame of reference for the assessment of personal motor qualities. The paradigmatic matrix relates to the universal aspects of a healthy body and their correlations to psychoanalytic, developmental, and neurobiological paradigms. Its theoretical premises integrate information from several channels such as
   - Clinical DMT processes
   - Baby observation
   - Developmental-psychoanalytic approach
   - Neuropsychoanalytic findings about the biological connections between emotive and motor circuits in the brain
2. To define a paradigmatic matrix of binary core-potentials of emotive motor processes. Each core-potential represents a physiomotor and emotive aspect and is used as a diagnostic marker in movement observation, notation, and analysis. The matrix as a whole represents the complex interweaving between the emotive motor core-potentials (see Part Two).

This chapter discusses EMOTORICS, a psychomotor model for the analysis and interpretation of emotive motor systems. It is based on the Body–Movement–Mind Paradigm (BMMP) (Shahar-Levy, 1996, 2001, 2004). *Paradigm* refers to a distinction between the phenomenology of individual emotive motor behavior and the universal biological qualities of emotive motor behavior.

According to BMMP-EMOTORICS the building blocks of emotive movement are

Universal archetypes of mother-child physical relations
Core-potentials and universal prototypes of emotive movement
A binary matrix of emotive motor psychodynamic markers i.e.,
　　22 Binary potentials
　　4 Dynamic modifiers

Activation and avoidance of activation of these potential units are used as diagnostic markers for emotive movement analysis as well as therapeutic intervention.

In the development of the model I relied on several complementary resources, including

Theoretical and clinical aspects of dance-movement therapy: Gordon
Benov, Bernstein, Krantz, Melson, & Rifkin-Ganor (1991); Sandel,
Chaiklin, & Lohn (1993); Capy (pers. comm.); Bernstein & Singer
(1982), Siegel (1984).

Observation and analysis of the moving body: Feldenkrais (1949),
Gesell (1977); Eshkol & Wachman (1958), Lowen (1958, 1967), and
Brown (1975).

Psychoanalytic paradigms: Freud (1965), Mahler, Pine, & Bergman
(1975), Winnicott (1974), Khan (1974), Kohut (1977), Rorty (1980)
Stern (1985), Haynal (1993).

Contemporary neuropsychoanalysis and brain researchers: Evarts
(1976), Ekman (1980), van der Kolk & van der Hart (1989), Le
Doux (1996), Damasio (1994), Panksepp (1998b, 2003).

In embarking on this project I did not try to modify or integrate the models of Effort/Shape (Jean Newlove (2003) or KMP (Kestenberg 1975, Kestenberg & Sossin, 1979, Kestenberg-Amighi et al., 1996). I evolved Emotorics from a perspective that differs from the Laban and Kestenberg systems, but because the body is the unifying element, there may be some similarities in particular concepts. However, the overall way of observation is quite different.

Part One: Paradigmatic Premises of Emotorics

Emotorics' diagnostic markers are based on a combination of premises, including the archetypal structure of the body in relation to space (premise 1), the nature of human movement as emotive movement (premises 2–3), archetypal stages of infant development (premises 4, 6), core-prototypes of the emotive movement (premise 5), neurobiological core-potentials of the emotive movement (premise 7, 8).

Archetypal Aspects of the Body Dynamics

I have not come across any paper that discusses the contribution made to our knowledge and experience of a patient from our looking at him or her in their person as a body as against looking at merely the verbal material and affective responses in the analytic situation.

Khan, 1974, p. 246

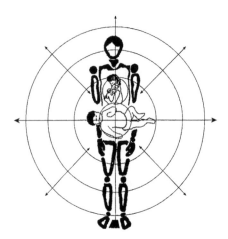

Figure 14.1 Body structure creates semi- and full circular contours that give the subjective illusion that it is the center of sphere-like space.

Body Structure

The human body contains universal properties such as the structure of differential joints and muscle organization and hierarchal constitution of flexible spine and limbs. The neuroanatomic configuration of the body determines the range of potential movement patterns. Certain movements are anatomically possible while other movements are anatomically impossible (Figure 14.1).

Due to the structure of the musculo-skeletal system (joint articulation) its movements create concentric contours. Every movement can be seen as either expanding away from the body or shrinking back toward the body. This creates a subjective illusion that oneself's body is the center of a sphere-like space.

From a similar point of view, the infant's physiomotor development can be seen as a process of activating its biological potentials for gradual motor expansion from its body to the surrounding space.

Gravity: The Universal Aspect of Physical Space

All movement, whatever its purpose may be … is in the last analysis an anti-gravity action.

Feldenkrais, 1949

Physical gravity is the hidden agent that shapes the body from moment to moment. Motor activity is always bound by the pull of gravity, which acts along vertical axes downward. The axis of gravity in itself is invisible, but

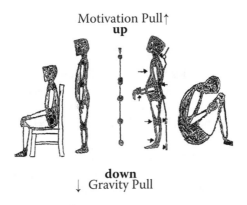

Motivation Pull↑
up

down
↓ Gravity Pull

Figure 14.2 Body postures are shaped by gravitational and motivational pulls.

the body's modes of coping with the pull of gravity can be inferred from postures and movements. Theoretically speaking, upward movements, i.e., counter-gravity movements, use more muscle effort than downward movements, which yield to gravity. To oppose the downward pull of gravity we need a strong counter pull upward. The sources of such a pull are the biological drives and the psychological energies of drives, emotions, and intentions. I use the term motivation as an inclusive concept of counter gravity pull along the same vertical axis. The dynamic relations between gravity and motivation determine the efficacy of one's motor behavior. To the observer they give information about the self's physical and emotional strength (Figure 14.2).

Interpersonal Gravitation: An Archetypal Aspect of Interpersonal Space
Interpersonal gravitation is a psychological pull between the self and others along horizontal axes. Unlike physical gravity which acts only in one direction (down) interpersonal gravity is bi-directional: it can work as a pull toward ("approach") or as a withdrawal from contact with objects and persons ("withdraw"). Significantly, the main parts of the motor system including the face, chest, arms and legs, are anatomically built to enable interactions along the horizontal axes.

*Archetypal Emotive Movement: The Interweaving among
Movement, Emotions, Perception, and Motivations*

I believe the sources of primary process core-consciousness are intertwined more intimately with intrinsic motor than with exteroceptively driven sensory processes within the brain.

Panksepp, 1998b, p. 115

An affect is therefore, at one and the same time a physiological modification, a visible expression (a communication), and a subjective experience (Haynal, 1993, p. 61).

Underneath motor behavior various emotive pulls are at work. The term "emotive movement" refers to the interconnectedness among movement, emotions, motivation, perception, body memories, and interpersonal relations. Emotive movement is the earliest form of psychophysical organization and self-expression.

From the first day, every motor pattern quickly assumes interactive-emotive overtones. Consequently, movement patterns are always emotive in the sense that underneath their functional level there are at work psychological states and emotive attitudes. Emotive excitation stimulates the motor system to active discharge.

Dance movement therapist and psychoanalyst Elaine Siegel (1984) wrote:

Affect is so strong a link in bridging the inner and outer world, psyche and soma so completely that it is the most complete approach tool which can be found. Affects are concrete, visible, felt, lived, and transmittable agents to the body–mind unity. They must be brought into their most evolved [i.e., secondary level and full expression] in order to become a vehicle both for discharge and self-observation. It is the incompleteness of affect that makes for trouble. (p. 74)

In deep analysis every movement is colored by feelings, emotions, memories, and motivations. In the words of Feldenkrais (1949), "to every attitude there corresponds not only an affective state but a muscular pattern of the face as well as of all muscles in general" (pp. 98–99).

Dynamic Aspects of Emotive Movement

Core-Modifiers of Emotive Movement

Freud had always emphasized that in the clinical situation *what* is most important and relevant is not what a patient hides but *how* he hides it. No human being can or ever does reveal the whole of their inner reality and truth. The question is whether their *privacy* constitutes relatedness to their true self or a paranoid and aggressive exclusion of others from any link with it (emphasis in original).

Khan, 1974, p. 218

Every movement, be it small or large, is modified by three categories of core modifiers.

- The energy modifiers
- The form modifiers
- The mode and rhythm modifiers

These modifiers, when examined carefully, give significant information about the mover's inner reality.

The Energy Modifiers

The energy modifiers reflect tension regulation, degrees of excitation, degrees of motor mobilization, attitude to gravity, and movement cycles between flow and inhibition. In general, they show how much energy a person uses in his emotive expression and in the pursuit of his or her wishes.

The Form Modifiers

The form modifiers reflect activation of body parts, body forms, and spatial axes and range of movement. Form modifiers relate to aspects of intentionality—what the person wishes to achieve.

The Rhythm and Mode Modifiers

The mode modifiers contain rhythm modifiers and differentiation modifiers.

- *Rhythm modifiers* reflect movement phrases in relation to time. Indirectly, they reflect degrees of enthusiasm and levels of coordination.
- *Differentiation modifiers* reflect body organization and regulation, learning abilities, attention regulation, and general level of differentiation and functioning—primary, secondary or high (Figure 14.3).

Archetypal Emotive Movement Cycles

Drives, emotions, and motivations memories create rhythms of excitation→activation→relaxation. Paradigmatically, there are two types of such cycles, namely, free flowing cycles and blocked cycles (Figure 14.4).

Free Flowing Cycles   Muscle activation is a rich source of pleasurable sensations. Free movement creates healthy sequences (cycles), which are characterized by ongoing transitions from neural excitation to active movement, which is followed by muscle relaxation. Motor activity cycles energize the whole body and reinforce feelings of self-esteem.

Blocked Cycles   Emotive motor cycles are affected by subjective emotions and motivations and by external encouragement or suppression. Systematic suppression of emotive motor discharge, especially in the early years of life, may have far-reaching pathogenic results. It may generate general anxiety and psychomotor conflicts. Pathologic cycles are characterized by blocked energy flow and undifferentiated muscle contraction. The result: rigid fixation takes the place of resilience. This is how Fenichel (1945) describes it:

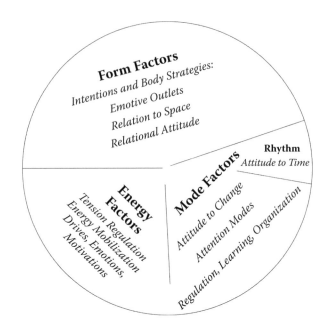

Figure 14.3 A graphic summary of the core modifiers.

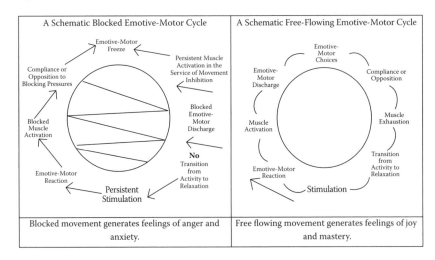

Figure 14.4 Blocked and free-flowing movement cycles.

The physical effects of the state of being dammed up emotionally are readily reflected in the muscular system. Pathogenic defenses generally aim at barring the warded-off impulses from movement ... thus, pathogenic defenses always means the blocking of certain movement. (pp. 246–247)

*The Human Body Stores Memories by Codes of Tension Contours, Movement
Patterns, and Habitual Postures*

The body keeps the score.

van der Kolk, 2000

The human body stores implicit and explicit *emotive motor memories* by
interwoven clusters of sensory, motor, emotive elements, and habitual relation to space, time, and objects (Shahar-Levy 1994, 2001). The fact that
the motor system stores primal, preverbal body memories in movement
patterns and body postures makes it possible to reconstruct—with utmost
cautiousness—the mover's inner state of mind on the basis of his body
shapes and attitudes.

However, because the earliest memories are stored in tension contours
and motor patterns, and because DMT techniques activate different layers
of stored tension and motor patterns, they can create powerful links to
hidden memory clusters. In such moments, a unique state of consciousness
appears in which memories are evoked in their full vividness.

The fact that the body keeps the score adds depth to the concept of emotive movement. The visual aspects of "the score," i.e., body form and spatial
shapes, may reflect the hidden presence of implicit memory clusters. As
such, they can be used as diagnostic markers.

Archetypal Interpersonal Settings

Personal movement patterns develop in an interpersonal world (Stern
1985). According to Emotorics, the infant's interpersonal world is characterized by two distinctly different physical settings:

- The parental envelope setting (Figure 14.5)
- The face-to-face setting (Figure 14.6)

*The Parental Envelope Setting: Selfbody in the Closed Space of a Parental
Envelope*

In the primal stage of human development an infant's tiny selfbody is held
by parenting others whose bodies, voices, smells, muscle tension, rhythms,
and movements form a physical parental envelope. Its body surface is subject
to various types of parental touch. This is a short phase of life in which the
human infant must wait for persons and objects to approach it. In its parental envelope, the baby depends on parental physical support because its
body cannot cope with gravity. Given its immature musculature, a young
baby cannot use its hands to reach out and grip objects. It depends on the
parental figures for satisfaction of food, hygiene, and mobility.

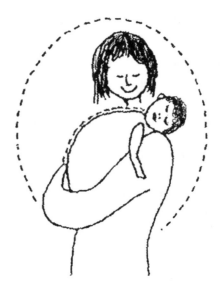

Figure 14.5 The parental envelope setting.

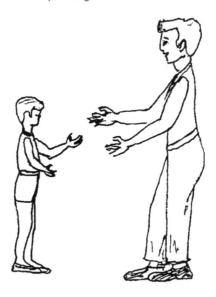

Figure 14.6 Face-to-face setting.

The concept of the parental envelope emphasizes the complex nature of infant dependence. It contains a twofold potential. An empathic envelope will assure a beneficial course of development. Empathic failures within the inescapable space of the parental envelope (i.e., in the earliest years) may cause many forms of cumulative traumata.

Paradigmatically, the parental envelope is "point zero" in the developmental timetable. In its pure form, it does not last more than a few months. However, its psychophysical marks are stored forever in the implicit body memory.

The Vertical Face-to-Face Setting: Selfbody vis-à-vis Other Bodies in an Expanding Space

The vertical face-to-face setting emerges during the second and third year of life, when the motor and postural skills reach maturation.

Relational gravitation within the parental envelope is very different from interpersonal gravitation in the face-to-face setting. In the space of the parental envelope, possibilities to detach and withdraw from the parental body are very limited. Indeed, they can be achieved mainly by postural manipulations within the infant self body. By contrast, in the face-to-face setting, locomotion and body separation opens diverse possibilities of interactions.

Core-Prototypes of Emotive Movement

From a paradigmatic point of view each relational setting is served by specific potentials and a specific psychomotor prototype. One prototype contains a group of core-potentials that are compatible with the envelope setting, while the other prototype contains a group of core-potentials that are compatible with the face-to-face setting.

- The parental envelope setting is served by the *attachment motor prototype* characterized by round body shapes and lack of spinal vertical support.
- The face-to-face setting is served by the *forceful-vertical prototype* characterized by ballistic-projective-forceful movements.

The [P-0] Motor Prototype—Compatibility with the Envelope Setting

This prototype contains potentials that are compatible with the physical conditions inside the parental envelope and the maturity level of the motor system, which is unable to maintain spinal-supported upright postures. The convergence of the two limiting factors, namely the physical boundaries of the parental envelope and the physiological immaturity of the motor system, creates a unique short period in human development in which the infant's language of emotive expression, interpersonal communication, and self-defense differs significantly from all aspects of later behavior. Typical movement qualities of the [P-0] motor prototype are

Little voluntary control and no cognitive intentionality
Trunk movement dominance.

Dominance of flexed postures. Flexion modes create round, soft body contours that enhance the physical interconnectedness between the infant's body and its parental envelope.

Dominance of gross motor movements.

Inability to fully cope with gravity.

Inability to maintain a vertical position.

Inability of the legs to give support to upright positions by proper grounding.

Generalized body activation. The body operates by the principles of "all at once" and "all or nothing." This is seen in tension fluctuation between generalized intense muscle contraction and total relaxation, as well as in generalized flexion or generalized (brief) extension.

Immature physical and mental differentiation.

Chronologically, this prototype is dominant during the first year of life. By the end of the first year, a more aggressive ballistic-forceful motor prototype becomes more and more prominent and the two prototypes interweave into complex patterns.

The [P-1] Aggressive-Forceful Prototype in the Service of the Face-to-Face Setting

In the second and third years of life forceful-ballistic movements and self spinal support are added to the envelope-compatible movements. These qualities give the young baby motor tools to build his or her spine and limbs as a preparation for the process of separation-individuation (Mahler et al., 1975). They also contain a potential of positive and negative aggression.

Typical movement qualities of the [P-1] motor prototype are

Extension of limbs and trunk is added to the repertoire of movement and posture.

Gross motor activity is the dominant mode of emotive expression in both prototypes.

Acquisition of vertical postures and spinal support.

Counter-gravity movements and postures.

Reaching out, expanding forceful-ballistic movements.

Independent grounding and locomotion.

Voluntary motor choices and intentional activity of the arms and legs.

Dominance of motor activation in discharge of emotions.

Dominance of motor activation in blocking emotive discharge.

Dominance of defense based on motor activation.

The two archetypal settings exist side by side during the first 2–3 years of life. Toddlers can shift quickly from one structure to the other. However, as the child grows, the face-to-face setting evolves as the dominant body organization in social interaction in school, at work, and in social meetings.

With the acquisition of the basic motor skills, forceful, counter-gravity movements become possible based on spinal support and vertical postures. For a healthy child, these movement qualities are associated with intense feelings of mastery and joy.

Thus, the "love affair with the world" (Mahler et al., 1975, p. 70) is at the same time a love affair with the body.

Archetypal Developmental Directionality

Psychomotor development is affected by individual life conditions. Yet, there is archetypal directionality common to all human beings. Every healthy human being develops from:

> The parental envelop setting to the face-to-face setting
> The dominance of the attachment prototype to the dominance of the forceful prototype
> Impulsive movement to voluntary, cognitively controlled movement
> Implicit psychomotor choices to explicit, cognitive choices

This potential to ascent from primary to higher levels applies to both the motor and the emotional aspects. The emotive motor behavior of a mature adult is supposed to be on a secondary level. However, unlike the physiomotor stages, which follow a biological-temporal maturation, the acquisition of higher psychomotor levels depends on the life experiences of the self. Primary patterns constitute the raw material for the secondary and higher level of functioning. But time alone does not assure the transformation from primary to high levels of functioning.

Archetypal Core-Potentials of Emotive-Movement

In Emotorics a distinction is made between archetypal core-potentials and personal emotive-motor patterns. Personal emotive movement patterns develop from universal biological core-potentials. The core-potentials are embedded in the archetypal properties of the body and its relation to physical and interpersonal space.

Theoretically, the potentials are defined as binary units, because they contain polar possibilities such as

> Muscle contraction vs. muscle relaxation
> Motor-flow vs. motor-inhibition
> Flexion dominance vs. extension dominance
> Compliance with gravity vs. opposition to gravity
> Forceful activity vs. avoidance of forceful motor activity

The concept of a specific system of binary core-potentials is based on the universal two prototypes of movement qualities. By definition, the core-potentials have physical as well as psychological-developmental aspects. The term "binary" designates a nonjudgmental approach. It treats opposites as complementary units in an interwoven matrix. Personal emotive motor patterns develop in a long process of reinforcement or suppression of potentials in the context of personal life circumstances.

Thus, the universal potentials themselves are positive in essence. Judgmental concepts such as "good" and "bad" are not relevant in regard to the biological potentials. The core-potentials are just biological raw material. Actual complex patterns appear on the level of personal emotive motor behavior as activation of specific potentials and avoidance of other.

Discrepancies between paradigmatic biological potentials and actual motor behavior offer potent diagnostic scales.

Motor Activity Is an Ongoing Process of Psychomotor Choices

Emotive motor behavior is a major channel of emotive discharge and expression, and of pre-symbolic thinking, an important way to gather information, to communicate, and to mentally organize one's environment. Its activity is an ongoing process of consecutive choices.

The motor system translates drives and emotions to practical moment-to-moment choices such as: Which body parts to use? How to move? Where to move? How much energy to spend? How much force to mobilize? What direction to take? What distance to take in relation to others? In addition, the infant's gross interpretations of immediate situations are summed up by the appraisal of which of its own movements are "safe" or "risky," "right" or "wrong." It learns quickly the "display rules" (Ekman, 1980, pp. 80–81) that dictate which emotions have parental permission to be expressed by motor activity and which emotions and behaviors must be repressed. As such, emotive motility is a precognitive mode of decision-making and a primary psychophysical organizer.

The anatomic structure of the body offers a basis for behavior based on choice. Body organs make endless invisible choices between degrees of muscle contraction vs. muscle relaxation, flexion vs. extension, shrinking vs. expansion. Emotive motor behavior is an ongoing process of choice-making. Each posture and every movement is only one choice out of many others.

Some choices are voluntary. The majority of these are implicit choices. They take place on a subliminal level and are neither accessible to the self's cognitive awareness nor to the outside observer. In the course of development, these voluntary cognitive choices are added to the procedural choices.

A premise that movement consists of sequences of choices assumes that human behavior has the potential to correct inefficient choices. This is an optimistic view of the role of therapy.

The Typology of Archetypal Interpersonal Settings and
Emotive Motor Prototypes Lays the Foundation for a
Binary System for Emotive-Movement Assessment

The two psychomotor prototypes and their core-potentials are used as a basis for the construction of a binary diagnostic model.

- The motor prototype that serves the Parental Envelope Setting is defined as Prototype Zero [P-0].
- The motor prototype that serves the Face-to-Face Setting is defined as Prototype One [P-1].

The two psychomotor prototypes are broken down to two groups of potential-units namely a group of [P-0] potential units and a group of [P-1] potential units. The [P-0] and [P-1] motor prototypes and potential units designate two consecutive stages of early development. Together, they constitute two parts of one system based on a quasi-binary principle.

General Remarks on the Binary Principle

The binary model has been chosen to emphasize the principle of reciprocal interweaving rather than splitting between seemingly contradictory segments of behavior. I borrowed the term from Gesell's (1977) description of the "spiral reciprocal interweaving" of flexion-extension and agonist–antagonist muscle activation and extended its application.

Analogous to the computer language, which is based on endless combinations of the digits 0 and 1, psychomotor behavior can be seen as the ongoing interactivity and mutual interweaving between [P-0] and [P-1] core-prototypes.

In a binary system there is no judgmental split between "good" and "bad" potentials. Both are raw material for a healthy psychomotor functioning.

Abstractly speaking, the binary principle reflects the modular functioning of biological systems. Hence, the modular nature of the binary principle makes it a suitable tool for the analysis of dynamic systems like emotive motor behavior.

In the next part the central tools and aspects of the binary system are described.

Part Two: The Binary Model for Emotive-Movement Assessment

The concept of interaction of opposites underlies the principle of change and progress.

Lowen, 1971

Motor subjective experience is always related to the surrounding space. The body's ability to alternate between expansion and shrinking as well as between approaching and withdrawal constitutes a system of binary potentials. The diagnostic system of Emotorics incorporates the concept of binary dynamics within the boundaries of a seemingly round space. (See the binary markers in Figure 14.7.)

The Paradigmatic Binary Matrix of Emotive Movement Analysis

According to the definition of the binary system, movement qualities of the two psychomotor prototypes are classified as two groups of 22 potential units.

Each potential unit contains a [P-0] pole and a [P-1] pole. The group of 22 [P-0] poles represents movement qualities of [P-0] prototype whereas the group of [P-1] poles represents movement qualities of [P-1] prototype.

Some of the potential units refer to movement qualities, some to body postures, some to axes in space, some to muscular mobilization, and some to perceptual schemes. The binary matrix of potential units is arranged in two notation charts: a binary table (Table 14.1) and a binary circular chart (Figure 14.7). The charts contain empty slots for each potential.

Binary Transitions Links and Interweaving between [P-0] Potential Units and the [P-1] Potential Units

Theoretically complex movement patterns are formed by processes of transitions and interweaving between P-0 and P-1 potential units. Binary transitions and interweaving reflect the combinatory processes by which the motor action units converge to complex patterns.

In healthy conditions, i.e., in flowing movement cycles, the transitions flow easily. In pathological conditions, i.e., in blocked movement cycles, the transitions are fragmentary or entirely constricted.

As an assessment tool, the binary potential units enable the therapist to perceive subtle body clues by which to make tentative working hypotheses about past subjective experiences and present body strategies, conflicts, fixations, and regressions.

The dynamic interweaving of binary potential units represents the mutual interweaving of particles in biological systems.

The binary core-potentials/action-units give the therapist external keys that unfold body strategies, conflicts, fixations, and regressions as they emerge in movement.

Graphically, the binary matrix is organized into two concentric rings and three sections representing the dynamic modifiers. The inner ring represents the [P-0] prototype and the [P-0] potential units while the outer ring represents the [P-1] prototype and the [P-1] potential units. Each ring contains 22 round slots (44 all together). Each core-potential has its marked slot. The numbers in the circle correlate to the numbers in the

Table 14.1 Binary Core Potentials

[P-0] Binary Poles			[P-1] Binary Poles		
No Visible Movement	**I**	**II**	**Visible Movement**	**I**	**II**
1. No muscle contraction			Muscle contraction		
2. Motor flow			Motor inhibition		
3. Weightiness			Forcefulness		
4. Low intensity			High intensity		
5. Pro-gravity alignment			Counter-gravity alignment		
6. Inward movement			Outward movement		
7. Trunk activation			Limbs activation		
8. Flexion			Extension		
9. Round/curved shapes			Straight-linear shapes		
10. Symmetry			Asymmetry		
11. Undulation, wavy movement			Ballistic, Projective movement		
12. Rotation			Regulated progression		
13. Bi-directional			Uni-directional		
14. Small range			Wide range		
15. Horizontal alignment			Vertical alignment		
16. Quick movement			Slow movement		
17. Fragmentary movement			Continuous movement		
18. Oscillations, Shifts			Fixation		
19. Repetition			Modulation, Variation		
20. Non-differentiation			Differentiation		
21. Indirect movement			Direct movement		
22. Diffused attention			Focussed attention		

The charts contain an empty slot for each core potential.

table. The binary circular chart represents the interweaving of the [P-0] and [P-1] prototypes, the core-potentials, and the dynamic modifiers in one comprehensive system.

Notation of Movement Processes in the Binary Chart

The plain binary profile contains the [P-0] and [P-1] potential units divided to the modifying categories. In addition, signs of transitional links between the [P-0] and [P-1] potential units are inserted according to the observed emotive motor behavior. Movement assessment according to the binary profile is based on four complementary aspects:

The Binary Potentials

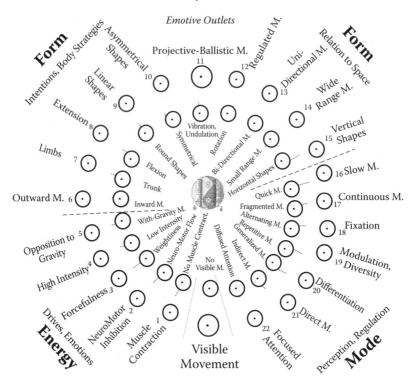

Figure 14.7 The binary circle.

1. Activation of the core-potentials in the [P-0] and [P-1] rings
2. Transitions between the [P-0] and [P-1] rings
3. Mutual interweaving and combinations (clusters) between [P-0] and [P-1] potential units
4. The balance between the dynamic modifiers

Activation of the core-potentials in the [P-0] and [P-1] rings
When we observe movement processes the first step is to note and notate the following:

Which potential units are activated and which are dormant?

When we insert the activation/non-activation sign into each relevant slot we receive a plain binary profile. The basic marks for notation are an empty slot with small dot for a dormant potential and a full slot for an activated potential (Figure 14.8).

Dormant Potential
Active Potential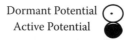

Figure 14.8 Potential activation.

The small dot signifies the premise that an archetypal potential is never extinct even when we do not see it. It is always present in the emotive motor system and can be reactivated if the right conditions are created.

The active/dormant signs enable us to see in a glance:

- How many core-potentials are activated in each ring
- How many core-potentials are activated in each modifying category
- Is there repetitive activation
- Is there excessive activation
- What potentials are systematically avoided, etc.

Transitions between the [P-0] and [P-1] rings
When the basic active/dormant signs are inserted in the respective slots of the binary circle they bring to the surface the quality of binary transition. The signs of transitions are inserted between the [P-0] ring and the [P-1] ring (Figure 14.9).

Mutual interweaving and combinations (clusters) between [P-0] and [P-1] potential units
The lines between activated potentials create combinations and clusters in the profile (Figure 14.10).

Dominant clusters may reflect emotive states such as conflicts, anger, anxiety, attraction, and joy (Figure 14.11).

Flowing Transitions

Blocked Transitions

Figure 14.9 Binary transitions.

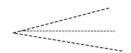

Figure 14.10 Signs of binary clusters.

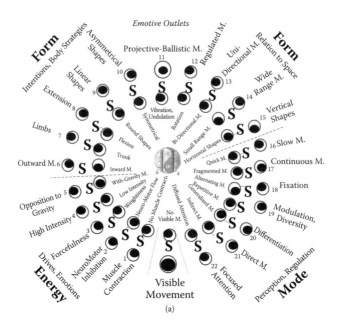

(a)

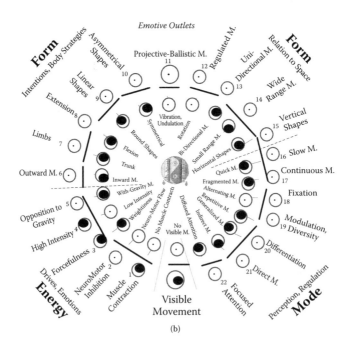

(b)

Figure 14.11 Types of [P-0] to [P-1] and [P-1] to [P-0] transitions; (a) flowing transitions; (b) blocked transitions from [P-0] to [P-1].

The [P-0]/[P-1] Balance between the Core-Modifiers
The potential units are divided into three categories of dynamic modifiers. Category Energy contains five potential units, category Form contains ten potential units and category Rhythm-Mode contains seven potential units.

The active/dormant signs in the [P-0] and [P-1] rings delineate the balance between the dynamic modifiers as well.

Contents of Binary Profiles
The binary chart can be used to notate diverse situations and diverse segments of therapeutic processes. To have a solid basis for analysis and interpretation, the therapist needs to prepare a series of binary profiles. Successive profiles bring to the surface cumulative information about the mover's emotive state. They also expose areas of fixation and areas of change in the course of therapy.

Various types of profiles can be made such as:

- A profile of one session
- A cumulative profile which combines several profiles from various time segments
- Differential profiles for the upper part and the lower part of the body
- Differential profiles for the limbs and for the torso
- Dyadic profiles
- Family differential profiles

Part Three: Differential Evaluation of Emotive Motor Behavior Based on Binary Profiles

Examples of personal binary profiles are described. The short vignettes below do not describe the therapeutic process. I took material from the process to illustrate the role of the binary diagnostic model in movement analysis during therapy.

Vera: A Victim of Medical Abuse

Vera was referred to me by a psychologist after two attempts to commit suicide. The therapist told me that her husband came home earlier than planned and found her in the bathtub covered with blood. He rushed her to the hospital. Her life was saved but she sank into deep depression. She was hospitalized for psychological treatment but remained totally unresponsive. Her therapist suggested that she try dance movement therapy. To her surprise, Vera accepted immediately.

At the appointed hour a tall, very beautiful woman stood at my doorstep. As we started talking I was impressed by her eloquence and sharp intelligence. She spoke about her dissociation from her body. She told me that a few months prior to the suicide attempts she had two miscarriages: one was spontaneous but the other was the result of medical intervention in the fifth month of pregnancy due to unexplained bleeding. She described this as a terribly painful experience. In her words, "I was lying there completely helpless with my legs forcedly apart. I looked at the doctors as they looked at me, or rather only at my bleeding vagina. I felt so humiliated. I felt raped. But no one noticed. After a week I was sent home as if nothing happened. It was then that I started to plan my suicide."

As she spoke, her body looked split: her face was turned toward me but the rest of her body was twisted diagonally away from my sight. Her torso was curved in, her legs and arms were flexed, closing over each other with great tension. It was as if she was trying to protect the lower part of her body. Vera talked freely but did not move. Her words came out monotonously without any sign of emotion.

I interpreted her choice of movement therapy as a wish to be released from her freeze. I suggested a gentle movement to loosen a little bit the tension in her hands. What followed was completely unexpected: Vera tried to follow the suggestion but immediately stopped and threw her body on the rug. As she was lying her body was curved in. She cried and kicked in the direction of an invisible object. Gradually, her crying turned to sobs until it stopped after about 10 minutes. She continued to lie restlessly on her side. When she came back to the place where I was sitting she complained of excruciating pain in her vagina.

Similar episodes repeated. Any movement would trigger the same painful experience. Her reaction was also the same: [P-0] movements (Figure 14.12).

The emergence of pain in the vagina was not accompanied by any images or cognitive memory. Vera thought that these were body memories of some kind of sexual abuse. The dominance of [P-0] movements led me to the hypothesis that the original trauma was medical rather than sexual. My working hypothesis was that the impingement occurred in the early stage of life before the appearance of the [P-1] prototype.

This is a typical picture of a baby whose motor apparatus is undeveloped. Such a baby cannot defend herself from outside penetration. No fight. No flight. Only contraction and freeze are possible as a body defense. At this age it is more plausible that the horrified memory came from some physical injury, perhaps medical.

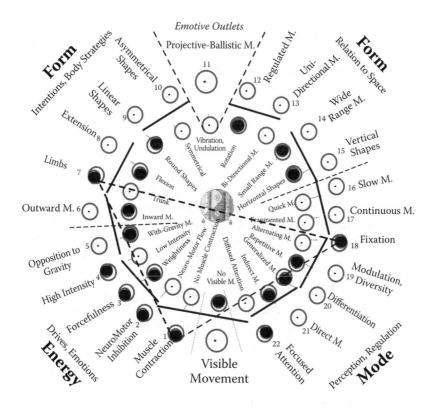

Figure 14.12 A cumulative binary profile of Vera's initial stage of therapy: motor defensive blocks.

Although she chose to come to movement therapy she resisted any kind of motor movement. Yet she was eager to talk about her body sensations, about her chronic unexplained (implicit) anxiety and about her dissociation from her body. Vera thought that she was a victim of unremembered sexual abuse. However, the two-prototype paradigm enabled me not to rush to simplistic conclusions. The dominant activation of [P-0] potentials and lack of [P-1] qualities in her movements seemed like an early body memory that retains the physical aspects of an experience (including the immaturity of the motor system) but not the content. I suspected that the original trauma was some very early medical impingement. In our verbal processing I insisted that the actual event is less important than the psychomotor defense against it, especially the tendency to freeze.

Our work focused on her bodily defense manipulations in an attempt to desensitize the body to the pain of an unexplained injury. We spoke about body conflicts, about body parts and their function in generating both pain and pleasure. She liked the idea but could not bring herself to move in the sessions. Instead, she decided to go to the gym twice a week.

On termination after 3 years, Vera's emotive movement did not change. Her defensive fixation and immobility persisted till the end. Yet she expressed her gratitude for the new connections she felt to her body (although not so much to her movement).

Six months after termination Vera called me and asked for a one-time session. When she sat down she said: "I had to tell you what happened to me. I went to a Yoga retreat and enjoyed it. In one of the meditations I suddenly "saw" a vivid image of myself as a small baby lying on my back and my mother doing something to my vagina. It was SO painful but I could not do anything. Then I came home and asked my mother if something like that really happened. She confirmed the memory, telling me that I had a terrible rash on my skin, so terrible that when she changed a diaper the skin came off with it. So you were right."

We examined our work in the light of the new information. The persistent cluster of catastrophic anticipation, horror, and helplessness in the face of her inability as a baby to fight or flight or to verbally express what she felt was present in the room. She was locked in memory cluster with no exit.

Nina: Emotive Motor Defense against Memories of Incest

Nina entered my studio with wide steps and emphatically upright posture. She threw her bag on the rug, measuring the distance between us. Then she sat down diagonally and said: "I want to be treated as a survivor and not as a victim." Nina had deep brown eyes and a piercing gaze. She was tall. Her movements were abrupt and forceful. She seemed very tense and suspicious. Her defensive strategy showed in her shifty eyes, in her over-contracted body, and in the many layers of clothes that she would wear even in the summer, although the summer in Israel is very hot. Nina told me that she has the need to keep her body intensely active and covered. She jogs every day; she dances three–four times a week (Figure 14.13).

In the initial phase of therapy the [P-1] forceful prototype was dominant. Nina did not allow herself any relaxed or "weak" position such as lying on the rug. She always started moving while standing upright and moving her arms in different directions. By doing so she seemed pushing away an invisible potential intruder.

One day after the active movements she sat down on the rug. With slow motions she started to scratch the rug with her finger. The

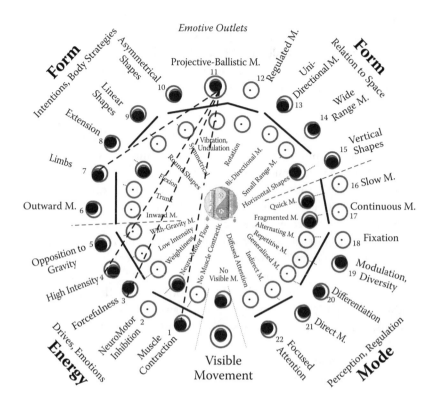

Figure 14.13 A cumulative binary profile of Nina's initial stage of therapy: motor defensive hyperactivity.

scratching movements intensified, and were followed by sobbing: "I feel his hairy back. I hate it. It makes me sick. I try to push him away or to pinch him with my nails, but he is so heavy and so strong." She fell down on her back and tried to kick something. Her face wrenched, her jaws crunched, and her hands tried to push away as if she was struggling with an invisible perpetrator. To me it looked like a videotape that had been edited so that instead of showing a drama of two persons, one had been erased. Yet the movements of the remaining one kept the drama with all its intensity.

Nina continued: "I feel his body on top of me. My wrists hurt. It is as if the old pain comes back. I tried so hard to escape my father's grip but he was stronger and he held my wrist tightly so that I shall not be able to hit him." Then she described how he would enter her room at night and rape her. It started when she was 4 years old and lasted till she was 14.

Her account fits what her movement qualities reflect. In her binary profile the [P-1] forceful prototype was dominant. At the same time, the [P-0] prototype receded to the background. It could not serve her well in a situation in which she had to keep her body in a fight mode against the lurking danger at home.

Comparison of Vera and Nina Based on Their Cumulative Binary Profiles

The two initial profiles show differences and similarities in Vera's and Nina's defenses against trauma; in both profiles there is a split between the [P-0] and the [P-1] prototypes. The direction of the split is different: Vera is locked in the [P-0] ring of potentials, while Nina is locked in the [P-1] ring of potentials. In both cases there are no transitions between the two.

In the course of therapy Vera's motor behavior did not change much. The initial profile remained the same at the end. By contrast, Nina made great progress from the initial motor dominance of excessive forcefulness [P-1] to [P-0] qualities such as lying motionless on the rug for a long time and eventually to the emergence of interwoven [P-1]/[P-0] movement patterns. Figure 14.14 shows the stages in a condensed graphic way (left to right).

Emotive movement patterns that appear in movement improvisation contain information encoded by motor sequences. The two-prototype model of Emotorics introduces typological–developmental coordinates to movement analysis. It enables the therapist to perceive subtle body clues in regard to the mover's emotive attitudes and body defense strategies.

A Final Word

A person who comes to therapy brings into the room a personal blend of anxiety and hope, of pleasurable and painful memories. The visible part of his or her drama is his or her body. We see body postures, we see movement patterns, and we see basic body attitudes to objects and space but we cannot see with our naked eyes the mental parts of a person's inner world.

Emotorics' binary model offers a method of organizing complex information about the mover's past history and present unresolved issues by markers of body, space, time, and relations arranged in binary coordinates. At the center of my efforts is the complex phenomenon of emotive movement.

Aron and Anderson (1998) consider the body an object for analytic observations rather than the physical embodiment of self agency. The role of the body as the active agent of the self is repeatedly ignored. For

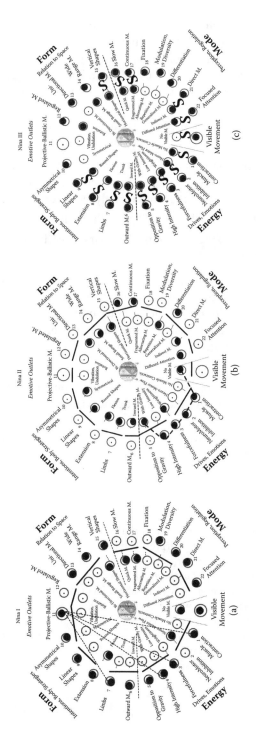

Figure 14.14 Stages in Nina's dance-movement therapy process.

instance, in his introductory words, Aron cites the typical supervisory advice: "Think body, think sex, think dirty."

It is a long erroneous tradition in psychoanalysis to ignore the role of the motor system and function. By contrast, in the last decades it is the brain researchers and neuroscientists who give motor behavior its more balanced place.

Brain scientist Evarts (1976) concludes his article "Brain Mechanisms and Movement" thus:

> Indeed, it seems possible that understanding of the human nervous system, even its most complex intellectual functions, may be enriched if the operation of the brain is analyzed in terms of its motor output rather than in terms of its sensory input. (p. 223)

A similar view is expressed some 25 years later by neurobiologist J. Panksepp (1998b):

> Contrary to traditional thinking on the matter, the above analysis affirms that affective consciousness may be more (at least as) integrally linked in evolution to endogenous motor-related processes than to incoming sensory ones. Emotional systems appear to be much more concentrated in frontal motor/planning than posterior sensory/perceptual regions. (p. 122)

These quotations support the view that when you think of the body you will connect it to emotive movement processes and not necessarily to "dirty" associations.

It is my aim to call attention to the complex role of the motor system in all areas of life and to add my contribution to refine our tools of movement understanding.

Endnote

1. This version of Emotorics is based on Shahar-Levy, A Body-Movement-Mind Paradigm for Analysis and Interpretation of Emotive Motor Systems. A comprehensive version of Emotorics came out in Hebrew under the title *The visible body reveals the secrets of the mind: A body-movement-mind paradigm for the analysis of emotive motility* (Jerusalem: Shahar-Levy. 1996, 2001, 2004). English and German versions are in preparation.

   Emotorics has been taught in all Israeli DMT training programs since 1985 and in the German Institute for Dance Therapy and Psychoanalysis (DITAT), in Bonn, Germany since 1996.

References

Aron L., & Anderson F.S. (1998). *Relational perspectives on the body*, Hillsdale, NJ: Analytic Press.

Averil R.J. (1980). Emotion and anxiety: Sociocultural, biological, and psychological determinants. In Rorty, A.O., *Explaining emotions* (pp. 37–68). Berkeley, CA: University of California Press.

Bernstein, P.L., & Singer, D. (Eds.). (1982). *Choreography of object relations*. Keene, NH: Antioch/ New England Graduate School.

Brown, B. (1975). New mind, new body. New York: Harper & Row.

Damasio, R.A. (1994). *Descartes' error: Emotion, reason and the human brain*. New York: Avon Books.

Damasio, R.A. (1999). *The feeling of what happens: Body and emotion in the making of consciousness*. New York: Harcourt, Brace.

Ekman, P. (1980). Biological and cultural contributions to body and facial movement in the expression of emotions. In Rorty, A.O. *Explaining emotions*. Berkeley, CA: University of California Press.

Eshkol, N., & Wachmann, A. (1958) *Movement notation*. London: Weidenfeld & Nicolson.

Evarts E.V. (1976), Brain mechanisms in movement. In: *Progress in psychobiology: Readings from* Scientific American. San Francisco: W. H. Freeman.

Feldenkrais, M. (1949). *Body and mature behavior*. London: Routledge and Kegan Paul.

Fenichel, O. (1945). *The psychoanalytic theory of neurosis*. New York: W. W. Norton.

Freud, A. (1965). *Normality and pathology in childhood*. London: Hogarth Press and the Institute of Psycho-Analysis.

Gesell, A. (1977). Reciprocal interweaving in neuromotor development. In Payton, O.H. and Newton, R. (Eds.) *Scientific bases for neurophysiologic approaches to therapeutic exercise*. Philadelphia: Davis.

Gordon Benov, R., Bernstein B., Krantz A., Melson B., & Rifkin-Ganor I. (1991). *Collected works by and about Blanche Evan unedited: Dancer, teacher, writer, dance/movement/word therapist*. San Francisco: Blanche Evan Dance Foundation.

Haynal, A. (1993). *Psychoanalysis and the sciences*. London: Karnac.

Khan, R.M. (1974). *The privacy of the self*. New York: International Universities Press.

Kohut, H. (1977). *The restoration of the self*. New York: International Universities Press.

Mahler M.S., Pine F., & Bergman, A. (Eds.) (1975).*The psychological birth of the human infant*. New York: Basic Books.

Newlove, J. (2003). *Laban for all*. London: Nick Hern Books.

Panksepp, J. (1998). *Affective neuroscience: The foundations of human and animal emotions*. New York: Oxford University Press.

Panksepp, J. (2000). The periconscious substrates of consciousness: Affective states and the evolutionary origins of the self. In S. Gallagher and J. Shear (Eds.) *Models of self*. Thorverton, U.K.: Imprint Academic.

Panksepp, J. (2003). At the interface of affective, behavioral, and cognitive neurosciences: Decoding the emotional feelings of the brain. *Brain and Cognition* 52, 4–14.

Rorty, A.O. (1980). *Explaining emotions*. Berkeley, CA: University of California Press.

Sandel, S., Chaiklin, S., & Lohn, A. (1993). *Foundations of dance/movement therapy: The life and work of Marian Chace*. Columbia, MD: Marian Chace Memorial Foundation.

Shahar-Levy, Y. (2001). The function of the human motor system in processes of storing and retrieving preverbal, primal experience. *Psychoanalytic Inquiry, 21,* 3.

Shahar-Levy, Y. (2004). *The visible body reveals the secrets of the mind: A body–movement–mind paradigm (BMMP) for the analysis and interpretation of emotive movement.* Jerusalem. Author's Hebrew edition.

Siegel, E.V. (1984). *Dance movement therapy: Mirror of our selves.* New York: Human Sciences.

Stern, D. (1985). *The interpersonal world of the infant.* New York: Basic Books.

van der Kolk, B. (2000). Trauma, coping and the body, Lecture, International Conference on Trauma, Jerusalem.

van der Kolk, B.A., & van der Hart, O. (1989). Pierre Janet and the breakdown of adaptation in psychological trauma. *American Journal of Psychiatry 146,* 12.

Winnicott, D. (1974). *Playing and reality.* London: Pelican Books.

Bibliography

Anzieu, D. (1989). *The skin ego: A psychoanalytic approach to the self.* New Haven and London: Yale University Press.

Blanck, G., & Blanck, R. (1974). *Ego psychology: Theory and practice.* New York: Columbia University Press.

Chodorow, J. (1991). *Dance therapy and depth psychology: The moving imagination.* London: Routledge.

Davis, M., & Walbridge, D. (1981). *Boundary and space: Introduction to the work of D.W. Winnicott.* New York: Brunner/Mazel.

Fisher, S., & Cleveland, S.E. (1968) *Body image and personality.* New York: Dover.

Fletcher, D. (1974). The use of movement and body experience in therapy. In: *Therapeutic process: Movement as integration.* Columbia, MD: Proceedings of Ninth Annual Conference, ADTA.

Kestenberg, J. (1965). The role of movement patterns in development. *Psychoanalytic Quarterly 34,* 1–36.

Kestenberg, J.S., & Sossin, K.M. (1979). *The role of movement patterns in development,* II. New York: Dance Notation Bureau.

LeDoux J. (1996). *The emotional brain.* New York: Simon & Schuster.

Levine R.L., & Fitzgerald H.E. (1992). *Analysis of dynamic psychological systems* New York: Plenum Press.

Loman, S. (1998). Employing a developmental model of movement patterns in dance/movement therapy with young children and their families, *American Journal of Dance Therapy 20,* (2), 101–115.

Loman, S., & Merman, H. (1996). The KMP: A tool for dance/movement therapy. *American Journal of Dance Therapy 18,* (1), 29–52.

Loman, S. with Foley, F. (1996). Models for understanding the nonverbal process in relationships. *The Arts in Psychotherapy 23,* (4), 341–350.

Lowen, A. (1967). *The betrayal of the body.* London: Collier MacMillan.

Lowen, A. (1958). *The language of the body*. New York: Collier Books.

Restak, R. (1988). *The brain*. New York: Bantam.

Schilder, P. (1970). *The image and appearance of the human body*. New York: International Universities Press.

Stein, R. (1991). *Psychoanalytic theories of affect*. London: Karnac Books.

Symington, J., & Symington, N. (1996). *The clinical thinking of Wilfred Bion*. London: Routledge and Kegan Paul.

CHAPTER 15

Cultural Consciousness and the Global Context of Dance/Movement Therapy

MEG CHANG

Contents

Introduction

For dance/movement therapy (DMT) to fulfill its stated purpose to facilitate body–mind integration with individuals and groups through creative body movement and dance, increased understanding of the role of social context for the dance/movement therapist is required. In a world where national boundaries change rapidly and cultural identities are fluid, where difference is the norm and emigration is a worldwide phenomenon (Suarez-Orozco & Qin-Hilliard, 2004), the dance/movement therapist needs an expanded capacity to respond to social conditions and knowingly embody cultural factors.

In this globalized environment, challenges to traditional values and ways of making sense of the world become the norm for both patients and dance/movement therapists alike (Kareem & Littlewood, 1992; Suarez-Orozco & Qin-Hilliard, 2004).

No longer an emerging profession, the field of creative arts therapies in general, and DMT in particular, is studied and practiced on six continents, with practitioners in at least 37 countries (Dulicai & Berger, 2005). Students travel to different countries to study DMT—frequently in a second language, and educators teach in other countries—frequently in English. International conferences assume commonalities of DMT praxis, i.e., a practice that combines established theories of dance and of the social sciences with the professional implementation of DMT skills. Such examples of shared theory and practice include application of nonverbal communication theories in observation and in assessing relationships with the centrality of dance and body movement in the service of health and well-being.

In preparing dance/movement therapists to address the life experiences of clients from around the world, formal education, professional training, and accepted clinical practices of DMT would benefit from including the sociocultural dimension (Jansen & van der Veen, 1997). Without first critically examining subtle forms of racial, ethnic, and cultural bias that exist in DMT education and practice, there is a danger of foreclosing communication among socioculturally diverse students and educators, between therapist and clients, and among community participants and facilitators of community-based healing arts events.

Through identifying and bringing racial, ethnic, and cultural issues into conscious awareness and seeking the personal and social roots of contested issues, mutual solutions can be discovered and danced. While not generally included in sufficient depth in DMT education and training, self-knowledge about, and intimacy with, the dance/movement therapist's own sociocultural identity increases his or her ability to work with clients, colleagues, and community members who are from different backgrounds. Such personal growth, in turn, has the potential to extend the scope and viability of the field.

DMT Principles and Practices

Historically, the clinical theories and models for dance/movement psychotherapy have been based on western European and North American concepts of mental health (Dokter, 1998; Sue, 1981, 2003). The field of dance/movement therapy in the United States and Europe was developed and became formalized as a discrete profession in the mid-twentieth century as an innovative intervention in mental health that synergized dance and psychology.

Foundational theories of psychological development that informed North American DMT were a focus on the individual or the nuclear family, emphasizing autonomy and independence along a linear progression towards adulthood (Erikson, 1963; Mahler et al., 1975). Psychodynamic psychotherapy was incorporated that similarly valued individual self-efficacy and assertiveness. A unitary ego-identity was espoused among the above distinctly Western Enlightenment principles, which culminated in a preference for patients who were verbal and self-disclosing, and initiated spontaneous communication in psychotherapy (Kareem & Littlewood, 1992; Dokter, 1998). Such psychological theories are examples of North American and European urban culture that became codified as the normative standard, influenced diagnosis, and subsequently guided therapy goals. As DMT became part of clinical treatment teams in psychiatric hospitals, the dominance of the medical model of diagnosis and treatment stimulated the codification of movement observation methods as counterparts to psychological evaluation and diagnosis (Stanton-Jones, 1992).

Cultural Bias—A Personal Account

A personal example of subtle and unintentional cultural bias demonstrates how theory influences practice. In our graduate DMT practicum class, we were practicing a resistance-pushing dyad exercise to establish one's sense of weight with another person. Each student was taking turns to push against the professor as a way to establish autonomy in relationship to her. It is possible that of all 15 students in the class I, as the only Asian, was unable to "stand up to" my teacher and push her off balance. In the discussion after the exercise, I was critiqued by the class for my inability to activate my strength (weight) effectively—admittedly not the first time my predilection for lightness had been noted. However, in this particular class example, the analogy was drawn that I must have some "problem with authority figures" because I could not activate my strong weight sufficiently to move the professor off place. With each person's contention of my nonconforming movement behavior, I felt increasingly inadequate, out of place in the class, and alienated from DMT; internally I began questioning my place in this field. Finally, the other professor present offered, "You know, I come from an Asian background, too, and we are taught never to disobey or challenge our parents, or authority figures. Maybe this is having an effect on Meg."

At this moment, with such acknowledgment of the significance of ethnicity in relationship to (my) multiracial identity, the contextual frame expanded. My unconscious *psychophysical habitus* (Chang, 2006) could be perceived, not as insufficient, but rather as embodying Asian-American cultural values. Once recognized, I felt understood as a student and no longer blamed for representing an identity—race and culture—over which I had little control.

The above vignette indicates that interpreting movement behavior depends in part on the cultural context of the viewer; how "culture is often communicated, internalized, and expressed on a non-verbal level" (Schelly-Hill & Goodill, 2005). This example indicates one way that subtle *ethnocentric monoculturism* (Sue, 2003) rather than conscious discrimination can bias the interpretation of movement. Movement observation is bounded by place and time, by culture and history; the meaning attributed to movement requires the social context to be properly understood (Birdwhistell, 1970).

Observation of Movement and Dance

Laban Movement Analysis (LMA) (Von Laban, 1975) is one system of movement analysis approved by the American Dance Therapy Association educational guidelines (American Dance Therapy Association, 2006) for graduate level training. However, scant research has been done on the generalizability of LMA across cultures.[1] "The Effort/Shape system ... developed out of Rudolph von Laban's analysis of twentieth-century European movement patterns. Given the demands of cross-cultural and intracultural research, no one system will be sufficient" (Desmond, 1997, p. 50). Dance theorist Jane Desmond suggests that movement observation will need to include both an individual's "micro [physical]" and also the sociocultural "macro [historical, ideological]" aspects of human movement analysis.

One preliminary phenomenological study (Tepayayone, 2004) found that cultural disparities influenced observers' interpretation of movement qualities, mover's personality, and movement behavior. The researcher found that when movement observers from one culture viewed dance/movement of a different culture, the observers had difficulty in rating the movement from the other's culture. Moreover, cultural images about dance influenced the way movement was perceived, e.g., "[The] traditional movement quality of Asian people [and] Brazilian dance ... would be more like a celebration, what you see in Carnival" (Tepayayone, 2004, p. 86). Even though the observers were consciously using a cognitive process to categorize the dance, they described emotional responses when rating the movement, i.e., "Brazilian mover[s] made them feel dizzy and uncomfortable" (p. 91). Finally, the rater's own level of cultural awareness and differences within ethnic/racial groups were found to influence their interpretation of dance movement from another culture.

Dance is central to DMT, and while it may be human to dance, to paraphrase anthropologist Judith Hanna (1979), the meanings ascribed to dancing, and the aesthetic standards of the dance are specific not only to each culture, but also within local subcultures. Rather than considering dance as a symbolic language that communicates similar aesthetics, emotions, and associations across all cultures, anthropologists look to the specific ways each culture constructs these meanings in their dance (Hanna, 1979, 1990, 1999, 2006; Fuller-Snyder & Johnson, 1999). In her seminal article "An Anthropologist Looks at Ballet as a Form of Ethnic Dance," dance ethnologist Joann Kealiinohomoku (1983) critiques dance historians for privileging Western modern dance and ballet as the only and highest aesthetic standard; their tendency to aggregate dances as "Native American" or "African" rather than specifically naming the region or nation, i.e., Lakota dances or Masai dances; and for designating non-Western dances as "primitive," "exotic," or "ethnic" when used as a euphemism for racially identified dances (Kealiinohomoku, 1983).

Given the history of the field, dance forms that predominate in the theory and practice of DMT are inescapably ethnocentric, because "all forms of dance reflect the cultural traditions within which they developed" (Kealiinohomoku, 1983, p. 533). As we know, the dance aesthetic underlying mainstream DMT is primarily derived from modern dance traditions of Germany, England, and the United States (Levy, 1992), with an infusion of Israeli folk dance choreography and sensibility in the 1960s and 1970s.[2] The dances of DMT "pioneers" Marian Chace, Blanche Evan, Trudi Schoop, Lillian Espenak, Mary Whitehouse, and Alma Hawkins (Levy, 1992), are distinctly culture-bound to time and place. These women were modern dancers with strong dance technique before they were therapists; they developed their dance therapy methods based on Western dance traditions of free improvisation, creativity, and individual expression (Manning, 1993; Evan, 1991; Schoop, 1974).

How we learn to observe and experience dance naturally predisposes us to how we understand the role of dance-as-aesthetic or dance-as-healing.[3] We in turn influence how our students, clients, or patients look at dance and their body(ies) in all their social and individual dimensions in the practice of dance-as-therapy. The entire range of unconscious associations to body movement—beginning with nonverbal movement observation— is an example of *psychophysical habitus* (Chang, 2006). This corporeal *habitus,* which includes aesthetic preferences, is an embodied and encompassing, unconscious and unavailable to linear thinking, mind and body prototype that is instilled preverbally (Bourdieu, 1977).

The *habitus* is specific to a cultural context of an individual or a profession (Bourdieu, 1991). Often, when the so-called universal nature of dance and hence of DMT is referenced, an assumption is made of a common shared *habitus.* On the contrary, as a distinct interdisciplinary practice of dance and psychology, DMT reflects a Western urban 20th-century heritage and aesthetic that may no longer be widely applicable, but rather needs to evolve in the practitioner's understanding in order to become more inclusive of the world and its representation in DMT.

Rationale for Building Intercultural Resonance

The *habitus* was defined by anthropologist/sociologist Pierre Bourdieu (1977) as the totality of physical habits and pre-dispositions that arise from specific geographies, local societies, and interpersonal relationships that reinforce "...the durably installed generative principle of regulated improvisations...[and] systems of relations, in and through the production of practice" (Bourdieu, 1977, p. 78). Because these systems are pervasive, the *habitus* is not readily available to conscious reflection. E. T. Hall's (1976) early comparative work on the immutable perception of time and use of space in the United States and Japan as the "hidden dimension" of culture comes to mind. "The *habitus*—embodied history, internalized as a second nature and so forgotten as history—is the active presence of the whole past of which it is the product...like a train laying its own rails" (Bourdieu in Lemert, 1999, p. 445).

Furthermore, Bourdieu (1991) asserted that professions as entities are identified with a characteristic *habitus,* "a special world ... endowed with its own laws of functioning" (p. 375), and that socialization of education systems produces a *secondary habitus* (Bourdieu, 1984). One recognizable tenet of DMT was expressed by a Korean dance therapy student. "I have personally experienced cohesion of myself through my body. I think problems can be solved through the body ... we are normally so dependent on words for self improvement." With this characterization she describes "the practical knowledge of the requirements that are inscribed in the very logic of the field in which they express themselves" (Bourdieu, 1991, p. 375). A case study of DMT education in East Asia found that DMT students sought a field whose rules include the aesthetic and creative use of dance in relationship to helping others, through a personal integration of the material in their own bodily experience, which is a key concept in DMT (Chang, 2002).

If dance reflects the local culture, as philosophers, sociologists, and anthropologists claim (Douglas, 1970; Lomax, Bartenieff, & Pauley, 1974; Polhemus, 1975; Bourdieu, 1984), then what do we as educators and therapists need to consider in our work with people from other race-ethnicities, cultures, or classes? What kind of education prepares the dance/movement therapist?

Nonverbal Aspects of Culture

Dance/movement therapy skills are taught through experiential and non-verbal methods, which are consistent with the logic of experiential dance education. "Other education systems depend on text—they always use textbooks and materials. In the case of dance therapy there is no text, only the body, and an open mind," is how one DMT student described her learning. However, educators Schelly-Hill and Goodill (2005) found in their qualitative pilot study with international students in the United States, that nonverbal aspects of culture and "hidden social codes" were the most difficult for non-American students to internalize: "jokes, spon-taneous cultural funny movements, gestures, postures, can make you feel not part of a group" (p. 5). Nonverbal interpersonal interactions are subject to cultural interpretation; what the Western dance therapist observes as an individual's idiosyncratic movement preferences may be the unconscious psychocultural habits of the body (Bourdieu, 1977; Gudykunst & Kim, 1992; Chang, 2002).

What we see when we watch movement is necessarily influenced by the psychophysical orientation of our culture, professional habits, and the diversity of our life experiences. For example, from a Korean perspective, looking down while performing the emotionally expressive *Salp'uri* dance has the attribute of being entranced and absorbed in the dance. This inward characteristic is highly valued, whereas an upward tilt of the head is seen as being flirtatious, Westernized, and improper (Loken-Kim, 1989). Unless the educator and therapist consciously acknowledge the culturally conditioned aspect of movement behavior, the tendency will be to mis-read the emotional intention, blame oneself, or find the student-client lacking when confronted with nonverbal codes of "the other" (Gudykunst & Kim, 1992).

Supporting Literature and Research Examples

The scope of research presented is drawn from case study research in teach-ing DMT in Korea and Taiwan (Chang, 2002), educating dance/movement therapists in the United States (Chang, 2000), and clinical practice in the

United States with patients from every race, many ethnicities, and numerous cultures that include all gender identities. These experiences are seen through the personal lens of my Chinese-American heritage. Rather than attempting to generalize from experiences of Korean, Chinese, Taiwanese, Thai, African-American, and Afro-Caribbean students and clients, these findings are preliminary. Ideally, comparative research and practice with other non-majority and non-dominant students and therapists will enrich the knowledge base of DMT. However, research generated by East Asian students and practitioners from Korea (Shim, 2003), China (Ho, 2005a; 2005b), Japan (Sakiyama & Koch, 2003), and Thailand (Tepayayone, 2004) does indicate similarities among related culture groups.

This research draws upon previous cross cultural work in DMT (Lomax, Bartenieff, & Pauley, 1974; Fuller-Snyder, 1999; Hanna, 1990, 1999; Lewis, 1997; Dosamantes, 1997a, 1997b; and Pallaro, 1997), as well as recent interest in intercultural DMT (Chang, 2002; Ho, 2005a, 2005b; Cummins, 2006). Such attention to race, culture, and ethnicity coincides with an increase in utilizing DMT in international work with survivors of trauma (Gray, 2001), as well as trends in internationalization of the field (Capello, 2006; Chang, 2002).

Unlike the pragmatic and student-centered education of the United States graduate dance therapy programs, the habitus of education in Korea is based on Confucian principles in which hierarchical relationships dictate not only educational systems, but all interactions. To attain the highly valued goal of social harmony, all interactions—including education—adhere to a strict hierarchy of relationships between men and women, older and younger, and "ruler and subject" that must be followed within the family, and by extension, between teacher and student. The prescribed order of relationships governs all interpersonal interactions from family to government (Reischauer & Fairbank, 1960).[4]

In a similar manner, Korean arts education is based on the Confucian hierarchy, in which duplication of the teacher's style by direct imitation is considered a demonstration of loyalty and respect from student to teacher; in fact students are expected to copy the master teacher until their own artwork is indistinguishable from the teacher's (Kristof, 1999). Because of Confucian attitudes respecting age, Korean dancers over the age of 60 are considered to be more socially appropriate and more accomplished at expressing strong emotions in dance (Loken-Kim, 1989). In addition, having attained age and status as a performer, Korean dance teachers expect their students to imitate their dance style, reproduce their choreography, and be unpaid dance company apprentices. In keeping with the tradition of following a master, a student's loyalty demands an exclusive relationship with the teacher and his or her dance style. These relationships exemplify the habitus in dance education, and by extension, of dance therapy and creative arts therapy education in Korea. When the student–teacher relationship is inculcated and maintained nonverbally, it is "generative and transposable; it can spawn different practices in sites away from that of its acquisition" (Usher, Bryant, & Johnston, 1997, p. 60).

Therefore, Korean and Chinese students will bring this unconscious Confucian valence or habitus to student-teacher relationships in peer-oriented Western DMT programs. Such dedication and learning is not infrequently interpreted by the non-Asian educator and fellow students as "passive," when the student seeks to reproduce the teacher's knowledge. From the Korean perspective, the student perceives the behavior as appropriate and respectful from a competent student. For these newly arrived students in the United States, their learning must include the unfamiliar skill of how to question the teacher and be a verbal presence in the Western-style classroom.

Initially, nondirective modern dance improvisations used to elicit learning about the self are seen as "*confusing*" because the teacher does not model the movement or prescribe an outcome. However, student-centered dance/movement directives can be valued for providing a chance to "*lead yourself*" in comparison with Confucian teacher-centered models where there is "*always a right answer.*"

Hoffman (1998), an anthropologist, states:

> Cultures differ greatly in the manner in which they define the relationship between self and other, the degree to which they distinguish between "mind" and "body" (or have separate categories for each), and in the way in which they conceptualize agency and motivation as external or internally directed. (Hoffman, 1998, p. 328)

She contrasts cultures that define the self as autonomous, individuated, and separate in comparison with those cultures in which a socially embedded self is more dependent on social situations, with fluid and flexible boundaries. Therefore, when an East Asian graduate student says, "My identity is not my personality. Who I am, is my family, my religion, how old I am, and where I go to school … things like that" would she be considered immature, or have poor ego boundaries in terms of conventional ego psychology? When applied to individuals and groups whose values and norms differ, something as intrinsic as identity is defined and lived in surprisingly diverse and culturally specific ways.

As clinicians, when we interact across language groups or between subcultures, we are compelled to recognize the disorienting and stimulating nature of cultural, racial, or ethnic difference. Confronting foundational disparities in the perceived nature of identity, family structure, or gender in clinical practice can heighten sensitivity and awareness in a practitioner who wants to understand different world views (H. Chaiklin, personal communication, October 16, 2006). The most favorable outcome is the "development of a dance/movement therapy profession that is genuinely international in character" (Schelly-Hill & Goodill, 2005).

Can DMT Be Practiced across Languages, Cultures, and Ethnic-Racial Differences?

Self-Awareness

In order for DMT to become more inclusive and available to the emerging global client, increased awareness of each dance/movement therapist's racial, ethnic, cultural, gender, and class background is a first step. Unless culturally ingrained beliefs and habits are brought to consciousness to be investigated, the therapist may relate with "unconscious avoidance of the client of difference based on factors such as fears, ambivalence or feelings of personal aversion" (Gaertner & Dovidio as cited in Dokter, 1998, p. 148). The ubiquity of prejudice is such that investigating one's own conscious bias(es) is a crucial factor in becoming an effective educator or therapist with an ethnic or racial group that is different from one's own (Carter & Qureshi, 1995). Systems of structured *racial identity development* (Sue, 2003; Helms, 1990) believe that racial identity is a key component of an individual's development of positive self-image. Knowledge of one's own racial/ethnic/culture/class history is analogous to self-assessment of movement style; it can be explored through the tools of dance.

One such model, as developed by Joi Gresham in the spring of 1995 at Lesley University, was "The Dance of the Ancestors." Originally situated in an education class, her semistructured creative dance process extrapolated *racial identity theory* (Helms, 1990; Sue, 1981, 2003) through a dance modality. As I have modified her work for dance therapists, participants are encouraged to imagine and physically recreate emblematic movements of their own ancestors (known or imagined). Embodied identification can be in the form of a typical ethnic folkdance, a personally constructed memory of an elder, by physically animating a photograph, or any other of a number of creative directives. From these dance sketches, choreographic elements reveal both formulaic and individual characteristics of one's forbears at the level of rhythm, use of space, and movement metaphors. By dancing a specific family member, the participant overcomes the stage of ignorance or naiveté about race and ethnicity (Sue, 2003, p. 172) while confronting the conforming or stereotypical aspects of his or her race and ethnicity. As a result of such direct and frequently uncomfortable experience, the dissonant and inconsistent elements of one's ancestry surface (p. 176). Exploring through dance directives, leads to introspection (p. 180) and finally clarity, or integrative awareness (p. 182) of how race, ethnicity, and culture are defined in one's body and movement. Such physicalized identity, combined with the dance/movement therapist's movement preferences, can be integrated with social or environmental contexts. A personal example is the way my English grandmother's verticality emerges through my tensely held straight spine when I am threatened or antagonized.

Through such self-identification of sociocultural background, participants understand how their own culture has influenced their perception of the world based on the accident of birth. And by interacting with all the other races and ethnicities represented in the group—directly or through the "ancestors"—group members come to understand how they are perceived by others. As a result, participants report heightened empathy for the life struggles of their patients who confront racial and cultural identity confusion or discrimination based on race or ethnicity. Adapting Gresham's conceptualization of embodied racial, ethnic, and cultural heritage to DMT training has helped dance therapy students and professionals grasp the salience of sociocultural identity within multicultural societies such as the United States and Western Europe.

Cultural Congruence

Following such a personal and embodied identification, *culturally congruent* and culturally inclusive psychotherapy models can be devised. At the Nafsiyat Intercultural Therapy Centre in London, England—a counseling center serving "black, ethnic minority groups, immigrants, migrants, and political refugees" (Kareem & Littlewood, 1992, p. xi), clinicians found that traditional psychodynamic theories that emphasized rigid boundaries and impersonal practices tended to intensify racial, ethnic, and cultural misunderstanding. As a result, alienation of all involved ensued. When, consciously or unconsciously, differences in the social-cultural backgrounds of therapist and client manifested in asymmetrical power relationships, clients reported that the psychotherapy was not effective, that they were not helped with their problems, and that their symptoms did not diminish (Kareem & Littlewood, 1992). Furthermore, when the therapist demonstrated ignorance of the client's culture, whether because of explicit prejudice or unexamined cultural misunderstandings, therapeutic interventions were disregarded and treatment was terminated prematurely (Acharyya, 1992; Gilroy, 1998).

Consequently, therapists at the Nafsiyat Centre developed the principle of *cultural congruence* to guide their practice (Acharyya, 1992; Gilroy, 1998). As defined, cultural congruence is complementary and collaborative; it occurs when the cultural and political context of both therapist and client is acknowledged and addressed in treatment. These reflexive principles are applied throughout the entire course of treatment, including diagnosis, and alignment of social-cultural differences is deliberately sought within the therapeutic relationship (Acharyya, 1992). An analogy in DMT would be to research music that represents clients' cultures, but more importantly, to critically examine the meaning of the music with the client rather than presume to know or intuit cultural references in another language. Further, the dance therapist must be alert to how each client's associations—to a samba, for example—will differ based on country of origin, gender, age, class, and education as well as from racial projections and cultural influences.

Mutuality

One indication of power differentials in treatment and cultural imbalance in teaching or in DMT practice is to detect whose definition of dance/movement predominates, and whether flexibility regarding the meaning of the dance and significance of movement interactions are mutually derived. Does the definition of the macro-culture or that of the micro-culture prevail? Similarly, the injunction to self-determination can be applied to any type of collective identity—whether racial, ethnic, or cultural. Rather than having interpretation imposed or meaning assigned by a dance/movement therapist who is not from a given culture group, it is important for native speakers to self-identify as cultural informants. Next, it is crucial to demonstrate respect for the member's opinions and suggestions—especially in reference to assessment and diagnosis—by implementing local knowledge. Similarly, is the practitioner alert for language use that acknowledges or excludes the life experiences of a particular race or gender, e.g., exclusive use of "husband" or "wife" when "partner" or "lover" would equally apply? Is the cultural aesthetic of one race, ethnicity, or culture privileged, including that of the group leader? While semantic responses can be learned, the transformative work comes from direct interaction, lived-experience, or case-based training and education.

A valid way to ground human movement behavior in the sociocultural environment acknowledges how "the social body constrains the way the physical body is perceived" (Douglas, 1970, p. 65). For example, movement observation systems based on Western standards for the body, relationships, and dance can be expanded to include subtle and rarefied Korean systems of nonverbal movement observation and sophisticated Japanese taxonomies of expressed emotions when working with these cultures. In this way, "Cultural variations in conceptions of the person must be mined for their implications for metatheory, theory, methods, and professional practices" (Gergen et al., 1995). Incorporating a global and international range of aesthetics and lifestyles would facilitate local, indigenous, and multicultural adaptations of movement observation, taxonomy, and diagnosis that then expand the body of knowledge of the field.

Conclusions and Next Steps

We live in a world of distinctive multiple cultures, a world in which multicultural contact is becoming normative, especially in urban areas where DMT is prevalent. Personal encounters and educational exchanges precipitate intercultural transmission as well as highlight cross-cultural points of friction. At such a time, revisioning the praxis of dance/movement therapy can ensure that our work reflects current psychocultural realities in order to be effective, conform to ethical guidelines, and consciously guide the evolving theories of DMT.

To meet this need, knowledge about cultural differences specific to DMT must be continuously acquired, critically examined, and then promulgated, lest a practitioner apply a broad-brush approach within a region or among apparently similar cultures. It would take more than superficial study, for example, to be sensitive to nuanced differences and apply useful similarities among Spanish speakers from the north of Spain with those from Mexico, Argentina, Chile, or, indeed, Guinea-Bissau. Even within one language or culture group, there may be different words, images, perceptions, and concepts about similar things. Historic legacies and social contexts that have deeply rooted significance for the local culture-bearer may be invisible to the outsider, however well-intentioned. Because of one's *psychophysical habitus*, a Westerner may see East Asian students' behaviors as excessively homogeneous and conformist in group classes, for example, while the East Asian person may be experiencing group harmony and respect for order and hierarchy.

Another area of challenge for the dance/movement therapist is to educate her or himself in becoming sufficiently aware of social structures, such as class differences, that impact interpersonal relationships. Exploration of embodied identity and cultural self-knowledge are ways to critically examine how race, ethnicity, culture, and class are first manifested in oneself and then influence the therapeutic milieu. As the field moves beyond the exclusively therapeutic domain—into community arts for example—an exciting opportunity exists for dance improvisation and self-expression in the creative arts to find new, more inclusive redefinitions beyond Western Enlightenment traditions. Aligned with an attitude of inquiry in which neither culture dominates, dynamic applications that are recognizable to a range of cultural actors, dancers, and artists can be generated.

The prospect of a global dance/movement therapy that sustains its disciplinary rigor and encompassing utility is best realized by questioning, selecting, and recombining the full range of theories-in-use to guide practices of DMT education and clinical practice in non-English-speaking environments. On the other hand, as DMT becomes a professional entity in many countries, the balance between its unique as well as ubiquitous aspects can invigorate the field. The creative habitus of DMT ensures that infinite ways exist to critically examine psychotherapeutic practices within the light of current intercultural needs, providing that even the notion of creativity can be reciprocal, provisional, and open to interrogation.

As dance/movement therapists in clinical practice engage in personal identity work and intentionally locate their own racial, ethnic, and cultural selves, they are better able to *meet the clients where they are* in their entire social and cultural contexts. As DMT educators and students interact in the spaces between cultures, opportunities for intercultural exploration can lead beyond stereotypes to self-identification if the dance/movement therapist is willing to be self-aware, self-educated, and develop an uncompromising critical attitude. In a way, this is the natural realm of creativity and art, and what other choice do we have as a profession, except to enlarge our curriculum to include the world and all its variations? And as colleagues, the field of DMT can only grow in scope and competence as we learn from each other, exchanging local wisdom of dance as healing.

Endnotes

1. One attempt to classify daily work actions around the world in parallel with local dance movements is the *Choreometrics* project based on LMA (Lomax, Bartenieff, & Pauley, 1974). Lomax's method has since been criticized by American anthropologists for its predictive, causal, and statistical approach (Kealiinohomoku, 1974; Seeger, 1994).
2. Israeli folk dance is itself a synthetic dance form according to Roginsky (2006).
3. For example, Korean dance therapy students told me that if they could perform emotional dances very skillfully for their psychiatric patients, that the patients would be healed. Such a notion is closely related to the way that *pansori* opera cleanses the audience with its shared conveying of sadness and joy.
4. For a more complete description of Confucianism, please see Reischauer & Fairbank, 1960.

References

Acharyya, S. (1992). The doctor's dilemma: The practice of cultural psychiatry in multicultural Britain. In Kareem, J. & Littlewood, R. (Eds.). *Intercultural therapy: Themes, interpretations and practice.* (pp. 74–82). Oxford, England: Blackwell Scientific.

American Dance Therapy Association (2006). *Committee on Approval procedural guidelines.* (Available from the American Dance Therapy Association, 2000 Century Plaza, Suite 108, Columbia, MD 21044.)

Benthall, J., & Polhemus, T. (1975). *The body as a medium of expression.* New York: E.P. Dutton.

Birdwhistell, R. L. (1970). *Kinesics and context: Essays on body motion communication.* New York: Ballantine.

Bourdieu, P. (1991). Epilogue: On the possibility of a field of world sociology. In Bourdieu, P. & Coleman, J. (Eds.). *Social theory for a changing society.* (pp. 373–387). San Francisco: Westview, Russell Sage Foundation.

Bourdieu, P. (1984). *Distinction: A social critique of the judgment of taste.* (R. Nice, Trans.). Cambridge, MA: Harvard University.

Bourdieu, P. (1977). *Outline of a theory of practice.* (R. Nice, Trans.). New York: Cambridge University.

Capello, P. P. (2006). Training dance/movement therapists: The international challenge. *American Journal of Dance Therapy 28*(1), 31–40.

Carter, R., & Qureshi, A. (1995). A typology of philosophical assumptions in multicultural counseling and training. In Ponterotto, J., Casas, J., Suzuki, L., Alexander, C. (Eds.). *Handbook of multicultural counseling.* (pp. 239–262). New York: Sage.

Chang, M. (2006). How do dance/movement therapists bring awareness of race, ethnicity, and cultural diversity into their practice? In Koch, S. & Brauninger, I. (Eds.). *Advances in dance/movement therapy. Theoretical perspectives and empirical findings,* pp. 192–205. Berlin: Logos.

Chang, M. (2002). Cultural congruence and aesthetic adult education: Teaching dance/movement therapy in Seoul, Korea. *Dissertation Abstracts International* (UMI No. 3052868).

Chang, M. (2000). Multicultural difference in dance-movement therapy: Pre-conference training seminar. 35th Annual American Dance Therapy Association Conference, Seattle, WA. October, 2000.

Cummins, L. (2006). *Awareness of racism: The responsibility of white dance/movement therapists.* Unpublished master's thesis, Pratt Institute, Brooklyn: NY.

Desmond, J. C. (Ed.). (1997). *Meaning in motion: New cultural studies of dance.* Durham, NC: Duke University.

Dokter, D. (1998). (Ed.). *Arts therapists, refugees and migrants reaching across borders.* London: Jessica Kingsley.

Dokter, D. (1998). Being a migrant, working with migrants: Issues of identity and embodiment. In Dokter, D. (Ed.). *Arts therapists, refugees and migrants reaching across borders.* (pp. 148) London: Jessica Kingsley.

Dosamantes-Beaudry, I. (1997a). Reconfiguring identity. *The Arts in Psychotherapy 24*(1), 51–57.

Dosamantes-Beaudry, I. (1997b). Embodying a cultural identity. *The Arts in Psychotherapy 24*(2), 129–135.

Douglas, M. (1970). *Natural symbols: Explorations in cosmology.* New York: Vintage.

Dulicai, D., & Berger, M. R. (2005). Global dance/movement therapy growth and development. *The Arts in Psychotherapy 32,* 205–216.

Erikson, E. (1963). *Childhood and society.* New York: W.W. Norton.

Evan, B. (1991). *Collected works by and about Blanche Evan.* San Francisco: Anne Krantz, Blanche Evan Dance Foundation.

Fuller-Snyder, A., & Johnson, C. (1999). *Securing our dance heritage: Issues in the documentation and preservation of dance.* Washington, D.C.: Council on Library and Information Resources.

Gaertner, S., & Dovidio, J. (1981). Racism among the well-intentioned. In *Manuals of Readings* (1991–1993). *Ethnocultural Issues in Social Work Practice.* New York University School of Social Work. Needham, MA: Gin.

Gray, A. (2001). The body remembers: Dance movement therapy with an adult survivor of torture. *American Journal of Dance Therapy 23* (1), 29–43.

Gergen, K., Gulerce, A., Lock, A., Misra, G. (Eds.). (1995). *Psychological science in cultural context.* http://www.massey.ac.nz/~alock/virtual/discuss.htm.

Gilroy, A. (1998). On being a temporary migrant to Australia: Reflections on art therapy education and practice. In Dokter, D. (Ed.). *Art therapists, refugees and migrants reaching across borders.* (pp. 262–277). Philadelphia, PA: Jessica Kingsley.

Gudykunst, W., & Kim, Y. (1992). *Communicating with strangers: An approach to intercultural communication* (2nd ed.). New York: McGraw-Hill.

Hall, E. T. (1976). *Beyond culture.* New York: Doubleday.

Hanna, J. L. (2006). The power of dance discourse: Explanation in self-defense. *American Journal of Dance Therapy 28* (1), 3–20.

Hanna, J. L. (1999). *Partnering dance and education: Intelligent moves for changing times.* Champaign, IL: Human Kinetics.

Hanna, J. L. (1990). Anthropological perspectives for dance/movement therapy. *American Journal of Dance Therapy 12* (2), 115–126.

Hanna, J. L. (1979). *To dance is human.* Austin, TX: University of Texas.

Helms, J. L. (1990). *Black and White racial identity: Theory, research, and practice.* Westport, CT: Praeger.

Ho, R. (2005a). Effects of dance/movement therapy on Chinese cancer patients: A pilot study in Hong Kong. *Arts in Psychotherapy 13* (11), 337–345.

Ho, R. (2005b). Regaining balance within: Dance/movement therapy with Chinese cancer patients in Hong Kong. *American Journal of Dance Therapy 27* (2), 87–99.

Hoffman, D. (1998). A therapeutic moment? Identity, self, and culture in the anthropology of education. *Anthropology & Education Quarterly 29*(3), 324–346.

Jansen, T., & van der Veen, R. (1997). Individualization, the new political spectrum and the functions of adult education. *International Journal of Lifelong Education 16*(4), 264–276.

Johnson, C., & Fuller-Snyder, A. (1999). *Securing our dance heritage: Issues in the documentation and preservation of dance.* Washington, DC: Council on Library and Information Resources.

Kareem, J., & Littlewood, R. (1992). (Eds.). *Intercultural therapy: Themes, interpretations and practice.* Boston, MA: Blackwell Scientific.

Kealiinohomoku, J. (1983). An anthropologist looks at ballet as a form of ethnic dance. In Copeland, R. & Cohen, M. (Eds.). *What is dance: Readings in theory and criticism* (pp. 533–549). New York: Oxford.

Kristof, N. (1999, May 12). Koreans, long copiers, try a new road to creativity. *The New York Times*, E2.

Lemert, C. (1999). (Ed.). *Social theory: The multicultural and classic readings.* Boulder, CO: Westview Perseus.

Levy, F. J. (1992). *Dance movement therapy: A healing art* (2nd ed.). Reston, VA: American Alliance for Health, Physical Education, Recreation and Dance.

Lewis, P. (1997). Appreciating diversity, commonality and the transcendent through the arts therapies. *The Arts in Psychotherapy 24* (3), 225–226.

Loken-Kim, C. (1989). Release from bitterness: Korean dancer as Korean woman. *Dissertation Abstracts International* (UMI No. 9032994).

Lomax, A., Bartenieff, I., & Paulay, F. (1974). Choreometrics: A method for the study of cross-cultural pattern in film. In *CORD Research Annual VI. New Dimensions in Dance Research: Anthropology and Dance: The American Indian.* Comstock, T. (Ed.). 193–212. New York: Congress on Research in Dance.

Mahler, M. S., Pine, F., & Bergman, A. (1975). *The psychological birth of the human infant.* New York: Basic.

Manning, S. (1993). *Ecstasy and the demon: Feminism and nationalism in the dances of Mary Wigman*, Berkeley, CA: University of California.

Pallaro, P. (1997). Culture, self and body-self: Dance/movement therapy with Asian Americans. *Arts in Psychotherapy 24* (3), 227–241.

Paulay, F., & Lomax, A. (1977). *Choreometrics: Dance and human history, the longest trail, palm play, step style.* Berkeley, CA: University of California Extension, Center for Media and Independent Learning.

Polhemus, T. (1975). Social bodies. In Benthall, J. & Polhemus, T. (Eds.). *The body as a medium of expression* (pp. 13–35) New York: E.P. Dutton.

Reischauer, E., & Fairbank, J. (1960). *East Asia: The great tradition.* Boston: Houghton Mifflin.

Roginsky, D. (2006). Nationalism and ambivalence: Ethnicity, gender and folklore as categories of otherness. *Patterns of Prejudice 40* (3), 237–258.

Schelly-Hill, E., & Goodill, S. (2005). International students in American dance/movement therapy education: Cultural riches and challenges. Presented at the 39th Annual American Dance Therapy Association Conference, Nashville, TN. October, 2005.

Schoop, T. (1974). *Won't you join the dance? A dancer's essay into the treatment of psychosis.* Palo Alto, CA: National Press.

Seeger, A. (1994). Music and dance. In Ingold, T. (Ed.). *Companion encyclopedia of anthropology.* (pp. 686–705). New York: Routledge.

Shim, M. (2003). *An exploration of ethnic identity through dance/movement therapy: A phenomenological study of the 1.5 and 2nd generation Korean American young adults.* Unpublished master's thesis, Drexel University, Philadelphia: PA.

Sakiyama, Y., & Koch, N. (2003). Touch in dance therapy in Japan. *American Journal of Dance Therapy 25*(2), 79–95.

Stanton-Jones, K. (1992). *Dance movement therapy in psychiatry.* New York: Routledge.

Suarez-Orozco, M. & Qin-Hilliard, D. (Eds.). (2004). *Globalization, culture and education in the new millennium.* Berkeley, CA: University of California.

Sue, D. (1981). *Counseling the culturally different: Theory and practice.* New York: Wiley.

Sue, D. (2003). *Overcoming our racism: The journey to liberation.* San Francisco: Jossey-Bass.

Tepayayone, W. (2004). *Culture, perception, and clinical assessment in dance/movement therapy: A phenomenological investigation.* Unpublished master's thesis, Drexel University, Philadelphia: PA.

Usher, R., Bryant, I., & Johnston, R. (Eds.). (1997). *Adult education and the postmodern challenge: Learning beyond the limits.* New York: Routledge.

Von Laban, R. (1975). In L. Ullmann (Trans.). *A life for dance.* New York: Theater Arts.

CHAPTER 16

Encouraging Research in Dance/Movement Therapy

LENORE W. HERVEY

Contents

Introduction

My area of interest has been the perception and experience of research by dance/movement therapists. I have been conducting research, teaching research to dance/movement therapy (DMT) students and working with the Research Subcommittee of the American Dance Therapy Association for many years. My research findings and professional experiences have compelled me to promote and develop research methods that resonate with the values, work experiences, skills, and ways of knowing of my students and colleagues. I have come to believe that promoting methodological diversity will facilitate participation in research. Despite the continuing call for quantifiable outcome and efficacy research results, which I also support, I still advocate for the greatest breadth of research options. The reader will no doubt perceive these biases toward a flexible and evolving understanding of research methodologies throughout this chapter.

The task of this chapter, to provide suggestions for how to encourage research in dance/movement therapy, leads me to a set of questions covering multiple perspectives. Understandably, greater attention will be given to those areas in which I have more experience and knowledge, and to those about which there are research findings. One way to consider the questions that arise from the need to promote research is to imagine focal areas, like spotlights of decreasing sizes. If we entertain large focal questions we need to consider the cultural and macrosystemic determinants of research production. At the microsystem end of this range we are examining questions about how the individual determines his or her professional behavior, even at an intrapsychic level. And of course there are the questions about how the larger systemic factors influence the smaller ones. To thoroughly address all the questions in this focal range would require a lifetime of work. My humble goal here is to identify the questions, stimulate thought about them, and offer suggestions about as many as I am able.

The Biggest Questions

To say that the production and publication of research in DMT depends on many complex, interactive, contextual factors is an understatement. But if we have to start sorting out these influences somewhere, it might as well be at the top. On the largest scale, how does a society, a government, or a culture encourage (or discourage) research in DMT? One of the most fascinating answers to explore is the culture-specific understanding of core concepts such as dance, science, health, illness, and healing. The implicit values placed on these ideas will influence attitudes toward theories and practices of DMT. For instance, how a culture perceives dance will influence how the practice of DMT will evolve. How that same culture understands healing determines how dance has been and will be used for healing. The idea of science—who does it, where, how and why—will determine what kind of research is considered valid and valuable. Understanding these cultural constructs will help researchers present their projects to the public and to funding sources in ways that resonate with cultural values and beliefs.

The political and economic climates of a system (an institution, a mental health services system, or a government) also sustain or transform the mechanisms by which research is supported. Bureaucratic power hierarchies determine who makes decisions and who simply responds to mandates. Policies establish how funding is generated and distributed. Political ideologies control what questions may even be asked. Researchers may be encouraged or seriously restrained by the systemic environments within which they find themselves. Again, researchers who use the language and address the values of any system will help its stakeholders understand how important research is to that system. Alternatively, activism to help create a more research-friendly environment is certainly an option that each researcher may have to consider.

Prevailing attitudes within the scientific and scholarly community also exert some control over what kind of research is published and by whom. In recent years there has been a notable broadening of methodological possibilities for research in the human sciences, which were once monopolized by positivist approaches. The fields of education, nursing, sociology, and anthropology have led the way for creative arts therapists to follow when they are ready. Ground-breaking qualitative and artistic methods are now welcomed in international journals such as *Qualitative Inquiry*. Knowing that there are journals that accept nontraditional research articles may encourage researchers in the creative arts to try their hands at developing and utilizing innovative methodologies.

Another factor that influences the production of research is the relationship of a practice or profession to historical events and social trends. For instance, the need of the medical system to care for traumatized veterans of World War II is acknowledged as a formative influence in the development of DMT in the United States (Levy, 1992). Also in the United States, the impending needs of a large population of aging "Baby Boomers" may soon result in the divergence of funds toward research supporting innovative treatments (such as DMT) for the elderly. Researching and responding to the impending needs of a society may place the profession in a position to address those needs through DMT.

Research also evolves with any particular profession over time. When a practice is young there are very few theories or consistent methods upon which to base hypotheses that could be tested through scientific method. Research in the form of case studies and qualitative descriptions of practice, accompanied by the initial development of theory, are most common. Such has been the case for DMT in North America over the past half century (Stark, 2002). Only when methods of practice are established and stabilized, and when theory is clearly articulated and recognized as clinically viable can hypotheses be developed and tested. This is a difficult stage to reach in the development of any human service field, as contextual factors such as those identified above require flexibility of practice in response to systemic change. These circumstances require clinicians and researchers to perpetually observe and describe adaptations in practice and evolution of theory. If the systems within which dance/movement therapists worked were predictable, and if practices were replicable, conducting research would be vastly simplified. Focusing on the aspects of treatment that do remain stable will set the research stage for less frustration and greater rates of completion.

Another systemic component that researchers must deal with is the institutional review board (IRB), a committee within an agency, university, or hospital whose job it is to ensure that research projects do not harm any human research subjects. The attitude of an IRB toward research may seem restrictive, oppressive, and challenging to the implementation of research projects. Because many researchers do not understand the function and operation of an IRB, they may see this body as the enemy, and may enter into dialogue with it defensively. The best way to get research proposals approved through the IRB is to develop a working relationship with it, and with its members. Try to understand the IRB from the inside, or better yet, try to become a member. It is true that some institutional review boards are more conservative than others, and in these cases, education of its members may help them understand forms of research that are outside of their realm of familiarity. (For more ideas about coping with an IRB see Oakes, 2002.)

Professional Organizational Support

One system that has a significant impact on research production and publication is the professional association. I will share how this has happened in the United States as one illustration that may have relevance for other countries. The American Dance Therapy Association (ADTA) was created in 1966 to support the development of the profession. Two essential founding and ongoing functions of the ADTA have been to support the development of a body of knowledge and "to provide recommendations for appropriate educational opportunities for those interested in obtaining training in dance/movement therapy" (Stark, 2002, p. 76). In her article tracing the evolution of the *American Journal of Dance Therapy*, Stark reported that "in the early years of our organization, research in dance/movement therapy was practically non-existent, *emerging only as graduate programs evolved*" (p. 76, italics added). Thus, we see evidence of the interdependent relationship among the professional organization, education, and research. The ADTA oversees the core content, quality, and stability of the graduate DMT programs, which in turn educate professionals, who then may produce a research-based thesis or choose to participate in research after graduation. Their ability to conduct research and interest in doing so depends in a very direct way on the quality of their education in research.

The ADTA has consistently been attentive to its role in promoting research in the field of DMT in a variety of ways. Its board of directors has been committed to providing publication venues for its members since its inception, in the form of conference proceedings, monographs, and a professional journal (Stark, 2002). The ADTA Board of Directors also created a research subcommittee, whose mandate was to support research in DMT. This group of four or five dance/movement therapists who are also researchers has been very active in response to its charge, especially since the late 1990s (Cruz & Hervey, 2001). Several endeavors have been very well received, such as free individualized consultation to ADTA members planning or conducting research, with help ranging from resource location to research design suggestions. The committee hosts continuing education workshops and a research poster session at every national ADTA conference. The subcommittee also maintains bibliographies, research tips, and useful research links on a research page of the ADTA website.

Less than a decade ago, as a representative of the research subcommittee, I recommended that dance/movement therapists rather than other professionals teach all the research courses in the graduate DMT programs, which was not the norm at the time. I believed this would provide role models for students, communicating that dance/movement therapists are researchers as well as clinicians. At the time of this writing, with slight variance from year to year, it is now customary for these courses to be taught by dance/movement therapists, many of whom are doctoral-level experienced researchers. Positioning DMT researchers in very visible roles such as educators and ADTA board members contributes to the acceptance of research as a valued and viable professional activity for dance/movement therapists.

The great majority of research in DMT is carried out by graduate students for their master's theses. In an effort to share this work with other researchers and to support the development of a solid and productive body of professional knowledge, several volumes of indexed thesis and dissertation bibliographies have been published (Leventhal, 1983; Fisher & Stark, 1992). The Marian Chace Foundation of the ADTA has also worked for years to make master's theses more available through a regularly published collection of abstracts indexed by author, subject, date, and graduate program. How to access theses from the various programs' libraries is also included in these publications. Most recently, the research subcommittee has initiated an effort to have all theses submitted by students in both hard-bound copies and on CD-rom, with signed releases of permission to reproduce, for easier and safer distribution through school libraries. Cataloging of theses in international databases such as *Worldcat* is also planned in the near future.

Education

We have considered how various large systems can encourage the production of research. Let us shift the focus of our questions to consider factors such as education and training and how they influence individual decisions to develop and pursue research interests. Many dance/movement therapists are educated from childhood in dance. In college, future dance/movement therapists often create their own hybrid curriculum of psychology combined with dance and liberal arts. In graduate school their training becomes specialized in DMT theory and practice, focusing on skills they need to be clinicians. Many receive additional postgraduate training in particular schools of psychotherapy or psychoanalysis, and various body-based practices. How does this kind of education influence the tendency to participate in research as a professional?

I have long been fascinated by the epistemology and skills promoted by dance training and how these can be utilized in research (see Hervey, 2000 for an extended discussion of this topic). Most dancers are probably strong in what Howard Gardner (1985) would call bodily kinesthetic intelligence, with strengths in musical and spatial intelligence as well. Dance/movement therapists also demonstrate significant interpersonal and intrapersonal intelligence in their work, which may be supported by training and experience in dance, a highly social art form using self and body as the primary tool in relation to space, time, and usually music. To encourage research it is important to support the idea that these skills and ways of knowing can be integral to research. Researchers must be permitted to develop new and innovative methods that use their strengths. Too often dance/movement therapists attempt research projects that rely on their least developed skills, and feel disinterested and discouraged in their efforts. Graduate education that exposes learners to a breadth of methodologies and supports their use for thesis research will begin to free the creative minds and bodies of dance/movement therapists to address problems in ways in which they feel confident and enthusiastic. In addition to more traditional quantitative methodologies, options include a range of qualitative methods such as arts-based (McNiff, 1998) or artistic inquiry (Hervey, 2000, 2004), case study, collaborative ethnography (Lassiter, 2005), evaluative (Cruz, 2004), transpersonal (Braud & Anderson, 1998), action, phenomenology, and heuristic (Moustakas, 1990). Research procedures that use dance/movement therapists' interpersonal skills, such as interviewing and focus groups, may prove especially valuable. Finally, consideration needs to be given to utilizing embodied phenomena, such as kinesthetic empathy and somatic countertransference, as valuable and much overlooked sources of data. I have repeatedly seen students heartily embrace research once they realize they can bring their whole creative, empathic selves to the process.

One factor that may strongly influence the production of research is the nature of the preparatory undergraduate education. Due primarily to communication via the World Wide Web, in recent years there has been greater awareness among college and even high school students about DMT as a potential career. As a result, according to educators in DMT graduate programs in the United States, more applicants are better prepared, with stronger undergraduate backgrounds in both dance and psychology. In a growing number of cases, undergraduate research and statistics courses are part of applicants' academic preparation.

In research that I have conducted on an annual basis with graduate DMT students, an attitude reflecting ambivalence or conflicted feelings about doing research consistently emerges (Hervey, 2000). Students feel excited or curious at the same time as they feel scared, overwhelmed, incompetent, or bored about doing research. In both this research and the ADTA membership survey (Cruz & Hervey, 2001), the feelings, beliefs, or attitudes expressed were based on minimal education and little or no experience with actually doing research, and so were mostly founded on anticipatory feelings or imagined experience. In many cases, responses were based on narrow and rigid ideas about what research can be. I have seen recent evidence among my students that familiarity with psychology and research methods before graduate school is promoting greater interest in research as a professional activity, and decreased ambivalence and anxiety associated with research courses and thesis writing. These trends may result in increased participation in research after completion of training.

In 2000, a survey of ADTA members gathered information about their attitudes, beliefs, education, needs, and experiences in relation to research (Cruz & Hervey, 2001). This survey found that although 84% of respondents received courses in research in their graduate programs, only 36% belived that their DMT education sufficiently prepared them for conducting research. Concerted effort has been made by the ADTA to improve the quality of research education in master's-level DMT programs. Although the content of research courses is left entirely to the individual graduate programs, recommendations have been made to the programs through the research subcommittee of the ADTA. Areas in which it may be especially important to prepare dance/movement therapists to do research are quantitative and qualitative methods of program evaluation, grant writing to apply for research funds, and applying to institutional review boards for research project approval. In relation to the last area, research training must include education about the ethical treatment of human research participants.

The purpose of graduate education in DMT is to train therapists of the highest quality, and so it is understandable that the emphasis is on learning clinical competencies. As has been discussed by Cruz & Hervey (2001) this focus strongly influences the identity and professional activities of dance/movement therapists. Most clinically based professions, such as counseling and the creative arts therapies, espouse a *clinician/researcher* identity to encourage research among their members. However, if research really is a priority to a developing profession, *researcher* as a discrete identity may need to be an alternative track in the training process. This would allow a small but valuable team of researchers to evolve, with training similar to their clinician colleagues, but with more courses in research and supportive skills such as grant writing and sophisticated statistical analysis.

One more finding regarding education and its relation to research is also worth noting. The ADTA research survey mentioned earlier found that many more respondents with doctorate degrees reported participating in, designing, and conducting independent research projects, and submitting or publishing research articles. Respondents with doctorates (regardless of the field) also tended to have a less restrictive understanding of research methods (Cruz & Hervey, 2001). These findings suggest that one way to encourage more research is to support doctoral-level education among dance/movement therapists.

Focusing on the Individual

The results of the ADTA membership survey indicated that the majority of respondents believed that research was essential to the survival of the profession, but in contrast they thought research had little relevance to their individual practice of DMT. Personal reasons for not conducting research included having too little interest, motivation, funding, skills, or collegial/workplace support to engage in research. These results are consistent with similar surveys conducted in related fields (Cruz & Hervey, 2001). So far, this chapter has addressed the ways that systems can support research, but perhaps is it equally important to consider how each of us as individuals can encourage investigation among our colleagues, students, and supervisees, and within our own professional lives. What determines dance/movement therapists' decisions to conduct inquiry? And what allows them to continue, complete, and publish their work once they have started? To encourage research we can try to understand the barriers and challenges individual researchers face at every stage of the process. Knowing how to support investigators through these challenges may reduce frustration and facilitate more successful efforts at production and publication of research. I would also like to make an argument for collegial collaboration on projects. Very few people have all the skills (or time) needed to complete an entire research undertaking from proposal to publication. Based on my own experience, I can personally attest that collaborating with colleagues, at the workplace or even long distance, can provide complementary skills as well as the commitment to another person to reach completion (Hervey & Kornblum, 2006; Cruz & Hervey, 2001). This kind of interpersonal support for research also uses the relational skills of dance/movement therapists and may make the whole research process feel more meaningful for everyone involved.

In dance/movement therapy, most potential enquirers are interns or clinicians who would like to (or must) produce research about their work. They sometimes begin with a question, but more often they start with a messy situation. Clinicians find themselves in such circumstances, about which they become passionate, fearful, curious, apathetic, confused, or frustrated, and over which they have almost no control. This lack of control often leads clinicians to believe they can't do investigation about their practice. This is just one of the *real* problems that clinicians face.

The traditional idea of a "research problem" also stumps clinicians who face the "problems" of their patients every day, and don't always understand the relationship between them and the larger questions that inquiry is supposed to address. This is one of the most basic barriers to clinically based research. Clinicians are most interested in the comparatively small interpersonal and unique issues that exist between themselves and each client, and this is where they function best, and receive their greatest professional rewards. It takes a significant change of focus to imagine how the individualized daily solutions to these therapeutic problems might be of generalizable value. Again, knowing there are inquiry options that focus on the depth and realities of the therapeutic interaction can help clinicians see research potential in their practice.

For example, keeping a journal for a period of time about one's feelings, experiences, dreams, or interventions as a clinician, and then examining that journal for themes (recurring challenges, descriptive words, metaphors, etc.) may present a clinician with an area of focus or a question. Beginning with something that is meaningful to the clinician, and examining that in relation to client issues or movement behaviors over time may start to reveal patterns and correlations that can be developed into more formalized inquiry.

Formulating a research question is one of the first steps toward transforming the clinical event into the development of a theory. It requires stepping outside the intimacy of the therapeutic relationship and being curious about subtle patterns and unfamiliar ways of perceiving the work. Asking a research question often requires that the clinician ask something of the therapeutic process that may not seem to directly serve the needs of each particular client. Making this shift in attention can create a conflict for the clinician whose focus has been on meeting clients' very particular needs, not the needs of his or her research project. Challenges and conflicts such as these can unconsciously sabotage clinicians' efforts to conduct investigation.

When attempting to formulate a question, researchers sometimes begin with very big issues that tend to get bigger. Or they ask many questions that tend to multiply, or two opposing interrogations that stubbornly refuse to become one.

However, it is the researcher's first task to wrestle this thing into a seemingly tiny formulation for a project that can be completed in less than one lifetime. Establishing the interrogation and the focus of the inquiry begins to distinguish it from other clinical or creative activities. Support or consultation from an experienced researcher may help clinicians step outside their clients' and their own dilemmas and see them as research problems, with accompanying realistic questions. Support from supervisors, including release time to carry out the project, would certainly be a factor in success.

Part of clarifying the focus is finding out who else has been in this situation before and has asked a similar question. Searching the professional literature informs the inquirer, and later the reader, about where this project fits in relation to others who have addressed the same problem. It also hopefully prevents traveling the same territory others have covered without learning what they have learned. A significant barrier to doing research is not having access to articles and books written on the subject. Although the internet has made access easier in some cases, affiliation with a university library provides the best support in getting references, especially those from outside the researcher's country. If he or she is working in a health service agency or institution, perhaps that agency can affiliate with a college or university that would allow the use of their resources and reference librarians. A good working relationship with a reference librarian can be immensely helpful. They are most often very knowledgeable and eager to be of assistance.

After identifying the question and the knowledge already constructed in the subject matter, there is need for the development of a plan for how it will be answered. The plan, or the design, is basically a description of what the data will be, how it will be collected from what source, how it will be analyzed, how the findings will be presented, and to whom. Researchers may find it helpful at this point to consider what unique skills they can bring to their task, and to use them as an integral part of their methodology. Again, there are research methods for every kind of learner, thinker, and doer. There is no reason to use methods that feel incompatible with who they are and what they do well. Dance/movement therapists need to consider what they can *perceive* and *describe* that other kinds of therapists cannot, such as change in movement qualities; subtle nonverbal communication in terms of shaping, proxemics, rhythms; and kinesthetic or somatic cues within the therapist's experience.

Research can also be made easier by recognizing to whom the therapist has easy access; in other words, who is available as a sample of participants or co-researchers. Patients are not the only possible research participants; staff, colleagues, administrators, and educators are too often overlooked as sources of data. Clinician researchers should also consider what kind of data may already be collected at their work site, what they have access to, and how it can be gathered as part of their clinical responsibilities. In other words, where will the information come from and what form will it take? Will it be client reports, the researcher's journals, clinical files from patient charts, video recordings of client movement, measurement of group member activity in response to a particular intervention, movement observations, or results of paper and pencil assessment tools? Will the data be numbers, words, images, or other artifacts of the clinical work?

Some of the best advice I've ever heard about doing clinically based research is to use research assistants and to collect data that can be gathered in 30 seconds or less. Jill Sonke-Henderson, co-director of the Center for the Arts in Healthcare Research and Education recommended that the artist/clinician should "never have a pencil and paper in his/her hand." If a research assistant can be present to collect the data, the artist/clinician is freed from the kinds of conflicts of purpose identified earlier. Finding tools for data collection that can be administered very quickly and simply also minimizes interference with the delivery of services. Sonke-Henderson described a tool that displayed two Likert-style rows of five "smiley faces," with facial expressions ranging from a frown to a smile. One row measured change in mood, the other change in stress. Research participants needed only to indicate, before and after the delivery of services, which face in each row reflected their present mood and stress level. With the help of an assistant, the entire data collection process took less than 30 seconds.

The next stage of research, data analysis, is the process of digging in, holding on, and waiting for meaning to arise from the information collected. It demands sustained attention to what at times seems like a chaotic compilation of meaningless stuff, and may require more anxiety-management skills than anything else. Collegial understanding and support during this phase would be especially encouraging. This stage of inquiry is also time intensive, so plans must be made to organize. Here is where release time for doing research is most critical.

The nature of the data will determine the method of its analysis. Quantitative data, or that which can be expressed in numbers, will require statistical analysis. Qualitative information, such as words from interviews, images, or movement analyses that cannot be measured, will require some kind of qualitative analysis. There are many excellent resources on the Internet and in print to support beginning researchers in their data analysis (see bibliography).

Finally the findings, or answers in relation to the research question, are organized into a form that effectively communicates to others. The editors of the *American Journal of Dance Therapy* have continually reported that one of the greatest obstacles to publication is the written quality of the articles submitted and the disappointment and frustration of authors who are asked to make revisions. Editors need to be discerning, and authors need to be prepared to make revisions. Colleagues can help by reading drafts or providing editing and emotional support to get articles back to the publisher after revisions are made. However, authors need to be prepared to hire independent editors to help them with their grammar, punctuation, APA style, and expression of ideas. Getting professional help of this sort is not anything to be ashamed of, and can be of tremendous assistance in developing a clear, coherent, expressive, scholarly "voice."

Thinking outside of the familiar inquiry box can inspire not only the creation of new methods, but new audiences and venues as well. There are many ways of sharing findings that may be more dynamic and have a greater impact and range than the traditional journal article. Artistic inquiry or performance-based research could result in shows at art galleries or live theatrical events. These formats can also be incorporated into conference presentations, research poster sessions, fundraising events, or institution sponsored celebrations.

Conclusion

From the social/cultural to the personal, there are various levels at which we can exert influence and understand the dynamics that impact the production and presentation of research. I, for example, find that understanding the motivations and frustrations of uniquely skilled and situated individual researchers, and offering them the support they need is the most effective action I can take. Each reader of this chapter, whether student, clinician, researcher, educator, manager, publisher, or administrator, has a particular perspective and sphere(s) of influence within which I hope he or she will take action to encourage research in dance/movement therapy.

References

Braud, W., & Anderson, R. (1998). *Transpersonal research methods for the social sciences.* Thousand Oaks, CA: Sage.

Cruz, R. F. (2004). What is evaluation research? In R. Cruz & C. Berrol (Eds.) *Dance/movement therapists in action.* Springfield, IL: Charles C Thomas. 171–180.

Cruz, R. F., & Hervey, L. (2001). The American Dance Therapy Association Research Survey. *American Journal of Dance Therapy, 23*(2): 89–118.

Fisher, A. C., & Stark, A. (Eds.) (1992). *Dance/movement therapy abstracts: Doctoral dissertations, master's theses, and special projects through 1990.* Columbia, MD: The Marian Chace Memorial Fund.

Gardner, H. (1985). *Frames of mind.* New York: Basic Books.

Hervey, L. (2000). *Artistic inquiry in dance/movement therapy: Creative alternatives for research.* Springfield, IL: Charles C Thomas.

Hervey, L. (2004). Artistic inquiry in dance/movement therapy. In R. F. Cruz & C. F. Berrol (Eds.), *Dance/movement therapists in action*. Springfield, IL: Charles C Thomas.

Hervey, L., & Kornblum, R. (2006). An evaluation of Kornblum's body-based violence prevention curriculum for children. *The Arts in Psychotherapy.* 33(2):113–129.

Lassiter, L. E. (2005). *The Chicago guide to collaborative ethnography*. Chicago: University of Chicago Press.

Leventhal, M. B. (1983). *Graduate research and studies in dance/movement therapy 1972–1982*. Philadelphia: Hahnemann University Press.

Levy, F. J. (1992). *Dance/movement therapy: A healing art*. Reston, VA. American Alliance for Health Physical Education. Recreation and Dance.

McNiff, S. (1998). *Art-based research*. London: Jessica Kingsley.

Moustakas, C. (1990). *Heuristic research*. Thousand Oaks, CA: Sage.

Oakes, J. M. (2002). Risks and wrongs in social science research: An evaluator's guide to the IRB. *Evaluation Review,* 24: 443–478.

Stark, A. (2002). *The American Journal of Dance Therapy:* Its history and evolution. *The American Journal of Dance Therapy,* 24(2):73–96.

Bibliography

Ansdell, G., & Pavlicevic, M. (2001). *Beginning research in the arts therapies: A practical guide*. London: Jessica Kingsley.

Cruz, R. F., & Berrol, C. F. (2004). *Dance/movement therapists in action*. Springfield, IL: Charles C Thomas.

Ely, M., Anzul, M., Friedman, T., & Garner, D. (1991). *Doing qualitative research: Circles within circles*. New York: Falmer Press.

Erlandson, D. A., Harris, E. L., Skipper, B. L., & Allen, S. D. (1993). *Doing naturalistic inquiry*. Thousand Oaks, CA: Sage.

Feder, B., & Feder, E. (1998). *The art and science of evaluation in the arts therapies*. Springfield, IL: Charles C Thomas.

Glesne, C. (1999). *Becoming qualitative researchers*. New York: Longman.

Grainger, R. (1999). *Researching in the arts therapies*. London: Jessica Kingsley.

Maykut, P., & Morehouse, R. (1994). *Beginning qualitative research*. Washington, D.C.: The Falmer Press.

Mertons, D. (1998). *Research methods in education and psychology*. Thousand Oaks: Sage.

Patton, M. Q. (2001). *Qualitative research and evaluation methods*. Thousand Oaks, CA: Sage.

Payne, H. (1993). *Handbook of inquiry in the arts therapies: One river, many currents*. London: Jessica Kingsley.

Sommer, B., & Sommer, R. (1991). *A practical guide to behavioral research*. London: Oxford University Press.

Strauss, A., & Corbin, J. (1990). *Basics of qualitative research: Grounded theory procedures and techniques*. Thousand Oaks, CA: Sage.

Afterword

I get up. I walk. I fall down. Meanwhile, I keep dancing.

—Rabbi Hillel
(http://infinitebody.blogspot.com/2008/11/love-art-isadora-duncan.html)

We would like to add some thoughts to the many ideas written in the previous chapters. We expect that after having read the book, the importance of dance and movement as therapy with persons of varied ages and psychological and physical problems has become clear for each of you.

People need and want to be recognized for their humanity and not merely by their disability. By means of dance and movement, professionals are able to address all the interrelated physical, cognitive, and emotional systems. Such interventions build on the strengths and creativity that individuals bring to their treatment and do not focus on the limitations.

There are many possible choices to be made in how one may interact with individuals and groups that will meet their interests and desires toward more satisfying ways of living. This requires a wide range of knowledge to be learned, experienced, and implemented by the therapist, but equally important is making use of creativity related to the art form itself. Spontaneity and drives toward health are a vital part of the potential for positive change and therefore are supported and encouraged in the therapeutic process.

Spontaneity is important on the part of both therapist and client as transitions concerning new learning may emerge because of the structures a therapist sets that provide the safety for allowing different experiences and behaviors. By following an intuitive or creative thought, the therapist may lead treatment in new and more productive directions.

The several authors have provided important and basic information offering suggestions on how to focus the dance/movement therapy work with particular groups and individuals with specific problems. Additional chapters have been written to support furthering one's work through the understanding of systems of observation of movement, the roots of the profession, and how to add to the knowledge base by taking a more active attitude and minimizing fears related to research.

It is hoped that the reader will utilize this information in many forms. Those who are in related fields can expand their abilities in being aware of and drawing upon the nonverbal aspects of behavior and thereby adding to their own store of knowledge. Those more directly involved with dance as therapy will be able to deepen their practice as they absorb the suggestions and ideas of experienced clinicians in order to use this knowledge to form their own perceptions in their practice.

The full breadth and depth of dance and movement in therapy can be recognized and employed by many. Dance has always been therapeutic to those who engage in and focus on its unique qualities. Dance adds to the possibilities of helpful interventions within the framework of therapy. Those who have offered their knowledge within this book have all had the experience of personal growth and change through this medium and understand the powerful impact made by the use of the body in movement and rhythm. We are convinced that all those who are similarly open to connecting to the bodymind will have much to gain.

Author Index

Subject Index

Note. f indicates figures, n indicates notes, t indicates tables.

A

ABI (acquired brain injury), see Brain injury rehabilitation
Abuse, 128, 287–290, 289f, 292
Acknowledging, 138, 139, 141
Acquired brain injury (ABI), see Brain injury rehabilitation
ADTA (American Dance Therapy Association), 9–10, 320–321
Affect, see Emotions
Affirmation, 187, 188
Aggression
  brain injury and, 200–201
  creativity and, 23
  developmental transitions and, 253–254
  expression of, 92
  motor prototype and, 278, 281
Alexander technique, 10
Alexithymia, 129
Alzheimer's disease, 182–183; see also Dementia
American Dance Therapy Association (ADTA), 9–10, 320–321
Amnesia, 196–197
Analogic communication, 27

Analysis of movement, see Emotorics; Observation
Anger
  case study, 173
  chaos and, 60
  expression of, 68–70
  thinking and, 63, 64
Anguish, 65–66
Anorexia nervosa, 127, 128–129, 138–139; see also Eating disorders
Anxiety
  case study, 151–155
  eating disorders and, 136, 138–139, 140
  expression of, 67–68
  neurotic styles and, 114–115
  schizoid personality and, 21–22
  tension-flow attunement and, 250
Archetypal aspects and structures
  affect system, 56–57
  body dynamics, 269–271, 270f, 271f
  core-potentials, 279–280
  developmental directionality, 279
  emotive movement, 271–272
  interpersonal settings, 275–279, 276f
Art, 17, 19–21
Artistic activity, 15, 18–19, 29n3; see also Creative process
Assessment, see Observation